AF706487

Constitutional Medicine of Korea

8체질의학

A Comprehensive Guide to Eight-Constitution Medicine including Theory, Acupuncture Technique, Clinical Cases, and Personalized Healing

Suk-Won Joo, K.M.D.

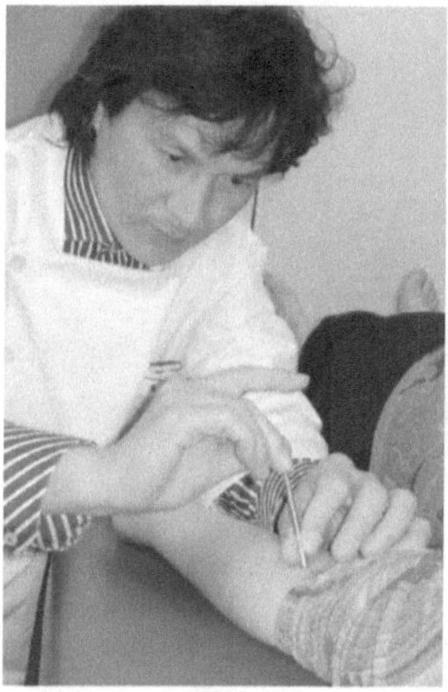

Dr. Suk-Won Joo, born in Korea, is a man of 8-Constitution Medicine dedicated solely to exploring and practicing this unique system of healing. It would be no exaggeration to say that his entire life's focus has been concentrated on the path of Eight-Constitution Medicine. From the dawn of the new millennium in 2000 to this very moment, every day of his medical journey has been etched into the heart of this profound system.

[Authored Works]

The Principle of 8-Constitution Medicine (2007)
Stories of the 8 Constitutions (2008)
What Is My Constitution? (2009)
Health Tips through Constitutional Diet (2010)
The 8-Constitution Diet (2012)
The Female and the Male (2013)
What Is Constitution? (2016)
Eight-Constitution Weight Loss Program (2016)
Dialogue on 8 Constitutions (2019)
The 8-Constitution Report (2020)
Complete Series on 8-Constitution Medicine (2023)
Health Strategies for Economic Downturns (2024)
8-Constitution Medicine: Core Principle and Constitution-acupuncture Treatment (2025)

[Contacts]
https://blog.naver.com/docj62
TEL: +82 2-423-7534

Copyright © 2025 Suk-Won Joo, K.M.D.

All rights reserved. No part of this book may be reproduced, stored, or transmitted by any means—whether auditory, graphic, mechanical, or electronic—without written permission of both publisher and author, except in the case of brief excerpts used in critical articles and reviews. Unauthorized reproduction of any part of this work is illegal and is punishable by law.

I learned the fundamentals
of Eight-Constitution Medicine
from the philosopher Doh-ol Young-oak Kim.

I learned the structure
of Eight-Constitution Medicine
from the creator of Eight-Constitution Medicine,
Dongho Do-won Kuon.

I realized the continuity
of mind and body
from the creator of Sasang Constitution-medicine,
Dongmu Je-ma Lee.

I verified these principles
through the patients
who visited Joowonjang Clinic of Korean Medicine.

This book is entirely inspired by these honorable figures.

I merely described their remarks
in terms of the language of mathematics.

Contents

Introduction to Joowonjang's work

by Philosopher Doh-ol Young-oak Kim[1]

Doctor Suk-won Joo is my disciple. He currently runs a local clinic called *Joowonjang Clinic of Korean Medicine* in Seoul, where he treats numerous patients. Many who suffer from various ailments experience what feels like magical relief through his medical treatments.

Suk-won Joo originally studied mechanical engineering at Korea

[1] My teacher Doh-ol Young-oak Kim is a world-renowned Korean philosopher in the fields of Chinese and Korean philosophy and public intellectual. He received his B.A. in Philosophy from Korea University, his M.A. in Philosophy from National Taiwan University, and an M.A. in Chinese Philosophy from the University of Tokyo. He later earned his Ph.D. in Philosophy from Harvard University. Upon his return to Korea, he was appointed Professor of Philosophy at Korea University in 1982, where he began his academic career in effect in Korea. In 1986, under the harsh oppression of the Doo-hwan Chun's military dictatorship, he resigned from his professorship after issuing a "Declaration of Conscience," stating that he could no longer teach students as a scholar and mentor—a courageous act that intellectually and politically enlightened the Korean people. In 1990, he entered the College of Korean Medicine at Wonkwang University to explore the fundamental principles of the human body through Eight-Constitution Medicine and obtained a degree and a medical license in Korean Medicine in 1996.

Under his academic influence, I also enrolled in the College of Korean Medicine at Dongshin University in 1993. When he established Doh-ol Academy, dedicated to educating young people who would lead future Korea, I joined the academy and studied Eastern and Western classics and philosophy under his guidance. After graduating from the College of Korean Medicine, I served as the director of Doh-ol Clinic of Korean Medicine, a clinic he founded in Daehak-ro, Seoul. There, I practiced as a doctor of Korean Medicine for three years, learning Eight-Constitution Medicine directly from him.

Doh-ol Young-oak Kim is widely regarded as one of the most influential scholars in Korea, significantly impacting various fields such as Eastern and Western philosophy, religion, culture, journalism, arts, and so on, through his extensive writings and lectures.

University, so I had no need to teach him anything in that field. However, he sought me out with profound philosophical questions that his life as an engineer could not satisfy. At the Doh-ol Academy, I taught him the Chinese classics, in which he excelled.

Unexpectedly, though, his true talent lay in singing. While he didn't perform Italian arias, he had an extraordinary gift for singing well-known pop songs. When he played the guitar and sang, all the students at the Doh-ol Academy contest were spellbound. They set aside their own talents, listening to him with rapt attention, as if their own light dimmed in his presence. When he sang *Imagine* by John Lennon (1940~1980) or *Vincent* by Don McLean (1945~), all desire for material things seemed to vanish—it felt almost as though you were walking along the Rhône River with Van Gogh. It was widely believed that his rendition of *Starry Starry Night* was even more moving than the original by Don McLean. No one disagreed.

One day, there was a gathering of about a hundred students in the Academy, and during a discussion session where they asked and answered questions among themselves, someone naturally directed a question to him: "How do you sing so well?"

Suk-won Joo's response was utterly shocking to everyone. He said, "Anyone can sing well, but it requires practice. If I want to sing a song, I must sing it 1,000 times with absolute precision before I let anyone hear it. I never make public a song that I haven't sung a thousand times. And while the quality of a song may depend on vocal cords and volume, a song that has been sung seriously over a thousand times becomes something worthy of being heard by anyone."

Although he was an engineering student, he would practice singing songs over and over again, pushing himself to the limit, on the hill of Aegineung ("Baby Tomb")—the tomb of King Jeongjo's concubine who passed away at a young age during the Joseon Dynasty—located on the campus of Korea University. In truth, his statement was not an unreasonable demand, but his claim—that one must sing a song at least 1,000 times to truly master it—shocked everyone who heard it. Whenever I reflect on the attitude we must uphold in life—that even the smallest tasks should be approached with professionalism—I am reminded of what Suk-won Joo said at Doh-ol Academy. Suk-won Joo, an engineering student, practiced each song 1,000 times!

Influenced by me, he entered a college of Korean Medicine in 1993. After graduating, I appointed him as the director of Doh-ol Korean Medicine Clinic, which I had just opened. As I had a lifelong principle of never becoming the "director" of any institution, I appointed the rookie doctor who had been my assistant as the "director," while I continued to work as a rankless doctor.

When I closed Doh-ol Clinic, all the patients followed him and called him "Joowonjang" (which means the director Joo in Korean, and, at the same time, Zhu Yuanzhang, the founder of Ming Dynasty in China), and his clinic title became Joowonjang Clinic. The name "Joowonjang" has no negative connotations, as it carries multiple overlapping meanings.

Professor Dong-hee Choi, who taught Kantian philosophy in the Department of Philosophy at Korea University, often mentioned a highly credible story that has been passed down in various regions of North Korea. According to this story, Zhu Yuanzhang was originally from that area, later advanced to China, and became an emperor. If you read the *Annals of King Taejo of the Joseon Dynasty*, it can be inferred that many Goryeo people (Koreans from late Goryeo Dynasty at that time) were part of Zhu Yuanzhang's entourage. In any case, it is clear that Zhu Yuanzhang was a man of remarkable ambition and an indomitable spirit.

Western civilization developed a new knowledge system called "Science" through the modern spirit that emerged during the Renaissance (the word "Science" literally means "knowledge"). The core of this knowledge system lies in a cognitive method called "Reason." The word "Reason" originates from "ratio," and its defining characteristic is "calculation," which involves quantifying all natural phenomena. The characteristic of quantification is that it does not accommodate qualitative feelings. René Descartes defined the hallmark of rationalistic truth as being "clear and distinct," explicitly excluding non-quantitative ambiguity.

However, the fundamental object of truth that humanity has pursued remains in a state of chaos. The system of clear and distinct truths, which was developed by abstracting scientific knowledge from this chaos, actually addresses only an extremely small portion of the vast, ultimate chaos.

It is universally acknowledged that the human body is the most advanced system among living organisms. However, reducing the entirety of this high-dimensional universe to rationalistic clarity can be a grave act of violence. Even if it serves a practical purpose, the utility of such clarity remains confined to only a small subset of physical phenomena.

Recently, the term "alternative medicine" has gained popularity, and in many countries, including the United States and Europe, a strong public opinion favoring alternative medicine is emerging. However, the term "alternative" inherently implies a hierarchy, suggesting that there is a master, and the subordinate role of the alternative is merely to replace the master when necessary. In this sense, the alternatives cannot truly replace the main body.

This indicates the alternatives still lack the real power, organization, and logic to supplant conventional systems. Yet, the persistent attention on the alternatives stems from their incredibly undeniable effectiveness, particularly as the limitations of Western medical treatments, rooted in rationalism, become more apparent.

Master Do-won Kuon is someone who has developed an entirely new medical system. He ventured to establish his own clear and distinct system within the chaotic complexity of the human body, a realm others hesitated to explore. Although his system employs a highly mathematical methodology, it employs his own unique "clear and distinct" approach, which is entirely different from the Western "clear and distinct" methods. The most fitting description of his life may be this: "Do-won Kuon is the founder of Constitutional Medicine and the new Pythagoras of 20th-century Joseon."

How did Do-won Kuon, the new Pythagoras, develop a new mathematical theory for the human body? Anyone seeking answer to this question should read this book by Suk-won Joo. His dedication to uncovering the physiology of acupuncture, with the same zeal as practicing a song 1,000 times to master it, deserves great appreciation.

A complete and holistic medicine can only be achieved by integrating Eastern and Western medicine. Furthermore, within Korean Medicine society itself, we must transcend narrow-minded divisions between schools and sects, abandoning mutual disapproval. Constitutional Medicine and the conventional Zang-Fu theory are not incompatible—they can communicate and coexist.

I, Doh-ol Young-oak Kim, was the first to introduce Master Do-won Kuon's Constitutional Medicine to international audiences. My own deep fascination with Do-won Kuon's Constitutional Medicine also drove me to make the bold decision to attend the College of Korean Medicine for six years, following Do-won Kuon's recommendation.

However, Doh-ol myself has yet to publish a comprehensive work on Korean Medicine. I am uncertain what direction my path of thoughts will ultimately take. Nevertheless, younger scholars should avoid exclusionary attitudes and instead exchange knowledge and encourage one another. By doing so, they can forge a new path to create an innovative medical system.

A medical doctor is constantly confronted with life and death—facing *Dasein* (presence) and reality of life that transcends dogma, medical systems, and scientific knowledge. Always, doctors must approach matters not from their own perspective but from the patient's point of view, never losing their benevolent heart.

The purpose of publishing Suk-won Joo's research and its precise findings is to pronounce that everyone must remain humble before the awe of life.

Doh-ol Young-oak Kim introduces
Dr. Suk-won Joo
In Doh-ol Research Institute of Naksongam

Author's Prelude

Humans are mathematical beings. This does not mean that humans think or act in mathematical ways. Rather, it means that humans are living organisms constructed based on mathematical principles. In essence, humans are mathematics itself.

The foundation of the human body's biological activities lies in the Zang-Fu, which means the 5 representative visceral organs in Oriental medicine. These activities follow the dynamic laws of Synchronizing (Interpromoting) and Antagonizing (Intersuppressing) governed by the Five Phases. The Five Phases structure of these Zang-Fu, symbolizing the human body, is rooted in the mathematical principles having the causational number 5.

Zang-Fu organs exchange Qi with one another to create and sustain the body's vital functions. This Qi exchange is also governed strictly by the mathematical principles.

Constitution refers to Zang-Fu Structure inherently given to humans. This Structure operates as the symmetrical system of mathematics meticulously designed to maintain dynamic equilibrium. Moreover, this structure can be mathematically represented with precision on a coordinate plane.

The types of Constitution can also be mathematically defined based on the definition of the Constitution's Zang-Fu Structure.

In the course of life, the human body can experience a disease. Disease occurs when there is an excessive imbalance among Zang-Fu organs, disrupting the dynamic equilibrium of the Constitution. The process of therapy—reversing this excessive imbalance and restoring the body to its original physiological state—also follows the mathematical principles.

From the beginning to the end of life, the entire process of the human body is rooted in the mathematics. Humans are mathematical beings.

This book delves into the original meaning of Eight-Constitution Medicine by analyzing Dongho Do-won Kuon's paper in 1965, *"A Study of Constitution-Acupuncture."* Through this exploration, I discovered the remarkable mathematical principles inherent in Constitutional Medicine. Additionally, I was able to clearly confirm the connection with Je-ma Lee's Sasang Medicine (Four-Constitution Medicine)—crucial to the development of Do-won Kuon's Eight-Constitution Medicine—through the original text of *Donguisusebowon* by Je-ma Lee.

This realization also deepened my understanding that history does not come for free. The fruits of Je-ma Lee's labor and sacrifice bore the results a century later, just as he had envisioned. However, it is ironic that Constitutional Medicine flourished in a way vastly different from what Je-ma Lee had imagined. His Yin-Yang model of the human body underwent a fundamental transformation into Do-won Kuon's Five Phases-based human body. As a result, Sasang Medicine and Eight-Constitution Medicine have diverged significantly. What began as a small difference grew into a monumental divergence over 100 years. "Creating and creating is called Changes (生生之謂易)!"

I made a concerted effort to consistently uncover and explain the mathematical principles underlying Eight-Constitution Medicine from the beginning to the end. Just as Ludwig Wittgenstein (1889–1951) became captivated by philosophy after reading Bertrand Russell's *Principia Mathematica* (co-authored with Alfred North Whitehead, 1861–1947), I—an expert in Eight-Constitution Medicine—was similarly enthralled after recognizing its mathematical principles. This realization sparked my unshakable passion for Eight-Constitution Medicine.

As a result of that effort, I published *Principles of Eight-Constitution Medicine* in 2007. Now, more than 17 years later, in 2024, I felt a strong need to create a revised edition that reflects my evolved understanding of Eight-Constitution Medicine, shaped by years of accumulated clinical experiences. Thus, this book, *Constitutional Medicine of Korea: A Comprehensive Guide to Eight-Constitution Medicine,* has been reborn.

This book not only reinforces the existing theoretical principles of Eight-Constitution Medicine but also expands its practical applications in the clinical practice. It introduces a new Formulae (Prescriptions) chapter for Constitution-Acupuncture, which is essential for patient treatment. These prescriptions act as high-performance bullets that Eight-Constitution Medicine practitioners earnestly need in their clinical practices, providing invaluable guidance akin to the rain in a drought.

Moreover, I have included a variety of clinical cases accumulated at Joowonjang Clinic of Korean Medicine. Readers will have the opportunity to witness firsthand how Eight-Constitution Medicine is applied in real treatments, bringing theory to life in an engaging and practical way.

It appears that Western medicine has never been truly scientific. While it presents itself as science, much of its framework consists of pseudo-sciences. There is no single, overarching principle that comprehensively explains the human body. Instead, it appears to be a collection of empirical, fragmented knowledge about disease treatments. From the perspective of scientists engaged in elite disciplines like physics and chemistry, the theories of Western medicine fall short of the rigorous scientific process of "formulating rational hypotheses – discovering laws – and experimental verification."

If Western medicine were truly a science, shouldn't there be a grand theory or general principle underpinning it? Consider the standard theories in physics, such as Newton's laws of motion, Einstein's theory of relativity, or the uncertainty principle in quantum mechanics. The only fundamental principle I have encountered in Western medicine is the cell theory. All branches of Western medicine—anatomy, histology, physiology, pathology, diagnostics, pharmacology, and so on—are rooted in the study of cells. However, from a scientific perspective, even this is difficult to be regarded as a principle, as it is merely a factual description of the material and physical form of the human body. While accurate, it is limited to a descriptive level, akin to a detailed realistic drawing. It seems like Western medicine harbors a baseless self-reliance, believing that endlessly delving into minute levels will uncover something profound. However, no overarching principles about the human body have emerged.

Behold the current state of Western medicine: how ineffective is it in treating chronic internal diseases, the most significant area on human diseases? Western medicine has been stagnant for a long time. A complete cure for core internal diseases—such as hypertension, diabetes, heart disease, thyroid disorders, and immune system diseases, etc.—remains elusive. Decades have passed while most people rely on lifelong conservative treatments that manage symptoms by controlling numbers or levels of physiological or pathological markers.

The treatment of cancer, one of the most significant human diseases, remains challenging. The efficacy of anti-cancer drugs, which are central to treatment, falls short of expectations when weighed against their severe side effects. Recently, the trend seems to focus on reducing cancer cells as a supplementary measure to cancer surgery. Western medicine appears to prioritize developing techniques rather than pursuing the foundational principle. As a result, internal medicine within Western medicine has been stagnant for a long time, with only surgery—supported by the advanced scientific tools and equipment—sustaining its reputation.

What about medical papers in the renowned academic journals like *Nature*, *Science*, *The Lancet*, or *Cell*, which set benchmarks for scientific discovery? Most studies focus on identifying substances associated with specific diseases, contributing simply to modest progress in drug development for money. Beyond incremental advancements useful for pharmaceutical profit, there are few significant discoveries that explore the fundamental principles. Western medicine lacks the comprehensive general principles that illuminate the life processes of the human body.

In contrast, Eight-Constitution Medicine offers the detailed mathematical principles—"Mathematical Grand Theory"—of the human body. It reveals an astonishingly intricate mathematical structure underlying human physiology, showing that the body operates according to the precise mathematical principles. Few would have imagined that the human body possesses such an elaborate mathematical organization. Eight-Constitution Medicine represents a new *Épistémè* for human species, offering a paradigm shift in understanding the human body and its functions.

Humanity is facing an unprecedented crisis in history due to the extreme global warming. Modern science, once pursued for the benefit of humanity, is now harming humanity itself. Modern science has lost its foundational justification for existence, as it primarily serves to maximize capitalist desires. Until now, science has been dominated by physics and chemistry, whose industrial and technological revolutions have brought us to this point. These advancements are now consuming the Earth itself, ruthlessly erasing the biological home of humanity. Consequently, we find ourselves confronting an immense environmental and ecological crises. Despite this, the world remains fixated on material gain and financial excess.

What we desperately need is a new science. Biology must bear the responsibility for this paradigm shift, as it holds the key to addressing these critical challenges and paving the way for the sustainable future.

It is time for Eight-Constitution Medicine to emerge as a leader in this new science. This is because the Earth needs "New Human" to recreate itself as a thriving home for life. This is a human grounded in life science, standing tall on the mathematical structure of Constitutional Medicine.

Since New Human is founded on the structure of "difference," represented by Constitution, this New Human inherently value diversity. New Human naturally acknowledges and embraces the differences between individuals, recognizing the unique differences between "you" and "me." This acknowledgment fosters a profound love for the coexistence of all beings.

With different Constitutions requiring different suitable foods, New Human naturally consume a variety of foods. This dietary diversity provides an anthropological foundation to combat the destruction caused by large-scale monoculture, fundamentally restoring biodiversity.

Since aptitudes vary according to Constitution, New Human can develop specialized skills and talents across diverse fields.

By following a diet tailored to Constitution, New Human can maintain health independently, reducing reliance on the profit-driven medical industry.

When illness arises, New Human can receive efficient and Constitutionally appropriate care, such as Constitution-acupuncture or Constitutional decoction. This allows one to avoid over-reliance on large-scale medical institutions, the medical industry, and financial capital (such as private medical insurance), granting access to more humane healthcare.

New Human is already equipped with a fundamental model, rooted in the principles of the Zangs and Fus that constitute the human body, to fundamentally counter modern civilization's tragic trajectory of exploiting the Earth for just a season before departing for "Mars." This model enables the realization of the sustainable Earth. We have no choice but to build a new civilization as envisioned by Constitutional Medicine for this New Human.

Eight-Constitution Medicine is a new form of humane biology, integrating the coexistence of diverse humans and the coexistence between humans and nature, all within the mathematical framework of the human body.

Preluded by the author, Suk-won Joo,
Director of Joowonjang Clinic
of Korean Medicine

CHAPTER 1

Zang-Fu Theory

THE HUMAN BODY IS AN EXTENSION OF THE ZANG-FU.
THE ZANG-FU EMITS INFORMATION.
THE ZANG-FU IS A MESSAGE.
THE HUMAN BODY IS ALSO A MESSAGE.

CHAPTER 1

Zang-Fu Theory

The human body is a system composed of "Zang-Fu" (장부, 臟腑), which refers to the visceral organs in Oriental medicine. The biological activities of the human body mean the transmission of organic information between the different Zang-Fu organs. All organs and tissues in the human body are part of this Zang-Fu system. The human body itself can be viewed as the Zang-Fu system.[2]

Zang-Fu is an abbreviation for "Six Zangs" and "Six Fus." The Six Zangs are Liver, Heart, Pancreas, Lungs, Kidneys, and Pericardium, while the Six Fus are Gallbladder, Small intestine, Stomach, Large intestine, Bladder, and Triple Burner (or Triple Energizer). The Zangs and Fus work together, with the Zangs representing Yang and the Fus representing Yin—a perspective that is quite contrary to the traditional concept.[3] Their interdependent relationships can be illustrated as follows:

---

[2] Master Do-won Kuon (1921~2022), the creator of Eight-Constitution Medicine, does not often use the word "Zang-Fu," but instead uses the term "organ." Although he does not seem to reject the comprehensive concept of Zang-Fu, he views it more frequently in terms of internal organs as materialistically understood in Western medicine. Therefore, he explains the Zang-Fu using Western medical terminology as Liver is the organ liver, Heart the organ heart, Pancreas the organ pancreas, Lungs the organ lungs, Kidneys the organ kidneys, Gallbladder the organ gallbladder, and Stomach the organ stomach. However, since the concept of "Zang-Fu" differs from the Western concept of "organ" which refers only to a specific organ, I will continue to use the same traditional terminology of Zang-Fu, except for special cases.

[3] In Eight-Constitution Medicine, the Yin-Yang relationship between Zang and Fu is different from the traditional view. Generally, the Zang is considered Yin, and the Fu is considered Yang, but in Eight-Constitution Medicine, the Zang is considered Yang, and the Fu is considered Yin. This will be discussed later.

- Liver (Yang) and Gallbladder (Yin) complement each other.
- Heart (Yang) and Small intestine (Yin) complement each other.
- Pancreas (Yang) and Stomach (Yin) complement each other.
- Lungs (Yang) and Large intestine (Yin) complement each other.
- Kidneys (Yang) and Bladder (Yin) complement each other.
- Pericardium (Yang) and Triple Burner (Yin) complement each other.

The Zangs and the Fus maintain complementary relationship based on Yin-Yang balance, so the Zangs and the Fus become a whole. If needed, I will group the Zang and Fu organs as above and refer to them as "Zang-Fu pairs," which include the Liver-Gallbladder, Pancreas-Stomach, Heart-Small Intestine, Lungs-Large Intestine, and Kidneys-Bladder. This complementary relationship is also known as "Exterior and Interior Relationship" (表裏關係), where the Yang Zang organ means the Exterior and the Yin Fu organ means the Interior.

This concept can be likened to a carriage, where the left wheel represents Yang and the right wheel represents Yin (vice versa). Together, they cooperate and balance each other to help the "carriage" called the human body gallop forward.

What is the function of Zang-Fu?

The function of each Zang-Fu pair is as follows[4]: Liver-Gallbladder creates[5] Wood Qi (Qi is a kind of life energy) and transmits it to the other Zang-Fu organs that need it, thereby regulating their functions. In the same way, Heart-Small intestine creates Fire Qi and transmits it to the other Zang-Fu organs that need it, thereby regulating their functions; Pancreas-Stomach creates Earth Qi and transmits it to the other Zang-Fu organs that need it, thereby regulating their functions; Lungs-Large intestine creates Metal Qi

[4] This function I am talking about is a premise and a declaration. In other words, it is equivalent to the axiom of mathematics. No proof is required. This is my original Zang-Fu theory, which I developed based on Do-won Kuon's paper in 1965.

[5] The word "create" means "to transform something into something new," not "to produce something from nothing."

and transmits it to the other Zang-Fu organs that need it, thereby regulating their functions; Kidneys-Bladder creates Water Qi and transmits it to the other Zang-Fu organs that need it, thereby regulating their functions.

The word "regulate" is important here. For example, saying that Liver and Gallbladder regulate the Wood Qi means that it can either increase (positive regulation) or decrease (negative regulation) the transmission of the Wood Qi. Therefore, the expression of Zang or Fu organ creating Qi and regulating the other Zang-Fu organs through the Qi should be viewed as a "symbolic" expression such as intangible information transfer, rather than a physical or a material process of actually creating Qi and transmitting it to the other Zang-Fu organs. I intentionally compared the function of creating and regulating Qi in the Zang-Fu organs to a material flow to facilitate the reader's understanding.

The concept of the Zang-Fu organs creating and regulating their own Qi is my very original idea in light of the existing conventional theories of Oriental medicine. The saying that Zang or Fu organ creates and regulates Qi clearly states the relationship between "Zang-Fu" and "Five Phases" (오행, 五行).[6] Still, Oriental medicine only says that Zang-Fu belongs to the Five Phases: Liver-Gallbladder belongs to Wood, Heart-Small intestine belongs to Fire, Pancreas-Stomach belongs to Earth, Lungs-Large intestine belongs to Metal, and Kidneys-Bladder belongs to Water. So what?[7] Just assigning them like this, there is no detailed medical discussion about the specific relationship or mechanism.

[6] Five Phases is a system composed of five Qis which are Wood, Fire, Earth, Metal and Water. The five Qis are in a mechanical or dynamic relationship, constantly influencing on one another.

[7] In Oriental medicine, this is called the "Five-Phase Classification." It refers to assigning humans and all things to the attributes of the Five Phases.

		Wood	Fire	Earth	Metal	Water
Zang	Yang (Yin)	Liver	Heart	Pancreas	Lungs	Kidneys
Fu	Yin (Yang)	Gallbladder	Small intestine	Stomach	Large intestine	Bladder

Figure 1. The Relationship of Zang-Fu, Yin-Yang, and the Five Phases

> The Liver-Gallbladder creates and regulates Wood Qi; the Heart-Small Intestine, Fire Qi; the Pancreas-Stomach, Earth Qi; the Lungs-Large Intestine, Metal Qi; and the Kidneys-Bladder, Water Qi. The words in parentheses indicate the traditional Yin-Yang assignment of Zang-Fu. In Eight-Constitution Medicine, the Yin-Yang relationship between the Zang and Fu is reversed.

Saying that each Zang-Fu organ is assigned to a certain Qi of the Five Phases and saying that each Zang-Fu organ creates and regulates a Qi of the Five Phases are two completely different things. The statement that each of the Zang-Fu organs is assigned to one of the Five Phases suggests that the Zang-Fu belongs to the Five Phases, implying that the Zang-Fu is subordinate to them. However, the statement that each of the Zang-Fu organs creates and regulates the Qi of the Five Phases suggests that the Zang-Fu encompass the Five Phases, as Qi originates from the Zang-Fu. I find this latter explanation much more reasonable, as Qi of Five Phases emerges from Zang-Fu and operates the human body. In conclusion, Liver and Gallbladder create and regulate Wood Qi, Heart and Small intestine create and regulate Fire Qi, Pancreas and Stomach create and regulate Earth Qi, Lungs and Large intestine create and regulate Metal Qi, and Kidneys and Bladder create and regulate Water Qi.

Pericardium and Triple Burner

Pericardium and Triple Burner have different functions compared to the other Zang-Fu organs. Pericardium and Triple Burner do not receive Qi from the other Zang-Fu organs (Pericardium and Triple Burner are not influenced by Five Zang-Fu organs). Instead, they serve solely to harmoniously regulate the interaction between Five Zang-Fu organs.

In Western medicine, there is a nerve pathway called the extrapyramidal tract, located in the medulla oblongata of the central nervous system (CNS). This broadly refers to a specific area related to motor nerves, which is distinct from the nerve pathway called the pyramidal tract that exists in the same medulla oblongata. The pyramidal tract is the area through which the commonly known motor nerves pass. So, through the motor nerves that go down through this path, we are able to perform volitional actions, such as holding a glass or kicking a ball. But this alone does not allow us to harmonize our movements. The act of holding a glass requires the movement of several muscles simultaneously. Therefore, several nerves that control them are mobilized together. Accordingly, harmonious control of these motor nerves is required.

The extrapyramidal system functions like a control tower, reflexively or unconsciously regulating movements such as muscular tension and relaxation based on the activity of the pyramidal system. As a result, numerous motor nerves can simultaneously coordinate the movement of complex muscles, ensuring that they function harmoniously and align with the intended purpose without conflict.

However, when degeneration or functional issues occur in the extrapyramidal tract, the coordinated movement becomes difficult, and the person's movements appear abnormal. Examples include Parkinson's disease, which causes muscle stiffness and unintentional tremors, as well as chorea, which leads to abnormal, dance-like movements. These are movement disorders related to the extrapyramidal system.[8] To use an analogy, Pericardium and Triple Burner function like the extrapyramidal system within the human body's system, coordinating the interactions of the other Five Zang-Fu organs.

---

[8] These diseases statistically tend to appear in people with Geumeum Constitution.

If I borrow another concept from Western medicine, Pericardium and Triple Burner are similar to the nervous system or endocrine system. Therefore, the activities of all organs and tissues are controlled and harmoniously coordinated by them to correspond to the biological activities of the human body. The countless and complex flows of Qi between the Zang-Fu organs are regulated at every moment to ensure that the desired biological activities are carried out smoothly without being biased toward one side.

Nevertheless, Pericardium and Triple Burner cannot be said to be the nervous or endocrine system itself. This is because Pericardium and Triple Burner are not actual organs; they exist only as intangible functions.[9] The Five Zang-Fu pairs rely on one another, receiving Qi from another Zang-Fu pair and each generating its own Qi. Each Zang-Fu pair has a limited function related to one of the Five Phases.

However, unlike the Five Zang-Fu organs, Pericardium and Triple Burner do not generate their own Qis by receiving Qis from the other 5 Zang-Fu organs. Instead, they function solely to harmonize the biological activities of Five Zang-Fu organs by independently generating their own Qis and regulating the Five Zang-Fu organs through them. They are like the "invisible hand" that governs the human body. Pericardium and Triple Burner are like the sun, which provides limitless energy to all the planets in the solar system—Mercury, Venus, Earth, Mars, Jupiter, Saturn, Uranus, and Neptune.

The fact that the Five Zang-Fu organs create Five Qis of Wood, Fire, Earth, Metal, and Water cannot be verified with the naked eyes. Of course, it cannot be detected even with high-performance precision machines such as an electron microscope, a computerized tomography (CT), or a magnetic resonance imaging (MRI). Five Qis are a premise that explains the functions of the Five Zangs and Five Fus.

---

[9] In the chapter "*Twenty fifth Nan*" (二十五難) of the medical classic of *Nanjing* (難經, Classic of Difficult Issues), there is the following reference to the Pericardium and Triple Burner: "It is said that there are 12 meridians, but there are only 11 meridians, so what is the other meridian? Ah! That one meridian is a different meridian called Xinzhu (心主, Pericardium), which branches off from Hand-Shaoyin (Heart meridian). This Xinzhu and Triple Burner form the Exterior and Interior relationship, and both have names but no form. That is why it is said that there are 12 meridians."

Western medicine is a theory of visceral organs

Western medicine is fundamentally "a theory of visceral organs." It focuses on the material structure of organs and their functions. These organs are composed of tissues which are subordinate, and these tissues are made up of cells, considered the smallest unit (Although the cells are composed of even smaller organelles, they are generally regarded as the basic units of life). In Western medicine, organs are functional units that operate based on the activities of cells, the basic units of living organisms. Being entirely grounded in the material foundation of cellular tissues, these organs are groups of substances which drive the biochemical reactions of numerous matters produced and distributed within them. Made of material, they are materialistic organs that accept material and change it to another material, or synthesize new material.

In Western medicine, the function of the liver refers to the function of hepatic cells. Hepatocytes detoxify harmful substances that enter the liver and convert or synthesize substances necessary for the human body's biological activities through biochemical reactions. The same applies to other organs. The heart, through a mechanical pumping action, functions to supply oxygen and nutrients to the entire body and remove waste products. This action is driven by the electrical conduction of nerve cells in the heart, which enables the strong contraction of cardiac muscle cells. The pancreas aids digestion by producing various digestive enzymes in exocrine cells and regulates blood sugar by secreting insulin and glucagon from endocrine cells. In the lungs, gas exchange occurs through alveolar cells, which facilitate oxygen uptake and carbon dioxide elimination. In the kidneys, glomerular and tubular cells filter the blood to remove metabolic waste products and regulate electrolyte balance throughout the body.

Of course, there are many other functions, but these are the most central. These functions are all very factual description learned through the real research on the cells of each organ. This means that they are described "as they are." Nevertheless, this is, in reality, quite far from being science in the strict sense. Isn't the history also about describing facts? Science is not merely the description of facts as they appear, but the discovery of the laws that exist behind those facts. I believe that Western medicine simply describes the phenomena that occur in the human body as they are observed. If you think of it as a painting, it is just a realistic painting. (I agree that an accurate description of this phenomenon is, of course, important and useful.)

Also, the visceral organs in Western medicine are just some of the many organs in the human body. Of course, their importance is higher compared to other systems, but this is not always the case. For example, the organ like the gallbladder is considered relatively unimportant, to the extent that removing it is seen as inconsequential. Similarly, it is believed that one of the two kidneys can be removed without significant issue. On the other hand, sensory organs such as the eyes, ears, nose, and mouth, as well as reproductive organs like the testes and ovaries, are considered more important. However, in Oriental medicine, the Zang-Fu organs are considered almost absolute. They represent the human body itself.

Western medicine is a study that researches various organs, including the substances entering and leaving them, and the substances produced by them. Therefore, I refer to Western medicine as "Human Geography," "Human Logistics," or "Human Geology." It is a study that thoroughly explores only the materials related to the human body. Essentially, it investigates only the body, which is matter, within the framework of Cartesian dualism proposed by René Descartes (1596–1650), who divided the human into "mind and body." In fact, there is a trend these days to view even the mind as a function of substances, specifically the cerebrum, which is part of the central nervous system. The mind is thus also attributed to the body.[10] Brain science may be one such field.

---

[10] This may be viewed from the perspective of "incarnated consciousness," which philosopher Maurice Merleau-Ponty (1908–1961) discussed in *Phénoménologie de la perception* (Phenomenology of Perception). This is because the mind, as an entity, can be discarded and understood as an exploration of the body itself. In fact, the idea that the mind emerges from the body has been taken for granted since ancient times in Eastern thoughts, where the Platonic dualistic thinking of phenomenon and reality was fundamentally absent.

I think the problem with current Western medicine is its obsessive focus on analysis on and on. There exists a fantasy that if all the minute pieces split apart are reassembled like

In his book *Critique of Pure Reason*, Immanuel Kant (1724–1804) clearly delineated the limits of what reason can comprehend by asserting that the "thing-in-itself" (Ding an sich) is unknowable. However, contemporary Western medicine seems to be repeatedly immersed in material substance, believing it can fully comprehend the "thing-in-itself." No matter how minutely we dissect and analyze it, it ultimately provides only an image of one aspect of the human body. Western medicine, in artistic terms, is a discipline that pursues hyperrealism. It charges forward as though there is a Plato's "unchanging Idea" embedded within matter.

In reality, modern philosophy long ago deeply reflected on the blind spots of traditional philosophical inquiry, which had pursued only the unchanging heavens. Since then, modern thought has shifted toward a philosophy of the earth that embraces "change," drawing heavily on core ideas from Eastern philosophy.

Oriental medicine is a theory of Zang-Fu

Oriental medicine is based on the theory of Zang-Fu. Because it has not developed the means to explore the human body down to the microscopic level, as Western medicine has, the cellular functions of organs have not been

---

a puzzle, a perfect picture of the human body will emerge. (Nowadays, modern Western philosophy seems to be completely immersed in our philosophy of "Change (易)", which affirms only the ever-changing real world.)

Among the words of Zhuangzi's friend Huishi (惠施) in the miscellaneous section of *Zhuangzi* (莊子), *Under the Heavens*, there is a phrase that says "zhi-xiao-wu-nei (至小無內)," meaning "the extremely small has no inside" (originally from "至大無外, 至小無內" which reads zhi-da-wu-wai and zhi-xiao-wu-nei: "The extremely large has no outside, and the extremely small has no inside"). If you pursue only the smallest thing, in the end, only nothing will remain. This suggests that you will literally reach the realm of "Form is Emptiness (色卽是空)."

The human body cannot be fully understood through the synthesis of its parts alone. This is quite evident when we consider that modern Western medicine remains at a standstill in the treatment of chronic diseases. What we need now is a new kind of medicine that views the human body as a whole. A good example is Eight-Constitution Medicine, which boldly establishes a macroscopic hypothesis of the human body structure, known as the "Zang-Fu structure of the Constitution," and mathematically formulates the biological principles of the body based on this, carefully verifying and confirming them through actual clinical trials.

discovered. Instead, through human sensations, intuitive insights, symptoms observed in patients, and basic human anatomy, a system was established that has some similarities to Western medicine but is fundamentally different overall. First, let's examine the functions of the Zang-Fu organs in conventional Oriental medicine, focusing on Five Zangs.

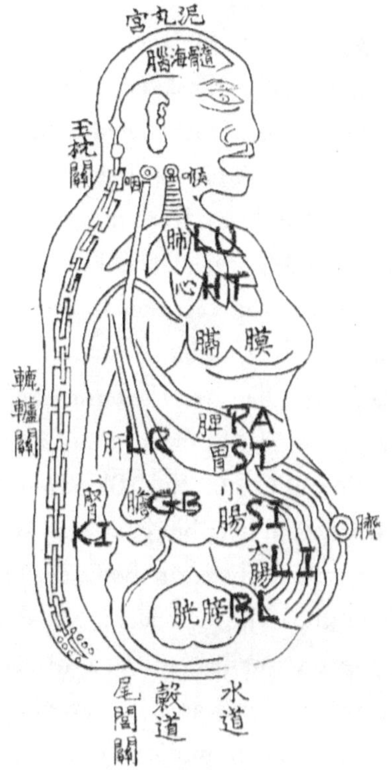

Figure 2. The Human Body in Traditional Oriental medicine

This picture represents a human anatomy called *Sinhyeongjangbudo* (신형장부도, 身形藏府圖) included in the most famous traditional book of Korean Medicine, *Donguibogam* (동의보감, 東醫寶鑑) by Jun Heo (허준, 許浚, 1539~1615), a royal medical doctor in Joseon Dynasty. Although it is quite brief compared to the human anatomy of modern Western medicine, the general location and structure of Five Zangs and Five Fus are roughly consistent. In the figure, LR is Liver, HT Heart, PA Pancreas, LU Lungs, KI

Kidneys, GB Gallbladder, SI Small intestine, ST Stomach, LI Large intestine, and BL Bladder. Additionally, important organs or parts that are not part of the Five Zangs and Five Fus are also depicted.

Let's look at Liver first. In Oriental medicine, the first word that comes to mind when thinking about the Liver is Gan-cang-xue (肝藏血), which appears in the chapter *Benshenpian* (本神篇, On the Origin of Spirit) of the medical classic of *Lingshu* (靈樞). Literally translated, it means that the Liver stores Blood. In Oriental medicine, this is interpreted to mean that the Liver stores blood and regulates blood flow. This seems to be based on a fairly simple level of anatomical knowledge. It is a basic fact that everyone feels the liver looks like a red lump of blood at first glance. However, there is little further specific mention of this Gan-cang-xue, that is, the Liver storing blood and controlling blood volume.

Instead, when it comes to the Liver, the term Gan-zhu-shu-xie (肝主疎泄) is more frequently mentioned, which means that Liver performs the smooth communication of the flow of Qi and Xue (Blood) in the human body. This is not limited to the anatomical liver but has a very broad extension encompassing all organs and tissues of the entire body, even the mental aspect.

As we have come to know through accumulated experience, the symptoms of Liver-related diseases usually manifest as discomfort in the right side, abdominal distension, and in severe cases, liver swelling or even hardening. It is thought that the inability to communicate well in these commonly occurring liver diseases was intuitively linked to the lack in the appropriate flow of Qi and Xue. Conversely, it was deduced that the Liver plays an important role in the communication of Qi and Xue in the human body. It is a kind of reasoning on physiology through pathology.

Also, when mentioning Heart, the term Xin-cang-shen (心藏神) from the chapter *Xuanmingwuqipian* (宣明五氣篇, On the Elucidation of the Five Qi) in the Chinese medical classic of *Suwen* (素問) is always included. This means that Heart retains the spirit, which, if interpreted, means that the spirit resides in Heart. The term Xin-zhu-shen-ming (心主神明) is also frequently mentioned, indicating that Heart governs the spirit and the things related to the spirit. These words clearly state that the primary function of Heart is to control the mental activities of the human body. This is quite different from the heart's function as a blood pump, as discussed in Western medicine. In Western medicine, the mental function of deliberation is now understood to be performed by the brain. It is not that similar views did not exist in Western medicine, but as a result of the development of science and detailed knowledge of the functions of brain nerve cells, views like these in Oriental medicine were abandoned.

Judging by the use of the expression "heart" as a symbol of love, it is clear that there was initially an aspect in the West that viewed the heart as the center of the mind. However, today it is only used in artistic genres such as poetry and music, and the heart is now seen simply as a pump. In Oriental medicine, however, since there was no means of scientific exploration, there was no way to understand the function of brain cells in mental activities, and thus Heart continued to be regarded as the center of mental activity.

If we look for something similar to the cardiac function of Western medicine, there is a term related to blood circulation called Xin-zhu-xue-mai (心主血脈). This means that Heart controls the blood vessels. However, it is closer to the meaning of controlling the vascular system that facilitates blood circulation rather than referring specifically to the pumping action of the heart.

In Oriental medicine, Pancreas has a function represented by the term Pi-zhu-yun-hua (脾主運化). Yun-hua out of Pi-zhu-yun-hua refers to movement and transformation. This means that Pancreas has a function that encompasses both the action of digestion, which transforms the food consumed into the digested ingredients, and the action of circulation, which distributes the resulting refined energy throughout the body.[11] Pancreas corresponds to

[11] The chapter *Jingmaibielun* (經脈別論, Separate Treatise on the Meridians) from the medical classic of *Suwen* (素問): "When food enters Stomach, it undergoes digestion and is filled with refined energy. When this energy reaches Pancreas, Pancreatic Qi breaks it down, and it enters Lungs located above (飮入於胃, 游溢精氣, 上輸於脾, 脾氣散精, 上歸於

a digestive system including the pancreas in modern Western medicine.[12] Considering the pancreas' ability to secrete digestive enzymes, this view is quite similar to the modern understanding. However, the concept of circulation, which delivers the refined energy obtained from this digestive process throughout the body, goes beyond the function of the pancreas as understood in Western medicine.

Another term for the function of Pancreas, which is closely related to blood circulation, is Pi-tong-xue (脾統血). This means that Pancreas controls the blood to ensure it does not escape from the vessels. The function of Pancreas mentioned here is completely unrelated to the anatomical pancreas in modern Western medicine.

Fei-zhu-qi (肺主氣) is one of the representative functions of Lungs in Oriental medicine. This literally means that Lungs control air, that is, breathing. Of course, this was not said with knowledge of the precise mechanism of gas exchange between oxygen and carbon dioxide as understood in modern Western medicine. It is simply a declarative statement that briefly expresses our live and clear experience. For people at that time, who could not distinguish between oxygen and carbon dioxide with their eyes, no further explanation

---

肺)." This briefly describes the process by which nutrients enter the circulatory system via the Lungs following digestion. Surprisingly, the understanding of the relationship between the digestive system and the circulatory system has existed since two to three thousand years prior.

[12] There is an argument that the Pi (脾) in Oriental medicine should be translated as "spleen," but this is clearly incorrect. The spleen in Western medicine functions to produce lymphocytes and destroy aged red blood cells, activities entirely unrelated to the Pi in Oriental medicine. When Japanese scholars introduced Western medicine, they mistranslated Pi as "spleen," and we continue to make this obvious translation mistake (even China is following this, as all English texts in Chinese medicine refer to Pi as "spleen"). These Japanese scholars even created a new Chinese character "膵臟" (cuizang) for the Western organ "pancreas" instead of using an existing one. Considering that the function of the *Pi* in Oriental medicine aligns more closely with that of the pancreas in Western medicine, Pi would logically correspond to the pancreas. Translating Pi as "pancreas" could have resolved this confusion, but the matters instead became convoluted and distorted. It appears that the Japanese scholars responsible for the translation did not fully grasp Oriental medicine, and now we continue to follow their lead. What a nonsense!

was necessary. In relation to the term Fei-zhu-qi, the term Fei-zhu-su-jiang (肺主肅降) is always mentioned. This means that the Lungs have the function of gathering Qi and sending it downward. This expression seems to have arisen because the Lungs are located in the Upper Burner (Shangjiao, 上焦) of the body. Qi goes through a cycle of constantly rising and falling in the human body, and it is thought that the Lungs are responsible for gathering the rising Qi and bringing it down so that it does not disperse. In Oriental medicine, Lungs are envisioned as a cold covering, like a pot lid, that covers the human body.

Shen-zhu-shui (腎主水) means Kidneys control the body's Water Qi. The overall function of the human body's fluid metabolism was attributed to the Kidneys. However, Oriental medicine tends to emphasize the Kidneys' reproductive function more than their role in fluid metabolism. The term Shen-cang-jing (腎藏精) literally means Kidneys contain essence, which clearly refers to the reproductive function of the Kidneys. The Kidneys are said to store Jing (精, essence). Jing is like a seed containing the vitality of life and carries the meaning similar to the sperm. In this case, the Kidneys (腎) correspond to the testicles in modern medical terms. Considering that male castration and the eunuch system also existed in the East, it was quite intentional that the reproductive function was attributed to the Kidneys, even though the connection between the testicles and reproduction was already clearly understood. From the perspective of the Zang-Fu theory, the testicles were simply seen as an organ attached to the Kidneys.

In Oriental medicine, the Zang-Fu not only refers to the organs, as in Western medicine, but also to a functional system that includes appendages and tissues related to the Zang-Fu organs. The Liver includes not only the liver itself, but also the muscles, fingernails, and eyes, and to a larger extent, the Gallbladder which belongs to the Fu. The Heart includes not only the heart but also the blood vessels, brain, tongue, and, broadly speaking, the Small intestines. The Pancreas includes not only the pancreas but also the muscles, mouth, and, to a larger extent, the Stomach. The Lungs include not only the lungs but also the skin, nose, and hair, as well as the Large intestines.

The Kidneys include not only the kidneys but also the bones, bone marrow, ears, and genitals, and they also include the Bladder. Therefore, in Oriental medicine, reflecting the concept of these functional systems, the Liver is also called the liver system, the Heart is called the heart system, the Pancreas is called the pancreas system, the Lungs are called the lungs system, and the Kidneys are called the kidney system.

Oriental medicine is a functional theory

The Zang-Fu theory in Oriental medicine is a system that is empirical in some ways and quite abstract in others. I believe that, based on basic anatomical knowledge, it has been synthesized through human emotions, intuitive insight, and clinical experience. It is systematically established by combining the functions of the actual Zang-Fu organs, understood through experience and insight, with a unique East Asian worldview. It is a thoroughly functional theory that focuses on the functions of real things. Sometimes it includes not only the Zang-Fu organ itself but also other related organs or tissues.

For example, as mentioned above, the Kidneys include the function of the testicles, which are part of the reproductive system. The Liver is associated with the circulatory system, controlling the flow of Qi and Blood. The Heart refers to the brain's mental activity, the Pancreas is responsible not only for digestion but also part of circulation, and the Lungs function to lower rising Qi, although this may seem unrelated to the anatomical lungs.

In Oriental medicine, the concept of the Zang-Fu system is ultimately a functional theory based on a symbolic deductive system called the Five Phases, rather than a substantive investigation of the actual organs. It is a symbolic functional theory that is rooted in real organs, while at the same time extending beyond them.

Therefore, there was not much substantive or noumenal exploration of the Zang-Fu system itself. This was rather unintentional, as there were almost no scientific means available at the time to explore the body. If there had been scientific development in the East similar to that of Western science, there would have naturally been a focus on exploring the physical body. If cells could be directly observed through a microscope and their activities clearly revealed, who would bother discussing the Five Phases and chanting about Yin and Yang? Wouldn't they have looked into it themselves and conducted rigorous research? However, since such means were not yet available in the East, they had no choice but to adhere to the tradition of functionalism. Although it was unfortunate, it also presented a fortunate opportunity to avoid being trapped in materialistic noumena and to preserve the macroscopic insight of functionalism into the organism called the human body.

Pi-zhu-sheng, Wei-zhu-jiang

Oriental medicine's functional theory of the Five Phases is now combined with Yin-Yang theory, blossoming into its unique theory of relationship. There is a famous saying in Oriental medicine: Pi-zhu-sheng, Wei-zhu-jiang (脾主升, 胃主降)[13], which means "the Pancreas governs the ascent, and the Stomach governs the descent." What kind of riddle is this?

We eat every day to survive. When we eat food, it goes through the process of digestion. It is mechanically broken down in the mouth, then turned into a porridge-like stuff by stomach acid and pepsin (which breaks down proteins into peptides) in the stomach, and further broken down by digestive enzymes in the duodenum and Small intestine. After all these processes, the food finally enters the body system through the epithelial cells of the gastrointestinal tract.

When the remaining nutrients and moisture are absorbed in the Large intestine, the food, which was an external foreign substance, finally enters our body and becomes part of it. Thus, the absorbed food transforms into

[13] Short for Pi-zhu-sheng-qing, Wei-zhu-jiang-zhuo (脾主升淸, 胃主降濁). The refined energy produced through digestion is called qing (淸, clear Qi), and the product remaining after the refined energy is extracted is called zhuo (濁, turbid Qi). The action of absorbing this clear Qi into the body and distributing it throughout the body is called Pi-zhu-sheng-qing (the Pancreas is to ascend clear Qi), and the action of transmitting the turbid Qi downward and expelling it is called Wei-zhu-jiang-zhuo (the Stomach is to descend turbid Qi).

nutrients in the blood for our body, is reborn as important substances like enzymes and hormones, and also becomes a component of our body tissue. Ultimately, the process of digestion is the process by which a foreign substance, such as the food, enters the body. For food to enter the sacred sanctuary of the human body, its strong polymer bonds must be broken down and reduced to small molecules or ions.

The poetic expression for this digestive process, where the food enters the body system, is Pi-zhu-sheng, Wei-zhu-jian.

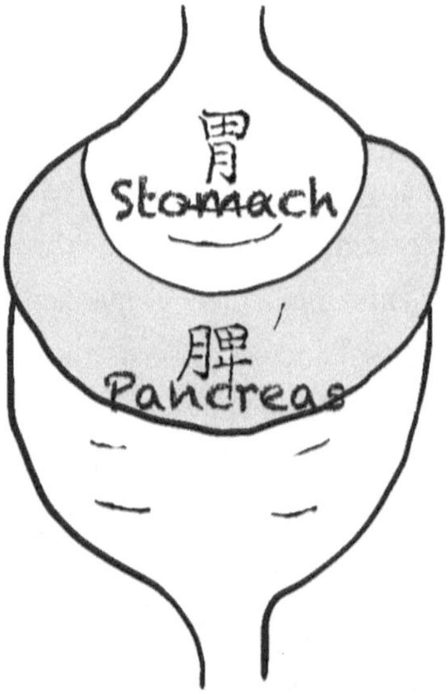

Figure 3. The image of Pancreas and Stomach in the traditional Oriental medicine

The image above shows an example of a traditional illustration. The Stomach is positioned in the center like a sack, with the Pancreas surrounding it. This is quite different from the actual anatomical structure of the stomach and pancreas. When the Stomach breaks down food and sends it downward, the Pancreas digests it and distributes the refined energy derived from it to the whole body.

For food to enter the body, it is broken into pieces by the teeth, destroyed by stomach acid, which is a strong acid with a pH of about 2, and further broken down into finer particles than dust by digestive enzymes. Simultaneously, it must be transported downward with subtle timing by the rhythmic peristalsis and segmentation of the gastrointestinal tract (GI tract). The chemical action that allows food to break down into fine particles and enter the body through the gastrointestinal tract is referred to as Pi-zhu-sheng (digestion), and the physical action that coordinates the timing of decomposition and gradually delivers the food downward is called Wei-zhu-jiang.[14] I think this phrase beautifully expresses the entire process of digestion through the Yin-Yang lens of ascending and descending.

What is important here is that the Pancreas in the phrase Pi-zhu-sheng does not refer to just one organ, namely the pancreas. Likewise, the Stomach referred to in Wei-zhu-jiang does not only refer to the stomach (the organ directly below the esophagus) as we refer to it today. In this context, Pancreas symbolizes the function that encompasses all the biochemical reactions occurring throughout the entire digestive process, and Stomach symbolizes the function that encompasses all the physical reactions throughout the entire digestive process.

---

[14] The entire digestive tract from the mouth to the anus is called the gastrointestinal tract. It is considered to be inside the body, so it appears to be internal, but strictly speaking, it belongs outside the body. From the mouth to the anus, it is outside the body, an extension of the external world. This is proven by the fact that all mucous membranes from the mouth to the anus are composed of epithelial cells. Food that has gone through digestion enters the body only after it is absorbed through the epithelial cells of the gastrointestinal tract.

Nutrients absorbed from the gastrointestinal tract enter the liver through the portal vein, where they are detoxified, synthesized into necessary substances, and then sent to the heart to circulate throughout the body. Only substances that are absorbed from the gastrointestinal tract and pass through the liver are recognized as part of the body, both in name and in reality. In other words, substances before passing through the liver are still considered foreign substances. Therefore, all substances that have not been detoxified and resynthesized in the liver are recognized as foreign and are attacked by the immune system.

To understand the human body, a clear understanding of what is inside and outside the body is required. These distinctions between inside and outside the body were taught through lectures by Doh-ol Young-oak Kim in Doh-ol Academy.

Thus, in the concept of Pancreas, it includes the action of enzymes like amylase in the oral cavity, the breakdown action of pepsin or gastric acid in the stomach, the activity of various digestive enzymes in the pancreas, the bile secretion of the liver and gallbladder, the action of other digestive enzymes in the duodenum and Small intestine, and the absorption process in the Large intestine. The Stomach also includes chewing in the mouth (mastication), swallowing in the esophagus, stomach peristalsis, the peristaltic and segmental movements of the small and large intestines, and even defecation from the rectum and anus.

Therefore, thinking of the Pancreas and Stomach as referring to specific organs is a serious distortion and misunderstanding caused by a poor understanding of Oriental medicine. In this way, Oriental medicine's view of the human body is very different from that of Western medicine.

Harmonic interaction of Heart and Kidneys

The Yin-Yang theory of Oriental medicine is reminiscent of the "archetype" in the collective unconsciousness mentioned by Carl Gustav Jung (1875-1961). An archetype is a primordial and fundamental image or symbol shared by humans, which can be said to represent a common unconsciousness that goes beyond individual experience. This is like a picture engraved in the human mind through the endless repetition of numerous human experiences. Yin-Yang is an archetypal symbol engraved in every corner and cell of our body through countless repetitions of night and day, or light and darkness, as a result of the Earth's rotation. The entire history of mankind, or rather the history of the evolution of all life, or even the entire geological history from the birth of the Earth to the present, is contained within it. I believe that the refinement of this Yin-Yang theory in the context of the organs is the love between the Heart and Kidneys, the harmonic interaction between the Heart and the Kidneys.

The Heart is Fire. The Kidneys are Water. The Heart is like the sun burning in the sky, and the Kidneys are like the water of the rivers and seas that nourishes the land. The flowing water of rivers and seas rises to the sky under the heat of the sun. It becomes invisible water, or vapor, and ascends to the heaven. Steam is water turned into fire. Water vapor rising into the sky meets cold air currents and changes back into its original form, water. The water turns into rain and returns to the earth. The earth, which had been burning with the heat of the sun, drinks the milk of the water from the rain and begins to move again. Life sprouts from the earth. The earth once again becomes a moist embrace, a womb that conceives new life. The Heart is Fire, and the Kidneys are Water. Just as the water of the earth communicates with the fire of the sky to create the cycle of nature, the water in our bodies also communicates with the fire in our bodies to create the cycle of life. This is the meaning of Shui-sheng-huo-jiang (水昇火降), which translates to "Water Ascending and Fire Descending."

Water should be above, and Fire should be below. This is because Water falls from above, and Fire burns from below. The source of the Water is the Kidneys, and the source of the Fire is the Heart. The Heart and Kidneys must interact in this way. The Water Qi of the Kidneys rises upward. Therefore, the Water Qi of the Kidneys should not consist solely of pure Water. There must be Fire in the Water. The Fire is what comes from the Heart. Only with that Fire can the Qi of the Kidneys rises.

The Kan-gua (坎卦) in *I Ching* (Book of Changes) symbolizes Water. The image of Kan-gua is '☵'. Look at this hexagram. In the top and bottom are Yin line "--", and in the middle is a Yang line "–". Yang is Fire, and Yin is Water. There is Fire hidden within Water. There must be Fire in Water for the Water to be alive. Water without Fire is dead Water, which is falling endlessly into the abyss.

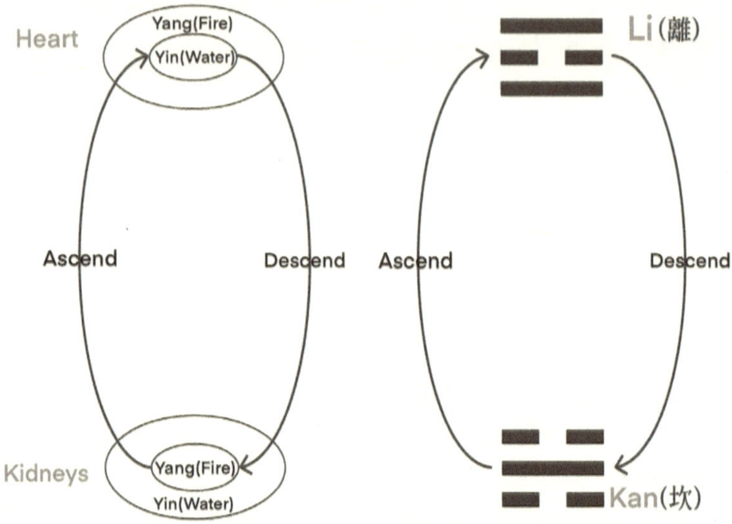

Figure 4. Shui-sheng-huo-jiang

> In terms of the Zang-Fu theory, Shui-sheng-huo-jiang is represented as the ascent of Kidney Yang (腎陽), a Fire within the Kidneys, and the descent of Heart Yin (心陰), a Water within the Heart. The Yang line in Kan-gua and the Yin line in Li-gua symbolize this.

On the contrary, Li-gua (離卦) in the *Book of Changes* symbolizes Fire. The trigram of Li-gua is '☲'. The top and bottom have Yang line '–', and the middle has Yin line '--'. This represents Water hidden within Fire. In this way, there must be Water within Fire so that Fire can descend to the Fire below. The Water in this Fire of the Heart comes from the Water of the Kidneys. Without this Water, the Fire would only rise into the sky. This Fire would also be a lifeless Fire-the Fire of death. It is the Fire of the deadly God whose circulation has been cut off. The Fire of the Heart rises endlessly to the sky, while the Water of the Kidneys falls endlessly into the abyss. This is a world of death where the cycle of circulation has collapsed. The Heart and Kidneys cannot interact with each other, becoming separated and falling apart, resulting in inharmonious interaction between the Heart and Kidneys.

The Fire within the Kidneys is called Kidney Yang. It refers to the Yang Qi within the Kidneys. In Oriental medicine, this Kidney Yang is also called Yuanyang (元陽), the original Yang. It is said to be the purest form of Yang Qi in the human body. Kidney Yang is the vital Qi that is the source of the Fire in the human body and is one of the most important physiological concepts in Oriental medicine. The Water in the Heart is called Heart Yin. It refers to the Yin Qi in the Heart. It is the symbol of the Water that nourishes the earth within the human body. The Heart and Kidneys interact and circulate in this way.

What we must remember here is that Water and Fire discussed in this context are entirely different from Water and Fire of the Five Phases. Water and Fire here are symbols of Yin and Yang, while Water and Fire of the Five Phases represent the two functional units among Wood, Fire, Earth, Metal, and Water that form a dynamic system of Synchronizing and Antagonizing (상생상극, 相生相剋) (the Synchronizing and Antagonizing of the Five Phases will be discussed in detail later). Therefore, the interaction of Water and Fire in Yin-Yang represents two aspects as a whole, while the interaction of Water and Fire in Five Phases represents just two Qis of the five Qis in a system.

In this way, Yin and Yang are a very relative aspect of human "subjective perception", where the interpretation of the system can change depending on the perspective and context. On the other hand, Five Phases are a system of the 5 constituent Qis that realizes a common purpose of the system. They represent the "objective law of the objects" that perform their given functions according to the law of the Synchronizing and the Antagonizing.[15]

Harmonious interaction of Pancreas and Kidneys

Je-ma Lee defined the four Constitutional types, "Sasangin" (사상인, 四象人), in his book *Donguisusebowon* (『동의수세보원』, 『東醫壽世保元』), categorizing them as follows: "Taeyangin" (태양인, 太陽人) has large Lungs and a small Liver; "Taeeumin" (태음인, 太陰人) has a large Liver and small Lungs; "Soyangin" (소양인, 少陽人) has a large Pancreas and small Kidneys; and "Soeumin" (소음인,

[15] Doh-ol Young-oak Kim, *Gichulhak Sanjo* (기철학 산조; 氣哲學 散調; *Impromptu of Qi Philosophy*) (Seoul: Tongnamu Publishing, 1992), pp. 57-58.

少陰人) has large Kidneys and a small Pancreas. He viewed the human body as a system of four main organs ("Four Zangs"): The Lungs, Pancreas, Liver, and Kidneys are arranged in a top-to-bottom structure within the body: the Lungs are located in the Upper Burner, the Pancreas in the Middle-Upper Burner, the Liver in the Middle-Lower Burner, and the Kidneys in the Lower Burner. Additionally, other organs, such as the Stomach, Small Intestine, and Large Intestine, are subordinate to these Four Zangs. The following presents Je-ma Lee's perspective on the human body.

Upper Burner	Lungs (폐, 肺)
Middle-upper Burner	Pancreas (비, 脾)
Middle-lower Burner	Liver (간, 肝)
Lower Burner	Kidnyes (신, 腎)

Figure 5. Je-ma Lee's perspective on the human body

> It is a human body with the Lungs, Pancreas, Liver, and Kidneys arranged in a top-to-bottom structure. The Lungs include the esophagus, tongue, ears, brain, skin, and hair; the Pancreas includes the stomach, breasts, eyes, thoracic spine, and muscles; the Liver includes the small intestine, navel, nose, lumbar spine, and muscles; and the Kidneys include the large intestine, external genitals, mouth, bladder, and bones. Among the Sasangin, Taeyangin and Taeeumin are defined as a pair associated with the Lungs and Liver, while Soyangin and Soeumin are defined as a pair associated with the Pancreas and Kidneys.

The above theory of Heart and Kidneys is accepted as the core framework for explaining the physiology and pathology of Soeumin and Soyangin in Je-ma Lee's *Sasang Medicine*. In Je-ma Lee's system, the Heart is considered the Central Supreme Ultimate (중앙지태극, 中央之太極), and is therefore excluded from the Four Zangs (폐비간신, 肺脾肝腎) that make up a Constitution. Instead, as the central Zang, it acts as the chief mediator that governs the other Zangs. Thus, the Heart of the Heart-Kidneys theory is replaced with "the Pancreas" in Soyangin (large "Pancreas" and small Kidneys) and in Soeumin (large Kidneys and small "Pancreas"). In other words, the Zang governing Fire became the Pancreas rather than the Heart.

The following discussion appears in Je-ma Lee's renowned book *Donguisusebowon*, in the section titled *Soeumin's Sin-su-yeol-pyo-yeol-byeong-lon* (少陰人腎受熱表熱病論), which translates to *A Discussion on Soeumin's Exterior Fever Disease Caused by the Kidneys Receiving Heat*. Pay attention to the hierarchical relationship between the Pancreas and Kidneys in Je-ma Lee's perspective of the human body in the table above. The Bladder mentioned in the below belongs to the Kidneys.

> Zhang Zhongjing (張仲景, 150-219)[16] discussed that Blood Accumulation Symptom in the Lower Burner was caused by the Yang Qi of Soeumin's Pancreas being suppressed by cold-pathogen (寒邪), and the Yang Qi of the Kidneys was also resisted by cold-pathogen. This occurs because the Qi cannot ascend directly to the Pancreas but accumulates in the Bladder.[17]

Also, in *Soyangin's Bi-su-han-pyo-han-byeong-lon* (少陽人脾受寒表寒病論), which translates to *A Discussion on Soyangin's Exterior Cold Disease Caused by the Pancreas Receiving Cold*, the following passage appears.:

[16] Zhang Zhongjing, whose adult name (字) is Zhang Ji (張機), is known as the author of *Shanghanzabinglun* or *The Treatise on Cold-pathogenic and Miscellaneous Diseases* (傷寒雜病論), which had a great influence on Je-ma Lee's Sasang Medicine. For detailed author information and text criticism, please refer to the following book by Doh-ol Young-oak Kim: *Korean Traditional Medicine of Yours and Mine* (Seoul: Tongnamu Publishing, 1993), Preface.

[17] "張仲景所論下焦血證, 卽少陰人脾局陽氣爲寒邪所掩抑, 而腎局陽氣爲邪所拒, 不能直升連接於脾局, 鬱縮膀胱之證也。" Je-ma Lee, *Donguisusebowon* (Seoul: Haenglim Publishing, 1993), p. 30.

This is an explanation of Blood Accumulation Symptom in the Lower Burner from Zhang Zhongjing's *Treatise on Cold-pathogenic and Miscellaneous Diseases*. His discussion of Blood Accumulation Symptom in the Lower Burner is accepted by Je-ma Lee as a framework for explaining the pathology of Soeumin.

> Zhang Zhongjing discussed symptoms such as bitter taste in the mouth, thirst, dizziness in the eyes, difficulty in hearing, discomfort in the chest and flanks, and sometimes alternating chills and fever. It is because the Yin Qi of Soyangin's Kidneys is deficient due to the heat-pathogen, and the Yin Qi of the Pancreas is also surrounded by the heat-pathogen, preventing it from descending to the Kidneys, becoming stuck at the flanks.[18]

Here, Je-ma Lee discusses the relationship between the Pancreas and the Kidneys in terms of the ascending and descending of Yin and Yang as a framework to explain the pathology of Soyangin and Soeumin. (Zhang Zhongjing's detailed explanations of conditions such as Blood Symptom in the Lower Burner and Shaoyang disease are beyond the scope of the subject, so they will be set aside for now.) You can see that the concept is exactly the same as the ascending and descending of the Qi of the Heart and Kidney, as previously mentioned. However, the only difference is that the Heart in the previous relationship between the Heart and the Kidneys is replaced by the Pancreas here as in the relationship between the Pancreas and the Kidneys.

In other words, for Soeumin, the Heart Fire from the interaction of Heart and Kidneys becomes the Pancreas' Yang Qi (Piyang), and influenced by this Qi, the Yang Qi of the Kidneys ascends upward, creating a cycle of Yin-Yang's rise and fall. For Soyangin, the Kidneys' Water from the theory of the interaction of Heart and Kidneys becomes the Yin Qi of the Kidneys. Therefore, the Yin Qi of the Pancreas descends due to the Yin Qi of the Kidneys, creating a cycle of Yin and Yang's ris and fall.

---

18 "張仲景所論少陽病, 口苦 咽乾 目眩 耳聾, 胸脇滿, 或往來寒熱之證, 卽少陽人腎局陰氣爲熱邪所陷, 而脾局陰氣爲熱邪所壅, 不能下降連接於腎局, 而凝聚膂間, 膠固囚滯之病也。" Je-ma Lee, *Donguisusebowon* (Seoul: Haenglim Publishing, 1993), p. 75. Soyang disease, one of the diseases in Zhang Zhongjing's *Treatise on Cold-pathogenic Diseases*, is accepted as a framework for explaining the pathology of Soyangin.

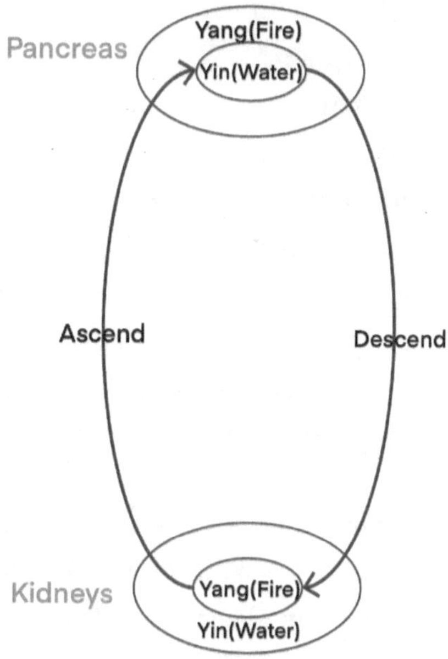

Figure 6. Pi-shen-xiang-jiao (비신상교, 脾腎相交)

> The physiological cycle of the Zang-Fu organs for Soeumin and Soyangin is symbolized in this way. The main axis of Zang either of Soeumin or Soyangin differs depending on the magnitude of the Zangs. For Soeumin, the Kidneys' Yang Qi (Shenyang) should ascend, and for Soyangin, the Pancreas' Yin Qi (Piyin) should descend.

In other words, the key issue for Soeumin is whether it can maintain the Pancreas' Yang (Piyang) alive, and for Soyangin, the key issue is whether it can keep the Kidney's Yin (Shenyin) alive. Therefore, for Soeumin, the core of its physiological activity is always to stimulate the Kidney's Yang to satisfy the Pancreas' Yang, and for Soyangin, the core of its physiological activity is to always stimulate the Pancreas' Yin to satisfy the Kidney's Yin.

This can be seen as the comprehensive resolution, within the framework of Constitutional theory, of the debate between Wenbulun (溫補論, Warming and tonifying theory) and Ziyinlun (滋陰論, Nourishing-Yin theory), which has caused centuries of controversy in the history of Oriental medicine. In other words, the theory of Soeumin refers to the Wenbulun, and the theory of Soyangin refers to the Ziyinlun.

That is, Je-ma Lee reinterpreted the traditional theory of Heart-Kidneys interaction as the theory that explains the physiology and pathology of Soyangin and Soeumin within the framework of his own Constitutional theory. To Je-ma Lee, Zhang Jingyue (張景岳, 1563-1640) and Zhu Danxi (朱丹溪, 1281-1358) were simply the ones who knew only one aspect but not the other. In Je-ma Lee's eyes, Jingyue and Danxi, the esteemed masters of Chinese medicine whom China takes pride in, were nothing more than physicians at the level of a frog at the bottom of a well (井底之蛙).

The Zang-Fu in Oriental medicine or Sasang medicine represents the primary entities—the central actors—of functional theory and relational theory. The terms like Heart-Kidneys, and Pancreas-Kidneys may partly correspond to the anatomical organs such as the heart, kidneys, or pancreas in Western medicine, but they do not carry only the Western anatomical or medical meaning. In any case, the concept of Zang-Fu in Oriental medicine is not an exploration of the thing-in-itself (*Ding an sich*, as mentioned by Immanuel Kant), regardless of whether it is an organ or not. It is nothing more than a symbolic event discussed abstractly within the framework of the cognitive relativity of Yin-Yang or the objective dynamics of Five Phases.

Western medicine is ontology

Western medicine is ontological, while Oriental medicine is functional. Maybe, this distinction is thought to have been determined by the discovery of human cells through the microscope by Czech anatomist Jan Evangelista Purkyně (1787-1869) in 1837. With the development of science, the West gained a deep understanding of the secrets of the microscopic world of the human body, which led to the development of Western medicine. Before that, Western medicine was relatively at a lower level than expected, compared to Eastern medicine. As seen in the various Zang-Fu theories discussed earlier, the level of Oriental medicine up until the 19th century was so advanced that

Western medicine could not match its sophistication and the vastness of its theories.

Thanks to the achievements in the anatomy that became prominent after the Renaissance, British medical scientist William Harvey (1578-1657) refuted the theory of Galen (Claudius Galenos, 129-199) and introduced a new theory that blood circulates throughout the body via the pumping action of the heart. Considering that the principles of blood circulation were only published in the 17th century, we can infer how underdeveloped their medical science was. This concept of blood circulation had already been a matter of common sense in the tradition of Oriental medicine, where the worldview of change was common knowledge, and it had been clearly recognized since ancient times.

Originally, before the development of modern science, the ontology of western philosophy denied the sense-data captured by the senses and focused on an unchangeable theory that existed beyond the object emitting the sense. It aimed to explore the essence, the Idea. Modern science has faithfully followed this tradition and directed all its efforts toward the exploration of the real object, that is, the body as substance. Now, Western medicine has moved beyond the cells and the organelles, delving deeply into the world of molecules. It seems as though a long time has already passed since we entered the era of molecular biology. There seems to be no room for debate that Western medicine's ultimate destination is what I would call "molecular medicine." (The world of atoms beneath it is part of physics, which goes beyond organisms.) Plato's "Idea" still seems to linger throughout all Western thoughts. The molecular medicine pursued by Western medicine appears to be the "substance" (*noumenon*), but in reality, I believe it is merely a microscopic "phenomenon." Therefore, as Immanuel Kant suggested, it may be a kind of *thing-in-itself* (*Ding an sich*), which can never be truly known by human reason. In other words, molecular medicine is nothing more than a highly detailed image—essentially, a form of hyper-realism—that humans create based on the human body.

Je-ma Lee's functional theory

Compared to Western medicine, Oriental medicine does not engage in ontological inquiry. Gan-zhu-shu-xie (肝主疏泄), Xin-cang-shen (心藏神), Pi-zhu-yun-hua (脾主運化), Fei-zhu-qi (肺主氣), and Shen-cang-jing (腎藏精) are all merely symbolic expressions of the functions of the Zang-Fu organs themselves, rather than discussions about their substance. Pi-zhu-sheng, Wei-zhu-jiang (脾主升, 胃主降), Xin-shen-xiang-jiao (心腎相交), and Pi-shen-xiang-jiao (脾腎相交) are all simply theories that describe the relationships between the Zang-Fu organs, taken to their limits. Under this poetic insight based on Yin-Yang and Five Phases, the history of Oriental medicine is a vast variation of clinical theory and practice regarding the functions of the Zang-Fu. And at the pinnacle of this functional theory is Constitutional Medicine.

> The Lungs exhale Air and Fluid, and the Liver inhale Air and Fluid. Therefore, the Liver and Lungs are the gates which exhale and inhale Air and Fluid. The Pancreas brings in Water and Grain, and the Kidneys send out Water and Grain. Therefore, the Kidneys and Pancreas are the storehouses that bring in and send out Water and Grain.[19]

This is what Je-ma Lee said about the physiology of the Lungs, Pancreas, Liver, and Kidneys in *Donguisusebowon*. The Liver and Lungs are seen generally as the Zangs involved in the respiration, while the Pancreas and Kidneys are seen generally as the Zangs involved in the digestion. However, there is no substantive discussion about the Lungs, Pancreas, Liver, and Kidneys themselves. Je-ma Lee's words seem difficult to understand from the perspective of modern medical science.

For Je-ma Lee, respiration is the act of inhaling and exhaling both Air and Fluid together. However, in his theory, the action of exhaling (呼, exhalation) is performed by the Lungs, and the action of inhaling (吸, inhalation) is performed by the Liver. This is a puzzling statement, as we know from Western

[19] 肺以呼, 肝以吸, 肝肺者, 呼吸氣液之門戶也. 脾以納, 腎以出, 腎脾者, 出納水穀之府庫也。Je-ma Lee, Sadanlon (사단론, 四端論), *Donguisusebowon* (Seoul: Haenglim Publishing, 1993), p. 9.

medicine that the lungs are responsible for both inhalation and exhalation, and the liver primarily performs functions such as nutrient synthesis, detoxification, enzyme production, and bile secretion. While it is generally possible to understand that the Pancreas, usually including the Stomach in Oriental medicine, brings in Water and Grain, it is quite difficult to comprehend that the Kidneys send out Grain because the Kidneys seem to partly function like the Large intestines of the digestive system.

As seen before, Je-ma Lee's theory is based on the reinterpretation of the traditional theory of Zang-Fu within the framework of Constitutional Medicine. The physiology and pathology of Soeumin and Soyangin, represented by the relationship between the Pancreas and Kidneys, are explained by the metabolism of Water and Grain, that is, roughly the framework of the digestive system (the previously discussed theory of the interaction between Pancreas and Kidneys can be considered a sophisticated version of this), and the physiology and pathology of Taeeumin and Taeyangin, symbolized by the relationship between the Lungs and the Liver, are explained by the metabolism of Air and Fluid, that is, roughly the framework of the respiratory system. This is where Lee Je-ma's unique perspective on Zang-Fu system is revealed. The Lungs, Pancreas, Liver, and Kidneys are all real organs, but the exhalation and inhalation of the Lungs and Liver, and the entry and exit of the Pancreas and Kidneys mentioned here, are all symbolic, functional theory.

Also, in Je-ma Lee's theory, the Lungs, Pancreas, Liver, and Kidneys do not simply refer to the lungs, pancreas, liver, and kidneys as in Western medicine, which is mentioned above. He summarizes the digestion, respiration, and other functions of the human body in the Zang-Fu Theory of *Donguisusebowon* as follows, considering the Lungs, Pancreas, Liver, and Kidneys as functional systems: the Lungs include the esophagus, tongue, ears, brain, skin, and hair; the Pancreas includes the stomach, breasts, eyes, thoracic vertebrae, and tendons; the Liver includes the small intestine, navel, nose, lumbar vertebrae, and muscles; and the Kidneys include the large intestine, external genitalia, mouth, bladder, and bones. That is, Four Zangs as functional systems explain all physiological processes in the human body.

This ultimately means viewing all organs and tissues of the entire body as a framework for Lungs, Pancreas, Liver, and Kidneys. The entire process of digesting food and circulating it throughout the body is accomplished through these four functional systems. Of course, Oriental medicine also has this functional view of the Zang-Fu system, but Je-ma Lee looks at the Lungs, Pancreas, Liver, and Kidneys in a completely different way from existing Oriental medicine, through the lens of his own philosophy. This can be said to be Je-ma Lee's very unique view of the human body.[20] His discussion of Zang-Fu theory is more of an ideal model than a real phenomenon. Using this model, the physiology of the human body is systematically explained.

However, Je-ma Lee only discusses the Lungs, Pancreas, Liver, and Kidneys within the framework of traditional Yin-Yang theory, and there is no theory of Five Phases regarding Lungs, Pancreas, Liver, and Kidneys. The concept of Five Phases exists only in the definition of Sasang Constitution, which is explained by the pairing of the Lungs and Liver, and the pairing of the Pancreas and Kidneys (they are the pairs of Zangs in Antagonizing relationships).[21] However, Do-won Kuon's Eight-Constitution Medicine is completely different from this.

Eight-Constitution Medicine: the essence of functional relationship theory

Eight-Constitution Medicine is the most refined example of Zang-Fu theory based on the theory of Five Phases. Of course, the anatomical Five Zangs and Five Fus themselves are not discussed at all here either. There is not a

[20] Je-ma Lee, *Donguisusebowon* (Seoul: Haenglim Publishing, 1993), pp. 20-21.

[21] What is interesting is that although Je-ma Lee defined each Constitution as a pair of Antagonizing relations within the framework of Five Phases, he did not say anything about the Antagonizing relations of Five Phases themselves. It is unclear whether this was intentionally avoided or whether the Constitution was defined as the pair of Antagonizing relations coincidentally, simply because the Lungs, Pancreas, Liver, and Kidneys were positioned vertically in the human body's structure. I find the latter more persuasive. This becomes clear when looking at the Four Fus paired with the Lungs, Pancreas, Liver, and Kidneys, namely the Esophagus, Stomach, Small intestine, and Large intestine. Here, only the anatomical upper and lower structures are considered, and the Antagonizing relations are not considered at all. It seems that Je-ma Lee had no interest in Five Phases at all.

single word about what they look like, where they are located, or what they are made of. The discussion focuses solely on the function of the Zang-Fu. The function is also very simple: the Five Zangs and Five Fus create and regulate the Qis of Wood, Fire, Earth, Metal, and Water. There is no classical discussions like Gan-zhu-shu-xie, Xin-cang-shen, Pi-zhu-yun-hua, Fei-zhu-qi, or Shen-cang-jing as in the traditional Oriental medicine. These may serve as ways to understand the Zang-Fu organs, but they do not provide the scientific explanation that unifies them all.

The Zang-Fu theory in Eight-Constitution Medicine refers only to the laws of relationships between Zang-Fu organs that create and regulate Five Qis. The Five Zangs and Five Fus exist as entities, but they are meaningful only as the central actors of the function of generating and regulating the Five Qis, and have no other significance. Therefore, even if there are no physical entities, it is irrelevant. What is important is only the law of communication between Five Qis that arises from the relationship of Synchronizing and Antagonizing (this will be discussed later). The Zang-Fu theory in Eight-Constitution Medicine contains only the theory of relationships. Noumenal theory does not exist here at all.

Isaac Newton (1642-1727) proposed the concept of a particle when describing his mechanics. The particle is like a point that has mass but no size. This is because, if an object has a magnitude, rotational effects may occur when the object is subjected to force, making the mechanics of motion more complex. So, initially, the motion of an object was described for the particle where such rotational effects were ignored. He also introduced the virtual concept of mass, which acts like a constant representing the inertia of a motion system.

In addition, Newton invented calculus to dynamically describe the motion of objects. Through the calculus, it became possible to calculate the instantaneous rate of change, which provides dynamic information about an object's movement at any given moment. Previously, motion was only approached geometrically, which meant only the position of an object at a certain point of time could be known, but not its instantaneous information of motion. This is why Newton's mechanics is called dynamics—because it describes a dynamic worldview.

He called the information about an object's motion its momentum and defined it as the product of the object's mass (m) and velocity (v) (momentum = mv). Ultimately, the instantaneous rate of change of momentum (dmv/dt) is force, leading to one of the most famous scientific laws, "F = ma" where F is force, m is mass, and a is acceleration.[22]

Perhaps Newton's law of motion, which changed the human history, became possible due to the introduction of the virtual concepts of particle and mass. However, such a particle can never exist under any circumstances because a being with only mass and no magnitude is impossible. But we intentionally ignore these limitations and create models by making hypotheses. This is called idealization. In other words, it is like a conceptual model introduced to describe the state of a certain system. In this way, science involves boldly assuming something that can never exist in reality, establishing an ideal model, and logically or mathematically developing the intended theory under that assumption. Through experiments, we then seek to prove that it matches reality.

Establishing a model, making assumptions, developing a theory logically based on those assumptions, ultimately deriving a law as a result, and finally verifying it through precise experimentation—this entire process is science and the scientific method.

The theory of Eight Constitutions is the scientific model of medical science

The Zang-Fu theory in Eight-Constitution Medicine represents a typical example of this idealized model. The Five Zangs and Five Fus in Eight-Constitution Medicine are the control centers that create and regulate Wood, Fire, Earth, Metal, and Water. They operate solely under the dynamic law of Synchronizing and Antagonizing. Beyond that, there are no other constraints. This Zang-Fu system does not physically exist; it exists only as an

[22] To be more precise, in this equation, velocity, force, and acceleration are not scalar quantities that have only magnitude, but vector quantities that have both magnitude and direction.

imagination. In this way, Eight-Constitution Medicine defines the Zang-Fu organs as the subjects of very simple functions and mathematically establishes the laws of Qi communication between them in an orderly manner. This is a classic example of an idealized scientific model.

The real question is what laws can be established from this idealized model, and how useful those laws are for humans. In other words, what therapeutic effects does it have as medicine, and what kind of utility does it provide for promoting health?

People who only know that the liver detoxifies, synthesizes nutrients, produces bile, and makes enzymes will criticize this as some kind of crazy story when they hear the story as the Liver produces Wood Qi. But in fact, they are pretty ignorant. Those who say such things, please bring back the particles that Newton talks about! No matter where you go in the world, you will never be able to find the Newtonian particles. Even if you searched through the entire universe, it would be impossible. Maybe it might be in the black hole. Questions about the existence of meridians or Qi are akin to questions posed by those unfamiliar with the principles of science. If you are one of those people, please verify whether Niels Bohr's (1885–1962) model of the hydrogen atom accurately represents real hydrogen, and let me know your findings. I wonder if you would go so far as to regard Niels Bohr as insane and label him a fraud. These are the ones who do not know that all the scientific truths we know have been established through hypotheses and models that could not actually exist at all. Before criticizing others, you should reflect on yourself.

The law of Qi communication between the Zang Fu organs

The Zang-Fu organs create and regulate Qi. When one of Five Zangs and Five Fus create its Qi, it inevitably requires the involvement of other Zang-Fu organs. In other words, a Zang-Fu organ cannot independently generate its own Qi—one of the Five Qis of Wood, Fire, Earth, Metal, and Water—without assistance from other Zang-Fu organs. For example, the Liver and Gallbladder require the Fire Qi of the Heart and Small Intestine, the Earth Qi of the Pancreas and Stomach, the Metal Qi of the Lungs and Large Intestine, and the Water Qi of the Kidneys and Bladder to generate Wood Qi (see Figure 7 below). Likewise, this relationship is true for the other four pairs of Zang-Fu organs as well. In this way, all Zang-Fu organs in the human body are interdependent. This is similar to how all animals and plants on Earth depend on one another to survive, forming a vast chain called an ecosystem. You are a being that always needs other beings. You are never able to live aloe.

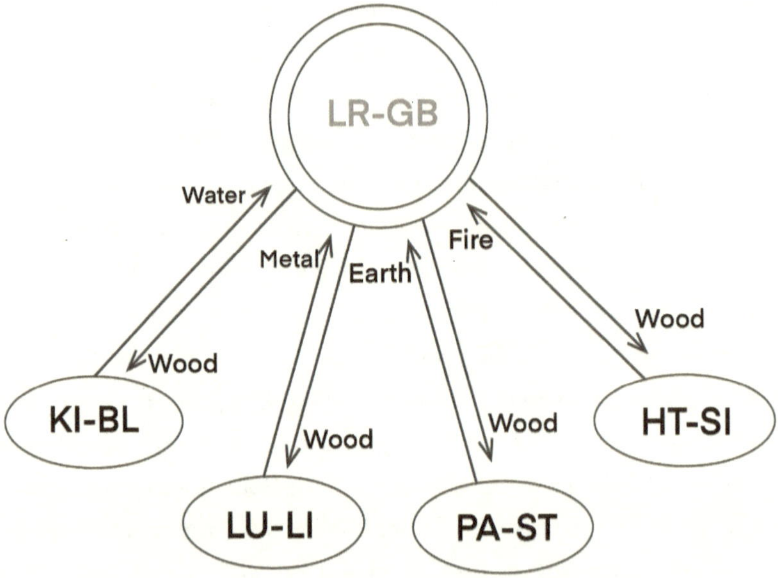

Figure 7. Flow of Qi centered on the Liver and Gallbladder[23]

The Liver and Gallbladder create Wood Qi and transmits it to other organs, and, at the same time, perform their own physiological functions by receiving the Fire Qi from the Heart and Small intestine, the Earth Qi from the Pancreas and Stomach, the Metal Qi from the Lungs and Large intestine, and the Water Qi from the Kidneys and Bladder.

[23] This is a reinterpretation of a picture from Do-won Kuon's thesis from 1965. See also: Do-won Kuon, *A Study Of Constitution-acupuncture*, 1965, p.17.

While Figure 7 illustrates the Qi relationships between the Liver-Gallbladder and the other four pairs of Zang-Fu organs, the following figure represents all the relationships among the five pairs of Zang-Fu organs. In other words, it shows all the Qis that are being communicated between these Five Zangs and Five Fs.

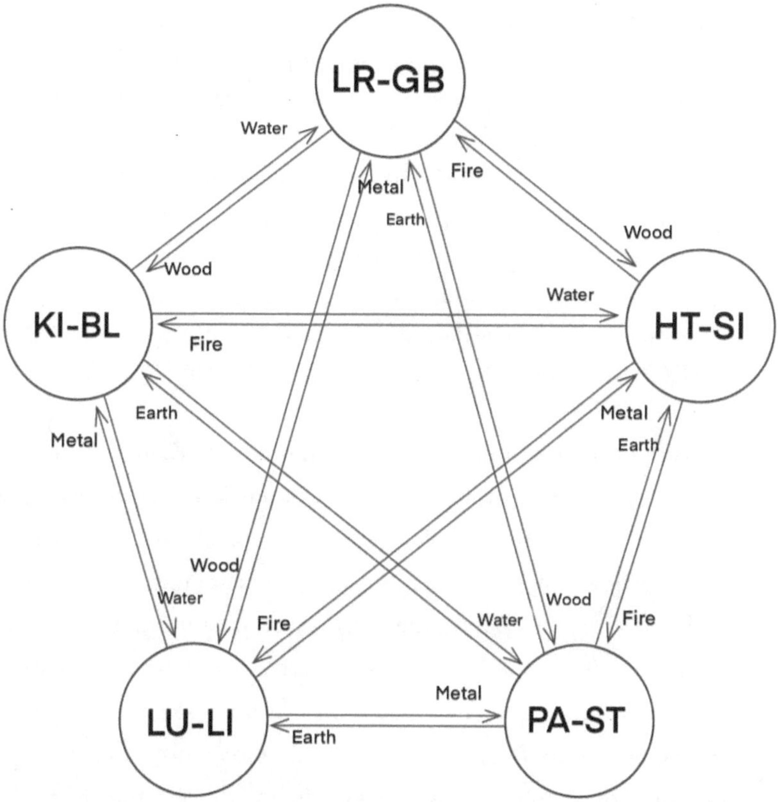

Figure 8. The flow of Qis between the Five Zangs and Five Zus

This diagram represents the relationship between the Five Zang-Fu organs, which I designed based on the hints from Do-won Kuon's Zang-Fu theory and meridian theory. My diagram depicts the flow of Qi between the Five Zang-Fu organs and serves as an important illustration that clearly explains the Synchronizing and Antagonizing relationships in Oriental medicine, which will be discussed in detail later. This is a crucial diagram that corrects the errors of the linear, one-way relationships of Interpromoting and Intersuppressing in traditional Oriental medicine, and it resolves the contradictions in physiology and pathology that often arise within it.

What is interesting is that, just as the gene model of DNA has the double helix structure, which is the core theory of modern Western biology, the flow of Qis between the Zang-Fu organs here also shows a structure of dual pathways, communicating Qis with one another. Similar to Newton's law of universal gravitation, where all the objects in the universe interact with one another through balanced forces, the law governing the interactions among the Five Zang-Fu organs—each communicating equally through Qi—is a natural physiological principle. This allows us to resolve the contradiction and rigidity of the unilateral Qi flow in Five Phases at once, which is one of the biggest blind spots in Oriental medicine. The more detailed diagram showing the flow of Qis between the Zang-Fu organs is shown later in Figure 17.

What is important to note here is that although the Zang and Fu organs cooperate closely with each other, there is no mutual exchange of Qis between the Zang and the Fu. This means that the flow of Qis between the Zang organs and the flow of Qis between the Fu organs are independent of each other. In other words, the Qi from the Zang organs does not transfer to the Fu organs, and the Qi from the Fu organs does not transfer to the Zang organs; therefore, they do not mix. The circulation of Qi among the Zang organs occurs exclusively within them, and similarly, the circulation of Qi among the Fu organs is confined to themselves.[24] This is like the left and right wheels

[24] This is proven by how the meridian acupuncture points are utilized during Constitution-acupuncture treatment. The "unit Formulae", to be discussed later, for the Zang organs are composed only of the acupoints from the Zang organs' meridians, and the unit Formulae for the Fu organs are composed only of the acupoints from the Fu organs' meridians. The two are never mixed. For example, according to the directional tonifying and draining method, the unit Formula for replenishing the Liver in Geumyang Constitution (금양체질, 金陽體質, Pulmotonia) uses the con-puncturing method (needling in the opposite direction to the meridian flow) on LU8 (經渠, Jingqu) and LR4 (中封, Zhongfeng), and the pro-puncturing method (needling in the same direction to the meridian flow) on KI10 (陰谷, Yingu) and LR8 (曲泉, Ququan). The unit Formula

of a carriage never meet each other. Nevertheless, the carriage, symbolizing the human body, functions smoothly because the left wheel, representing the Zang organs, and the right wheel, representing the Fu organs (and vice versa), work together in harmony. The human body is a stereo system of the Zangs and Fus.

Relationship of Synchronizing and Antagonizing

There is a dynamic law of Qi interactions that maintains the overall balance of the human body's system. From the perspective of interactive influence, it is as dynamic as Newtonian mechanics. That is what we call the Law of Interpromoting (상생, 相生, Xiangsheng) and Intersuppressing (상극, 相剋, Xiangke). I believe the term Interpromoting and Intersuppressing can actually be quite misleading. This is because the Interpromoting is often interpreted as bringing benefit to the other party, and the Intersuppressing is often understood as bringing harm to the other party. While this isn't entirely wrong, it's only half true. If you interpret the Interpromoting as purely benefiting the other, it might be understood as merely doing good to the other party. If you interpret the Intersuppressing as suppressing the other, it might be seen as only harming the other party. But that's not the case.

---

for replenishing the Gallbladder in the same Constitution applies the con-puncturing method to LI1 (商陽, Shangyang) and GB44 (足竅陰, Zuqiaoyin), and the pro-puncturing method to BL66 (足通谷, Zutonggu) and GB43 (俠谿, Xiaxi). The Zang and Fu acupoints here are treated completely separately. In other words, there is no unit Formula that combines both the acupoints of Zang and Fu organs, such as "LU8 (Jingqu), LR4 (Zhongfeng), BL66 (Zutonggu), and GB43 (Xiaxi)." This will be explained in detail in Chapter 3, which discusses the principles of unit Formulae.

To be precise, Interpromoting means synchronizing or resonating. In other words, when one increases, the other also increases, and when one decreases, the other also decreases. Intersuppressing, in contrast, mean antagonizing or opposing. In other words, when one increases, the other decreases, and when one decreases, the other increases. Therefore, Interpromoting does not necessarily strengthen the other, nor does Intersuppressing always suppress the other. On the contrary, Interpromoting can weaken the other, and Intersuppressing can strengthen the other. This is a very important concept in understanding Constitutional Medicine. Of course, it is also crucial for understanding Oriental medicine as a whole.

There is also a significant difference between the traditional law of Interpromoting and Intersuppressing and that observed in Eight-Constitution Medicine. Traditionally, the law of Interpromoting and Intersuppressing is primarily unilateral in its movement, whereas in Eight-Constitution Medicine, it is thoroughly bilateral. The traditional law of Interpromoting is *Wood creates Fire, Fire creates Earth, Earth creates Metal, Metal creates Water, and Water creates Wood,* which makes up a cycle of "Wood → Fire → Earth → Metal → Water → Wood", referring to an unilateral movement cycle. Similarly, the traditional law of Intersuppressing is *Wood suppresses Earth, Earth suppresses Water, Water suppresses Fire, Fire suppresses Metal, and Metal suppresses Wood,* also referring to an one-way movement cycle of "Wood → Earth → Water → Fire → Metal→ Wood."

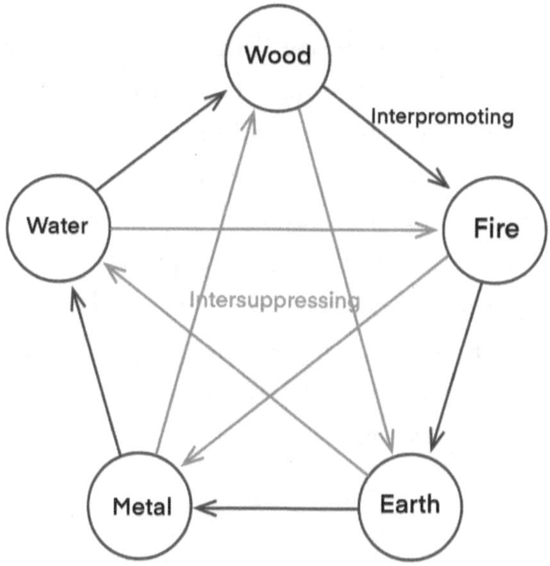

Figure 9. Traditional Interpromoting and Intersuppressing

In traditional Oriental medicine, Interpromoting relationship is one-way as Wood → Fire → Earth → Metal → Water → Wood, and Intersuppressing relationship is also one-way as Wood → Earth → Water → Fire → Metal → Wood.

However, in Eight-Constitution Medicine, both directions are admitted, showing a quite different aspect. In other words, in terms of Interpromoting, not only do *Wood creates Fire, Fire creates Earth, Earth creates Metal, Metal creates Water, and Water creates Wood* exist, but *Fire creates Wood, Earth creates Fire, Metal creates Earth, Water creates Metal, and Wood creates Water* also exist in the same way. Similarly, in Intersuppressing, not only do *Wood suppresses Earth, Earth suppresses Water, Water suppresses Fire, Fire suppresses Metal, and Metal suppresses Wood* exist, but *Earth suppresses Wood, Water suppresses Earth, Fire suppresses Water, and Metal suppresses Fire* also exist at the same time. Therefore, the circle of Interpromoting can be expressed as "Wood ⇄ Fire ⇄ Earth ⇄ Metal ⇄ Water ⇄ Wood," and the circle of Intersuppressing can be expressed as "Wood ⇄ Earth ⇄ Water ⇄ Fire ⇄ Metal ⇄ Wood."

Master Do-won Kuon presented this two-way relationship of Interpromoting and Intersuppressing. This is because it affects both sides of Phases equally.[25] This is also a very important concept that is indispensable in understanding the Eight-Constitution Medicine. Without this concept, the "Unit Formulae"[26] that follows in the next chapter cannot be derived. This concept is what made Eight-Constitution Medicine possible.

Looking at his concept of the reciprocal Interpromoting and Intersuppressing, I made new terms for it, which I think suits his idea the best, that is, the Relationship of Synchronizing and Antagonizing. The Synchronizing means the bilateral Interpromoting, and the Antagonizing means the bilateral Intersupressing.

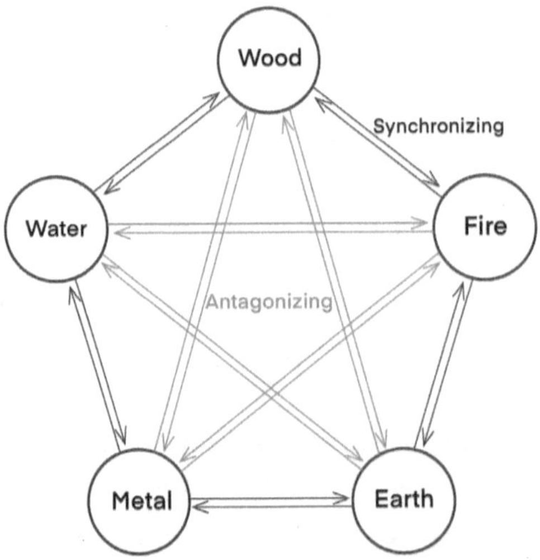

Figure 10. Synchronizing and Antagonizing of Eight-Constitution Medicine

> This two-way Synchronizing and Antagonizing is the greatest revolution in the history of Oriental medicine.

---

[25] "The word 'mutual' here in the present thesis means not that only one side performs either the accelerating or restraining actions, while the corresponding one is only acted by it, but that both sides perform the actions together." Do-won Kuon, *A Study Of Constitution-acupuncture*, 1965, pp.24-25.

[26] This is a term I coined. It will be discussed later in "Chapter 3, Principles of Unit Prescription."

This two-way Relationship of Synchronizing and Antagonizing is actually a natural outcome of the Qi communications between the Five Zang-Fu organs discussed earlier. Since each of the five Zang-Fu organs interdependently receives Qi from the other organs to generate its own Qi, it naturally follows that the relationships of Interpromoting and Intersuppressing extend bidirectionally. I have termed this the "Relationship of Synchronizing and Antagonizing." As depicted in Figures 8 and 10, the Qi communication pathways between the Five Zang-Fu organs are bidirectionally wide-open.

Even in general Oriental medicine, the concept of reverse Intersuppressing, such as "Xiangwu" (相侮), is sometimes discussed—for example, the relationship of Wood suppressing Metal (木剋金, Mu-ke-jin) instead of the commonly recognized relationship of Metal suppressing Wood (金剋木, Jin-ke-mu). However, this is introduced as an exception to explain a special pathological situation.[27] Unlike in Eight-Constitution Medicine, there is no full-fledged discussion of the theory of Interpromoting and Intersuppressing in the bilateral direction (like the Relationship of Synchronizing and Antagonizing) in physiology and pathology.

And there is not a single word about Interpromoting in the reverse direction. However, in Chapter 69 of the ancient classic *Nanjing*, it says, "What is deficient should be replenished by replenishing its mother, and what is excessive should be drained by draining its child. It is right to replenish first and then drain."[28] Here, "draining its child for what is excessive" can be seen as a small clue to the reverse interpromoting.

Draining its son to drain the excessive Zang or Fu can be seen as a reverse Interpromoting. However, because they only view the Interpromoting one-way, they take an ambiguous attitude as if draining the child would lead to a

---

[27] This is called Mu-huo-xing-jin (木火刑金, Wood-fire punishes Metal). Wood symbolizes the Liver, and Metal symbolizes the Lungs. This is a pathological theory explaining that when Liver-fire becomes overly active, it damages Lung-yin, causing fever in the Lungs (肝火犯肺, Gan-huo-fan-fei). Typically, this results in symptoms such as pain in the chest and sides, coughing, chest tightness, sore mouth, bloodshot eyes, and in severe cases, hemoptysis (coughing up blood).

[28] Chapter 69, *Nanjing* (難經·六十九難): 虛者補其母, 實者瀉其子。當先補之, 然後瀉之。

leakage of the mother's Qi. In the end, it looks as if the child stole the mother's Qi. The expression that the child steals the mother's Qi arises because only the one-way Interpromoting from mother to child must be maintained. Looking at these things, it seems that there was at least some recognition of two-way Interpromoting in the traditional Oriental medicine, too. However, it was not generalized as in Eight-Constitution Medicine but remained a special, partial theory.

I believe that the one-way relationship of Interpromoting and Intersuppressing generally accepted in Oriental medicine is wrong. How can only one-way relationships exist in the system of human body? All tissues and organs of the human body are interconnected like a network and constantly interact with one another. This interaction is similar to Newton's law of universal gravitation. The same principle can be applied to the interactions between the Zang-Fu organs of the human body. The concept of the bilateral action of Synchronizing and Antagonizing is akin to the Universal Law of Gravitation in human biology, that is, in medicine.

Why five?

There is a unique paper by former Professor Kwang-seop So from the Theoretical Physics Research at Seoul National University, titled *"Mathematical and Physical Model of the Five Phases."* As a physicist, he analyzes the concept of the Five Phases using the methods of mathematical physics in the paper, where he highlights several characteristics of the Five Phases system.

First, he explains that circularity is characterized by a cycle in which both Interpromoting and Intersuppressing each form a closed circuit.

Secondly, he discusses the symmetry of Interpromoting and Intersuppressing, meaning that even if the double-ring cycle of Interpromoting and Intersuppressing (in the shape of a pentagon and an inscribed star) switches the position of Interpromoting and Intersuppressing, the same structure remains, that is, the double ring of a pentagon and a star, possessing the ame closed circuit.

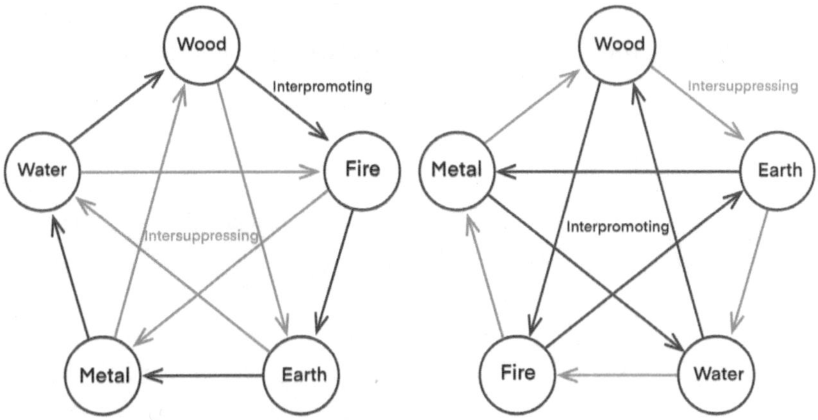

Figure 11. Symmetry of Interpromoting and Intersupressing

> On the left is a diagram of the traditional Interpromoting and Intersupressing. The cycle of Interpromoting from 'Wood → Fire → Earth → Metal → Water → Wood' and the cycle of Intersupressing from 'Wood → Earth → Water → Fire → Metal → Wood' coexist. If you switch the positions of Interpromoting and Intersuppressing, you get the diagram on the right. On the outside, there is a ring of Intersuppressing, represented as 'Wood → Earth → Water → Fire → Metal → Wood,' and on the inside, a ring of Interpromoting, represented as 'Wood → Fire → Earth → Metal → Water → Wood.' Even if the positions of Interpromoting and Intersuppressing are switched, the double-linked structure remains intact.

Thirdly, he mentioned on direct action, where each of Five Phases directly interacts with the other four Phases in Interpromoting and Intersuppressing.

Fourthly, the reason why it is composed of Five Phases was explained—it is because it is a minimal system that simultaneously satisfies the three conditions mentioned above. An even number would break the symmetry and circularity of Interpromoting and Intersuppressing, and an odd number would violate the direct interaction between all the Phases. I believe this is an excellent insight that offers a very important perspective in the interpretation of the Five Phases system. It is a truly incisive analysis tha helps us understand how the worldview called Five Phases was formed in East Asia.[29]

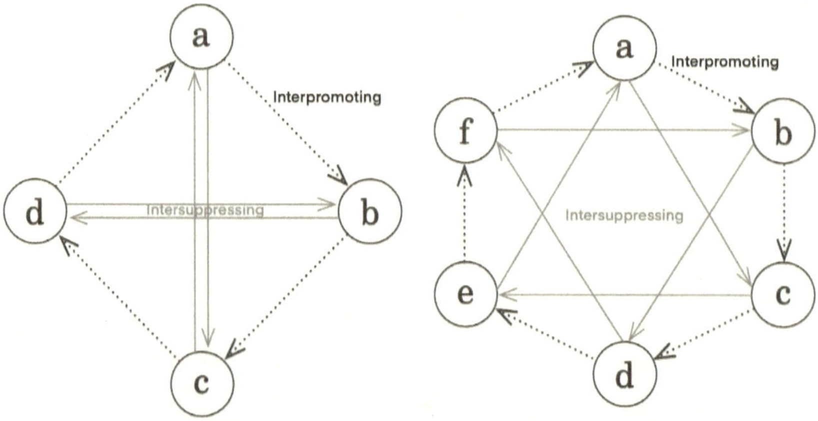

Four Phases Six Phases

Figure 12. Even Phases

In the case of four Phases, Interpromoting forms a loop of a→b→c→d→a, but the Intersuppressing becomes a⇄c and b⇄d, dividing the loop into two. In the case of six Phases, Interpromoting forms a ring of a→b→c→d→e→f→a, but the Intersuppressing is also divided into two rings, a→c→e→a and b→d→f→b. Essentially, all even Phases violate circularity and symmetry of Interpromoting and Itersuppressing.

[29] Kwang-seop So, "Mathematical and Physical Model of Five Phases," *Science and Philosophy Vol. 4*, (Seoul: Tongnamu Publishing, 1993), pp. 39-45.

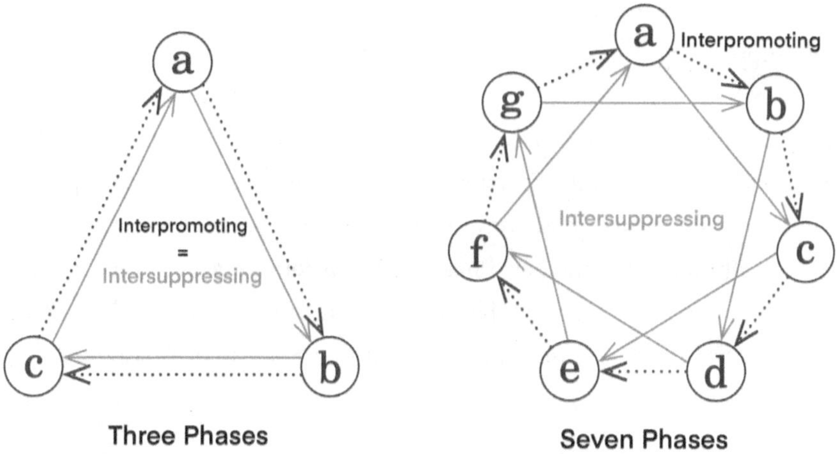

Figure 13. Odd Phases

In the case of three Phases, both Interpromoting and Intersuppressing become a→b→c→a, forming only the same loop, so they cannot fundamentally form a mutually beneficial relationship. In the case of odd-numbered Phases with fewer than 5 Phases, a mutually beneficial relationship is impossible. In the case of seven Phases, Interpromoting forms a ring as a→b→c→d→e→f→g→a, and Intersuppressing also forms a ring as a→c→e→g→b→d→f→a. Circularity exists. However, the condition that all Phases must interact directly with each other is not satisfied. For example, from "a"'s perspective, "a and d" as well as "a and e" do not have a direct Interpromoting or Intersuppressing relationship, as shown in the figure. All odd Phases with more than 5 Phases do not satisfy direct functionality. Therefore, it is disadvantageous in constructing the simplest minimal system.

The Five Phases are the simplest yet most detailed scientific model of the East Asian universe and human body, designed as a minimal system in which Interpromoting and Intersuppressing act directly between all Phases, while at the same time maintaining symmetry in the cycles of Interpromoting and Intersuppressing.

Professor Gwang-seop So's perspective provides a very important clue to understanding the East Asian view of the universe. It also presents a fundamental and core deep structure that is indispensable for understanding the view of the human body in Oriental medicine. We are so accustomed to uncritically accepting the Five Phases as an obvious premise and proceeding with our thinking from there. However, the question of why the Five Phases exist is actually a very important issue that should never be overlooked.

Five Phases system: the law of objects

The Five Phases system is not merely a categorization tool for humans to understand themselves and their environment. It is not simply about grouping things into five origins or classifying them as having the nature of wood, fire, earth, metal, or water. Nor is it a superficial reduction that attempts to comprehend objects by dividing them into plausible elements, like the Buddhist earth-water-fire-wind system or Western theories such as the three-element, four-element, five-element, or eight-element theories. Such concepts are merely common cultural understandings that exist across the world and within any civilization. The Five Phases theory is by no means a worldly five-element theory that claims all things are created from five basic elements. If that were the case, then everything except the 118 elements in the chemical periodic table should be discarded.

The Five Phases are the result of the human cognitive process, which conceptualizes the order of movement of objects as five forms of functions. It is an idealized scientific model that conceptualizes this world as a minimal system, where the relationships of Interpromoting and Intersuppressing are symmetrically established, and interactions occur only through direct engagement with each constituent Phase of the system.

In this context, there is no noumenal interest in the constituents of the world. The ontological question of what Wood, Fire, Earth, Metal, and Water are composed of is entirely meaningless. Similarly, the taxonomic interest in classifying what belongs to Wood, Fire, Earth, Metal, or Water holds no essential meaning.

It's better to disregard Wood, Fire, Earth, Metal, and Water as constituent elements of the system; it doesn't matter if they are labeled A, B, C, D, or E. In fact, considering them as mathematical variables without semantic meaning might be more appropriate. Their existence is inconsequential; it's preferable to think of them as non-existent since they exist solely as functions. They are not entities but functions. What matters is the action within the system. Ultimately, the significance lies in the laws governing the interactions among Wood, Fire, Earth, Metal, and Water—how they influence each other and how they contribute to the system's overall purpose. The significance of Professor Gwang-seop So's theory, which views the Five Phases from the perspective of functional system theory and mathematically demonstrates their causality, cannot be overstated.

However, it must be noted that his adherence to the traditional one-way view of Interpromoting and Intersuppressing is a limitation in this context. In applying system theory in this paper, he interprets the cycle of Interpromotion as positive feedback and the cycle of Intersuppression as negative feedback. While this interpretation is not entirely incorrect, in the actual human body, physiological functions and pathologies do not strictly follow the order of Wood → Fire → Earth → Metal → Water → Wood (which is a Interpromoting cycle), or Wood → Earth → Water → Fire → Metal → Wood (which is a Intersuppressing cycle). Some processes occur selectively, while others occur in a complex, random manner, crossing between Interpromoting and Intersuppressing.

This indicates that the given sequences are not blindly followed, as they might be in a simple automatic control system. Such feedback mechanisms do not apply to the human body in Oriental medicine. This type of feedback primarily pertains, for example, to the hormonal control system in Western medicine, which generally involves negative feedback. Moreover, in Eight-Constitution Medicine, as previously mentioned, Interpromoting and Intersuppressing are bilateral, which significantly differs from Professor Gwang-seop So's model. I believe that this bilaterality is not exclusive to Eight-Constitution Medicine but should serve as the foundation for a general theory of Oriental medicine with universal applicability.

In his paper, Professor Kwang-seop So designates the Five Phases—Wood, Fire, Earth, Metal, and Water—as state variables S_1, S_2, S_3, S_4, and S_5, respectively. He defines the time rate of change for these state variables and formulates a differential equation accordingly. This equation is derived from the traditional unidirectional Interpromoting and Intersuppression relationships.

$$
\begin{gathered}
dS1/dt = \alpha S5 - \beta S4 \\
dS2/dt = \alpha S1 - \beta S5 \\
dS3/dt = \alpha S2 - \beta S1 \\
dS4/dt = \alpha S3 - \beta S2 \\
dS5/dt = \alpha S4 - \beta S3 \\
(\alpha, \beta > 0, \text{constants})
\end{gathered}
$$

In the Five Phases model, the state variable S_1, representing Wood, receives an Interpromoting effect from S_5 (Water) and an Intersuppressing effect from S_4 (Metal). Consequently, the instantaneous rate of change for S_1 can be expressed as: $dS_1/dt = \alpha S_5 - \beta S_4$ where α and β are proportionality constants. Applying similar unidirectional Interpromoting and Intersuppressing interactions to the instantaneous rates of change for the remaining state variables S_2, S_3, S_4, and S_5 yields a system of differential equations. The formulation of differential equations can vary depending on the system's perspective; however, Professor Kwang-seop So opted for the simplest equations for convenience in his approach.

I do not believe that this differential equation fully describes the system of the Five Phases because it is based on a unidirectional Interpromoting and Intersuppression relationship, rather than a bidirectional Synchronizing and Antagonizing relationship. Therefore, considering the bidirectional Synchronizing and Antagonizing relationships discussed previously, Professor Kwang-seop So's differential equation should be reformulated as follows.

$$dS1/dt = \alpha S2 - \beta S3 - \gamma S4 + \delta S5$$
$$dS2/dt = \alpha S3 - \beta S4 - \gamma S5 + \delta S1$$
$$dS3/dt = \alpha S4 - \beta S5 - \gamma S1 + \delta S2$$
$$dS4/dt = \alpha S5 - \beta S1 - \gamma S2 + \delta S3$$
$$dS5/dt = \alpha S1 - \beta S2 - \gamma S3 + \delta S4$$
$$(\alpha, \beta, \gamma, \delta > 0, \text{constants})$$

In the equation above, state variables with a plus sign indicate the effect of Synchronizing actions, while those with a minus sign represent the effect of Antagonizing actions. Therefore, the instantaneous rate of change of S_1 (dS_1/dt) is influenced simultaneously by the synchronizing effects of S_2 and S_5 ($\alpha S_2 + \delta S_5$) and the antagonizing effects of S_3 and S_4 ($-\beta S_3 - \gamma S_4$). This relationship is expressed as: $dS_1/dt = \alpha S_2 - \beta S_3 - \gamma S_4 + \delta S_5$.

Applying the same method to determine the instantaneous rates of change for the remaining variables S_2, S_3, S_4, and S_5 results in a system of differential equations involving these five variables. Solving this system allows for accurate predictions of the states of the Five Qis—Wood, Fire, Earth, Metal, and Water—at any given time under specified conditions.[30]

If the Five Phases system had been interpreted by introducing the concept of two-way Interpromoting and Intersuppressing, that is, Synchronizing and Antagonizing, the differential equation model of the Five Phases that he proposed could have been a more realistic and practical model. It would have been even better if the perspective of Eight-Constitution Medicine, which reflects the Constitutional relationships of all Five Zangs and Fus, had been applied here as well.

Zang-Fu system is an idealized system that applies the Five Phase relationship as a minimal system of Synchronizing and Antagonizing to the human body. The Liver and Gallbladder create and regulate Wood Qi; the Heart and Small Intestine Fire Qi; the Pancreas and Stomach Earth Qi; the Lungs and Large Intestine Metal Qi; and the Kidneys and Bladder Water Qi. In general Oriental medicine, this creative and regulatory function is

[30] Kwang-seop So, "Mathematical and Physical Model of the Five Elements," *Science and Philosophy Vol. 4* (Seoul: Tongnamu Publishing, 1993), pp. 46-56.

often vaguely attributed to the Five Phase properties of the Zang-Fu organs. Such terminology tends to overlook the intricate processes involved in Qi generation within these Zang-Fu organs and the specific laws governing Qi communication between them, which will be elaborated upon later. Although this may seem like common knowledge, a closer examination reveals a lack of substantive content, rendering the explanation as nebulous as fog. Science demands precision.

The true meaning of the law of Synchronizing and Antagonizing

Each Zang-Fu organ uses the Qi delivered from the other four Zang-Fu organs to regulate the generation of Qi within itself. Therefore, a Zang-Fu organ's ability to regulate its Qi depends on the ability of the other four Zang-Fu organs to regulate their Qis. For example, the ability of the Liver and Gallbladder to regulate Wood Qi depends on the Heart and Small Intestine's ability to regulate Fire Qi, the Pancreas and Stomach's ability to regulate Earth Qi, the Lungs and Large Intestine's ability to regulate Metal Qi, and the Kidneys and Bladder's ability to regulate Water Qi.

For instance, if the production of Water Qi in the Kidneys and Bladder increases, the production of Wood Qi in the Liver and Gallbladder will also increase as it receives that Water Qi. Conversely, if the production of Water Qi in the Kidneys and Bladder decreases, the supply of Water Qi will decrease, leading to a reduction in the production of Wood Qi in the Liver and Gallbladder.

Therefore, the law of Interpromoting and Intersuppressing of the Five Phases applies equally to the Five Zangs and Five Fus which create 5 Qis. That is, there are relationships of Interpromoting where the Liver promotes the Heart, the Heart promotes the Pancreas, the Pancreas promotes the Lungs, the Lungs promotes the Kidneys, and the Kidneys promotes the Liver, along with their Intersuppressing relationships where the Liver suppresses the Pancreas, the Pancreas suppresses the Kidneys, the Kidneys suppresses the Heart, the Heart suppresses the Lungs, and the Lungs suppresses the Liver.

This same relationship is established not only between the Five Zangs but also between the Five Fus. For instance, the Gallbladder promotes the Small intestine, the Small intestine promotes the Stomach, the Stomach promotes the Large intestine, the Large intestine promotes the Bladder, and the Bladder promotes the Stomach. There are also Intersuppressing relationships where the Gallbladder suppresses Stomach, Stomach suppresses Bladder, Bladder suppresses Small intestine, Small intestine suppresses Large intestine, and Large intestine suppresses Gallbladder.

The Interpromoting and Intersuppressing relationships between Zang-Fu organs in Eight-Constitution Medicine are bilateral. Therefore, in addition to the traditional relationships of Interpromoting and Intersuppressing, there are also reverse-direction relationships, such as the Heart promoting the Liver, the Pancreas promoting the Heart, the Lungs promoting the Pancreas, the Kidneys promoting the Lungs, and the Liver promoting the Kidneys.

Similarly, reverse-direction Intersuppressing relationships are established, such as the Pancreas suppressing the Liver, the Kidneys suppressing the Pancreas, the Heart suppressing the Kidneys, the Lungs suppressing the Heart, and the Liver suppressing the Lungs.

The same bilateral relationships apply to the Five Fu organs. Reverse-direction Interpromoting relationships include the Small Intestine promoting the Gallbladder, the Stomach promoting the Small Intestine, the Large Intestine promoting the Stomach, the Bladder promoting the Large Intestine, and the Gallbladder promoting the Bladder.

Likewise, reverse-direction Intersuppressing relationships include the Stomach suppressing the Gallbladder, the Bladder suppressing the Stomach, the Small Intestine suppressing the Bladder, the Large Intestine suppressing the Small Intestine, and the Gallbladder suppressing the Large Intestine.

In general Oriental medicine, the law of Interpromoting and Intersuppressing between Zang-Fu organs has traditionally been limited to simply applying the law of Interpromoting and Intersuppressing of Five Phases. However, in Eight-Constitution Medicine, the law of Qi communication between Zang-Fu organs is presented in more detail. For example, when it is said that the Liver-Gallbladder promote the Heart-Small Intestine, the specific mechanism can be explained as follows: the Wood Qi generated by the Liver-Gallbladder is transmitted to the Heart-Small Intestine, thereby enhancing the Fire Qi in the Heart-Small Intestine. Conversely, when it is said that the Heart-Small intestine promotes the Liver-Gallbladder, this can be understood as follows: the Fire Qi generated from the Heart-Small intestine is transmitted to the Liver-Gallbladder, thereby enhancing the Liver-Gallbladder's ability to generate Wood Qi (See Figure 7). In addition, the fact that the Liver-Gallbladder exert the greatest influence on the Pancreas-Stomach can be explained by the Wood Qi generated from the Liver-Gallbladder being transmitted to the Pancreas-Stomach, suppressing the function of producing Earth Qi in the Pancreas-Stomach. Conversely, the fact that the Pancreas-Stomach suppress the Liver-Gallbladder can also be interpreted as the Earth Qi produced by the Pancreas-Stomach being transmitted to the Liver-Gallbladder, thereby suppressing the production function of Wood Qi in the Liver-Gallbladder. In this same way, all the mutually influential relationships between the Five Zang organs and the Five Fu organs can be explained (See Figure 8).

Core functions of the meridians

The Qi communications between these Zang-Fu organs take place through pathways called meridians. The meridians generally refer to Primary Meridians (12 main meridians) and Collaterals.[31] All Qi flows in the human body occur through these meridians and collaterals. The Primary Meridians are the most important pathways in the human body, representing the main channels or standard channels of the body. Collaterals are branches that split off from the Primary Meridians, distributed in more superficial areas than the Primary Meridians. If the Primary Meridians are like main lines, Collaterals are like branch lines. Therefore, if the Primary Meridians resemble big blood vessels such as the aorta in Western medicine, the Collaterals resemble tiny

[31] If the meridians are further subdivided, there are Primary Meridians (twelve main meridians), Eight Extraordinary Meridians, Collateral meridians, Sinew Meridians, Divergent Meridians, Cutaneous Regions, and Minute Collaterals.

blood vessels like arterioles or capillaries. Since the Collaterals depend on the Primary Meridians, the Primary Meridians are, of course, crucial.

There are 12 meridians in the Primary Meridian system. Since these exist in pairs on the left and right of the body, there are a total of 24 meridians. Each meridian is connected to a single organ or system in the body and flows through the tissues and skin that the meridian controls. Since there are six Zangs and six Fus in the human body, there are 12 meridians. These meridians are largely divided into Yin meridians and Yang meridians. Yin meridians usually flow inside the human body, and Yang meridians flow outside the human body (with some exceptions). In traditional Oriental medicine, the Yin meridians are associated with the Zangs, and the Yang meridians are associated with the Fus.

Therefore, the Yin meridians include the Liver meridian, Heart meridian, Pancreas meridian, Pericardium meridian, Kidney meridian, and Lung meridian, while the Yang meridians include the Gallbladder meridian, Small intestine meridian, Stomach meridian, Large intestine meridian, Bladder meridian, and Triple Burner meridian.[32]

All meridians connect the torso with the extremities. Out of 12 Primary Meridians, six meridians are connected to the hands, and the other six meridians are connected to the feet. Specifically, the three Yin meridians in the hands are connected to the three Yang meridians, and the three Yin

---

[32] However, according to Do-won Kuon, in Eight Constitution Medicine, the traditional associations of Yin and Yang are reversed: the Fus are considered Yin, and the Zangs are considered Yang. He explains that when humans stand upright in the course of evolution, the Yin meridians, which was oriented toward the ground, faces forward, and the Yang meridians, which was oriented toward the sky, faces backward, leading to a reversal of Yin and Yang. In this context, he altered the Yin-Yang classification based on his own unique meridian theory. However, this reversal of Yin-Yang has somewhat insignificant clinical implications in actual practice. Eight-Constitution Medicine is not a theory of the vertically ascending and descending Yin and Yang like Je-ma Lee's theory, but rather a theory of the horizontally interacting Five Phases. This can be understood when looking at the prescription theory in Eight-Constitution Medicine. A brief tip is that in the "Unit Prescription," which is the basic unit of Eight-Constitutions' acupuncture treatment, the acupuncture points of the Zang and Fu meridians are never mixed within any single Unit Prescription. This means that the acupoints are managed independently according to the Zang-system, and independently according to the Fu-system, regardless of whether the Zang or Fu organs are classified as Yin or Yang.

meridians in the feet are connected to the three Yang meridians in the feet. The three Hand Yin meridians include the Lung meridian, Heart meridian, and Pericardium meridian, while the three Hand Yang meridians include the Large intestine meridian, Small intestine meridian, and Triple Burner meridian. The three Foot Yin meridians include the Liver meridian, Pancreas meridian, and Kidney meridian, while the three Foot Yang meridians include the Gallbladder meridian, Stomach meridian, and Bladder meridian.

Each of these 12 meridians is connected to one of the Zang or Fu organs and regulates that organ, while, at the same time, all the meridians are interconnected, forming one large circulatory network. This is called the flow of the 12 meridians. As Qi flows through these 12 meridians, it passes through the acupuncture points of each meridian. Acupuncture points are like gateways through which the Qi of each meridian enters and exits. The flow of the 12 meridians are as follows:

> Lung Meridian (torso → fingertips) ⇢ Large intestine Meridian (fingertips → torso) ⇢ Stomach Meridian (torso → toes) ⇢ Pancreas Meridian (toes → torso) ⇢ Heart Meridian (torso → fingertips) ⇢ Small intestine Meridian (fingertips → torso) ⇢ Bladder Meridian (torso → toes) ⇢ Kidney Meridian (soles of feet → torso) ⇢ Pericardium Meridian (torso → fingertips) ⇢ Triple Burner Meridian (fingertips → torso) ⇢ Gallbladder Meridian (torso → toes) ⇢ Liver Meridian (toes → torso) ⇢ Lung Meridian.

These 12 meridians travel back and forth between the torso and the extremities, forming a continuous circuit from the Lung meridian to the Liver meridian, nourishing the whole body, and are closely connected to the six Fu organs and six Zang organs. In short, the meridians are the paths along which the Qis including the five Qis of Wood, Fire, Earth, Metal, and Water move. In other words, the Qis generated in the Zang-Fu organs are supplied to the entire body through the meridians, and adversely, they regulate the Zang-Fu organs through the meridians distributed throughout the body.

However, I think that the Qi flow of these 12 meridians is highly imaginary. This is because, in reality, the flow of Qi does not follow the predetermined path in a sequential manner. As seen in the example of the Synchronizing and Antagonizing of the Five Phases, the flow of Qi moves directly and invisibly through the direct lines between the Zang-Fu organs. In clinical practice, for instance, when Constitution-acupuncture is performed, the transfer of Qi occurs instantaneously, like lightning, from the Liver to the Lungs or from the Pancreas to the Kidneys. It is not at all necessary to pass through the designated flow of 12 meridians step by step to reach the target. In the same way, the flow of Qi is not one-directional as previously described. Of course, the reverse movement occurs in the same frequency.

Additionally, while the pathways of the 12 meridians are traditionally understood to perform the Qi flow uniformly from a Zang to a Fu, and the Fu to a Zang serially in the designated order, this has not been empirically substantiated in Eight-Constitution Medicine. It is clinically observed in Eight-Constitution Medicine that the Zang organs exchange Qi exclusively among themselves, and similarly, the Fu organs exchange Qi only within their group. The Zang and Fu are like parallel railroad tracks that run alongside each other forever without any connection.[33]

This transmission and regulation of Qi is specifically carried out by approximately 361 acupuncture points in the body's meridians. However, controlling the flow of Qi between Zang-Fu organs does not require mobilizing all of these 361 acupuncture points. There are special acupuncture points that regulate only the Zang-Fu organs, and these are Five Transport Points (五輸穴, Wushuxue). Now, let's take a closer look at how Qi moves along the meridians.

The Zang-Fu organs create Five Qis of Wood, Fire, Earth, Metal, and Water. The Five Qis created by these Zang-Fu organs are exchanged only through Five Transport Points among the numerous acupuncture points that exist on each meridian. These points are special locations on the meridians that regulate the flow of Qi between the Zang-Fu organs, possessing

[33] This only applies to the exchange of Qi between the Zang-Fu organs through Five Transport Points (Wushuxue, 五輸穴). That is why Do-won Kuon refers to it as "Zang-Fu Points."

the properties of the Five Phases: Wood, Fire, Earth, Metal, and Water. That's why Do-won Kuon refers to them as Zang-Fu Points. Let's simply call these points Wood point, Fire point, Earth point, Metal point, and Water point.[34] Each meridian belonging to a Zang or a Fu has these five acupoints (a total of 60 acupuncture points). Below is a detailed illustration of these specific points.

Five Transport Points of Zang Meridians

Meridian	Wood (1)	Fire (3)	Earth (5)	Metal (7)	Water (9)
Liver (I)	**Dadun** (LR1)	Xingjian (LR2)	Taichong (LR3)	Zhongfeng (LR4)	Ququan (LR8)
Heart (III)	Shaochong (HT9)	**Shaofu** (HT8)	Shenmen (HT7)	Lingdao (HT4)	Shaohai (HT3)
Pancreas (V)	Yinbai (SP1)	Dadu (SP2)	**Taibai** (SP3)	Shangqiu (SP5)	Yinlingquan (SP9)
Lung (VII)	Shaoshang (LU11)	Yuji (LU10)	Taiyuan (LU9)	**Jingqu** (LU8)	Chize (LU5)
Kidney (IX)	Yongquan (KI1)	Rangu (KI2)	Taixi (KI3)	Fuliu (KI7)	**Yingu** (KI10)
Pericardium (III')	Zhongchong (PC9)	Laogong (PC8)	Daling (PC7)	Jianshi (PC5)	Quze (PC3)

[34] Five Transport Points refers to the five acupoints—Jing (井), Ying (滎), Shu (輸), Jing (經), and He (合)—located below the elbow and knee joints of the human body. These acupuncture points are each endowed with the properties of the Five Phases, and therefore can be used to regulate the Zang-Fu organs through the principles of Synchronizing and Antagonizing. In the meridians belonging to the Zang organs, the Jing, Ying, Shu, Jing, and He acupoints correspond to the Phases of Wood, Fire, Earth, Metal, and Water, respectively. Meanwhile, in the meridians belonging to the Fu organs, they correspond to Metal, Water, Wood, Fire, and Earth, respectively.

Five Transport Points of Fu Meridians

Meridian	Wood (2)	Fire (4)	Earth (6)	Metal (8)	Water (10)
Gallbladder (II)	**Zulinqi** (GB41)	Yangfu (GB38)	Yanglingquan (GB34)	Zuqiaoyin (GB44)	Xiaxi (GB43)
Small intestine (IV)	Houxi (SI3)	**Yanggu** (SI5)	Xiaohai (SI8)	Shaoze (SI1)	Qiangu (SI2)
Stomach (VI)	Xianggu (ST43)	Jiexi (ST41)	**Zusanli** (ST36)	Lidui (ST45)	Neiting (ST44)
Large intestine (VIII)	Sanjian (LI3)	Yangxi (LI5)	Quchi (LI11)	**Shangyang** (LI1)	Erjian (LI2)
Bladder (X)	Shugu (BL65)	Kunlun (BL60)	Weizhong (BL40)	Zhiyin (BL67)	**Zutonggu** (BL66)
Triple Burner(IV')	Zhongzhu (TB3)	Zhigou (TB6)	Tianjing (TB10)	Guanchong (TB1)	Yemen (TB2)

Figure 14. Zang-Fu Points (Five Transport Points)

In relation to this, there are conventions of signs for the Zang-Fu organs, meridians, and acupoints as follows. These were designed by Master Do-won Kuon.

Signs for Zang-Fu organs and meridians:

> Liver = I, Heart = III, Pancreas = V, Lungs = VII, Kidneys = IX, Pericardium = III'
>
> Gallbladder = II, Small intestine = IV, Stomach = VI, Large intestine = VIII, Bladder = X, Triple Burner = IV'

(Master Do-won Kuon used Roman numerals as symbols for Zang-Fu organs and added a prime sign ['] to distinguish the meridians from the

Zang-Fu organs. However, I am using Roman numerals as symbols for both the Zang-Fu organs and their meridians according to the situational context. For Pericardium and Triple Burner, a prime is added to the Roman numeral to differentiate them.)

Signs for Zang-Fu Points:

> Zang-system: Wood point = 1, Fire point = 3, Earth point = 5, Metal point = 7, Water point = 9
>
> Fu-system: Wood point = 2, Fire point = 4, Earth point = 6, Metal point = 8, Water point = 10

The usage of the signs is as follows: For example, III5 in the Zang meridian is HT7 (Shenmen), the Earth point of the Heart meridian, IX3 is KI2 (Rangu), the Fire point of the Kidney meridian, VI8 in the Fu meridian is ST45 (Lidui), the Metal point of Stomach meridian, and X10 is BL66 (Zutonggu), the Water point of Bladder meridian (refer to the Zang-Fu acupoint table earlier). The same applies to other cases. You can write by combining the Roman numerals for the meridians and the Arabic numerals for the Phases according to the rows and columns in the table. This notation will be used later to simplify recording "Unit Formulae" or "Compound Formulae."

The following is a diagram drawn using the symbols mentioned earlier, illustrating the Zang-Fu acupuncture points and their locations on the meridians, which are mainly used in Eight-Constitution Medicine. The Heart meridian (III), Lung meridian (VII), and Pericardium meridian (III') travel from the torso to the fingertips, while the Liver meridian (I), Pancreas meridian (V), and Kidney meridian (IX) travel from the toes to the torso. Additionally, the Small intestine meridian (IV), Large intestine meridian (VIII), and Triple Burner meridian (IV') travel from the fingertips to the torso, while the Gallbladder meridian (II), Stomach meridian (VI), and Bladder meridian (X) run from the torso to the toes.

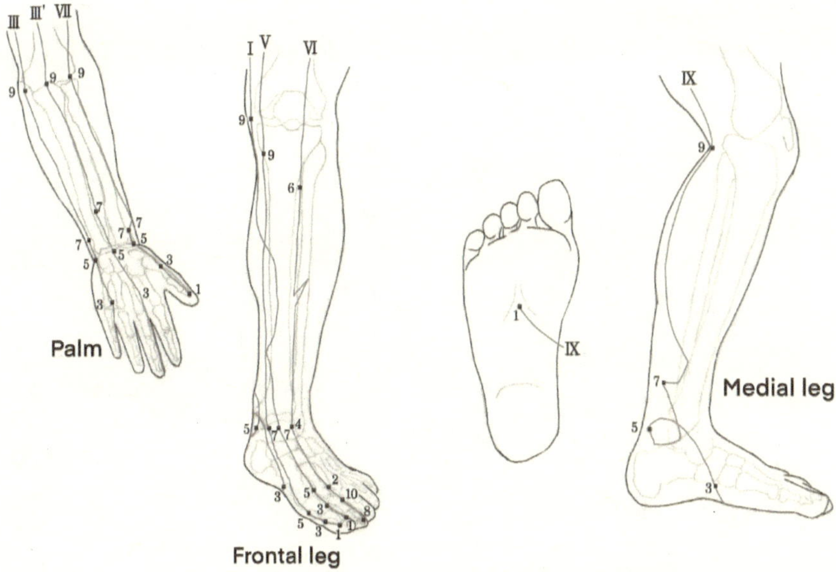

Figure 15A. Zang-Fu points of Zang Meridians

This is a picture of the Zang-Fu points belonging to the Liver Meridian (I), Heart Meridian (III), Pancreas Meridian (V), Lung Meridian (VII), Kidney Meridian (IX), and Pericardium Meridian (III'). The Arabic numerals represent the properties of the Five Phases for each acupoint, and from the extremities of the limbs, they have the attributes of Wood (1), Fire (3), Earth (5), Metal (7), and Water (9). The Wood point of the Heart Meridian is located approximately 0.1 cun (about 2mm) away from the radial corner of the little finger's nail, so it is shown at the tip of the little finger in the back-of-the-hand diagram in Figure 15B. Similarly, the Wood point of the Pericardium Meridian is located approximately 0.1 cun away from the radial corner of the middle finger's nail, so it is shown at the tip of the middle finger in the back-of-the-hand diagram in Figure 15B.

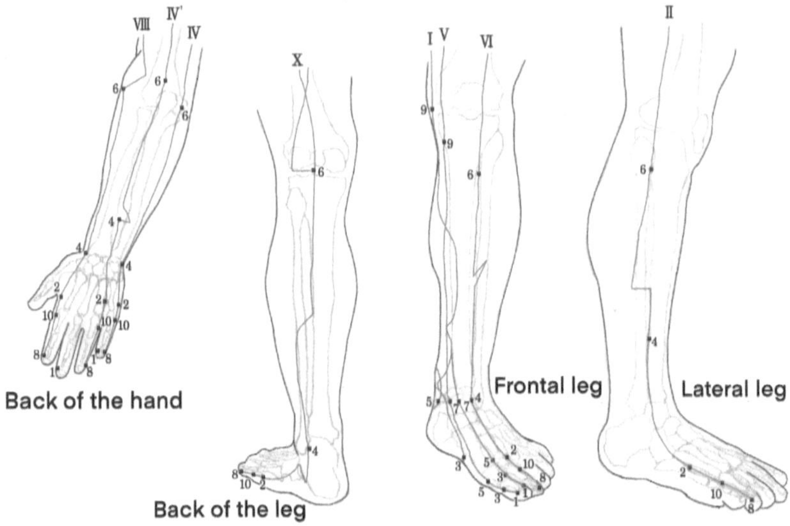

Figure 15B. Zang-Fu points of Fu Meridians

> This is a picture of the Zang-Fu points belonging to the Gallbladder Meridian (II), Small intestine Meridian (IV), Stomach Meridian (VI), Large intestine Meridian (VIII), Bladder Meridian (X), and Triple Burner Meridian (IV'). From the extremities of the limbs, it has the attributes of Metal (8), Water (10), Wood (2), Fire (4), and Earth (6).

These five acupoints present in each meridian are composed of one transmitting acupoint and four receiving acupoints. Transmitting acupoint is a point that have the same property as the Phase (one of the Five Phases) of the corresponding Zang-Fu organ and function to send the Qi created in that organ to other organs. In contrast, receiving points are the other four acupoints that have different properties from that of the organ and function as acupoints to receive Qis created and transmitted from the other four organs.[35]

---

[35] "Among the five visceral points the self-point, which has the same number with that of the self-meridian, is the very transmissive point which has only the function for sending the influential factor of the self-organ to the other four organs. And the remaining four points are the receiving ones which have only the roles for getting for the self-organ the influential factors from the four other organs which are the same numbers with those

The birth of a new diagram of Synchronizing and Antagonizing relationship

Let's explain using the Liver meridian as an example. The Liver is a Zang that creates and regulates Wood Qi. Accordingly, the Wood point LR1 (Dadun) of the Liver serves as the transmitting acupoint, while the other four acupoints—LR2 (Xingjian), LR3 (Taichong), LR4 (Zhongfeng), and LR8 (Ququan)—corresponding to the Qi of Fire, Earth, Metal, and Water respectively, function as the receiving acupoints. The Wood Qi released from the Wood acupoint of the Liver meridian is transmitted through this acupoint to the receiving acupoints of the other four Zang organs, while the Fire, Earth, Metal, and Water Qi delivered from the other four Zang organs are received through the corresponding acupoints in the Liver meridian for each respective Phase. This process explains the specific flow of Qi, as illustrated previously in Figure 7.

In other words, the Wood Qi generated in the Liver-Gallbladder is released through the Wood acupoint, which serves as the transmitting acupoint of the Liver-Gallbladder meridians, and is then transmitted to the Wood acupoints of the other four Zang-Fu organs—namely, the Wood acupoint of the Heart-Small Intestine meridians, the Wood acupoint of the Pancreas-Stomach meridians, the Wood acupoint of the Lung-Large Intestine meridians, and the Wood acupoint of the Kidney-Bladder meridians (see Figure 16 below). And Fire Qi, transmitted through the Fire acupoint of the Heart-Small Intestine meridians, is received through the Fire acupoint of the Liver-Gallbladder meridians. Similarly, Earth Qi, transmitted through the Earth acupoint of the Pancreas-Stomach meridians, is received through the Earth acupoint of the Liver-Gallbladder meridians; Metal Qi, transmitted through the Metal acupoint of the Lung-Large Intestine meridians, is received through the Metal acupoint of the Liver-Gallbladder meridians; and finally, Water Qi, transmitted through the Water acupoint of the Kidney-Bladder meridians, is received through the Water acupoint of the Liver-Gallbladder meridians.

---

of their own." Do-won Kuon, *A Study Of Constitution-acupuncture*, 1965, p.14. The influential factor Kuon refers to here means what I call Qi.

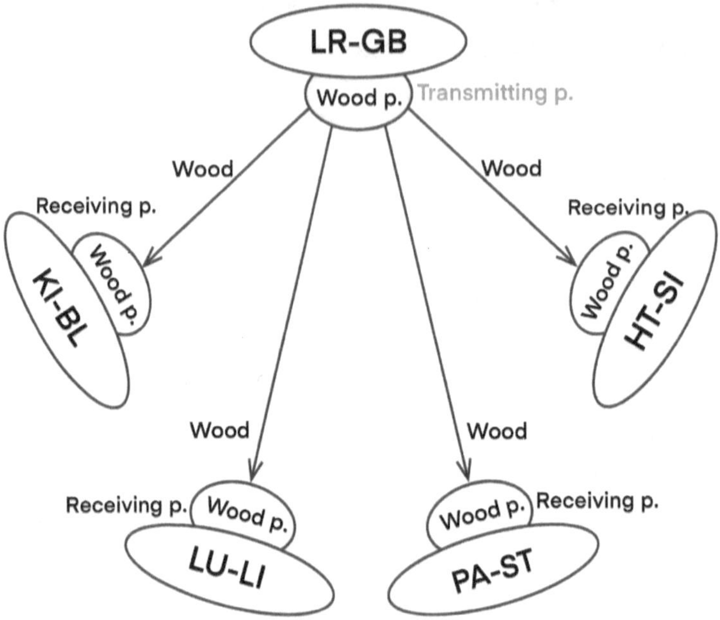

Figure 16. How to transfer Wood Qi from the Liver-Gallbladder to the other Zang-Fu organs (In the figure, "p" stands for acupoint.)

At the same time, the other four pairs of Zang-Fu organs also exchange the Five Qis of Wood, Fire, Earth, Metal, and Water in the same way. The Fire Qi of the Heart-Small intestine is transmitted to the receiving Fire acupoints of the other four Zang-Fu pairs through the transmitting Fire acupoint. Similarly, the Earth Qi of the Pancreas and Stomach is transmitted to the receiving Earth acupoints of the other four Zang-Fu pairs through the transmitting Earth acupoint. The Metal Qi of the Lungs and Large intestine is transmitted through the Metal acupoint, the transmitting acupoint, to the receiving Metal acupoints of the other four Zang-Fu pairs, and lastly, the Water Qi of the Kidneys and Bladder is transmitted to the receiving Water acupoints of the other four Zang-Fu pairs through the transmitting Water acupoint.

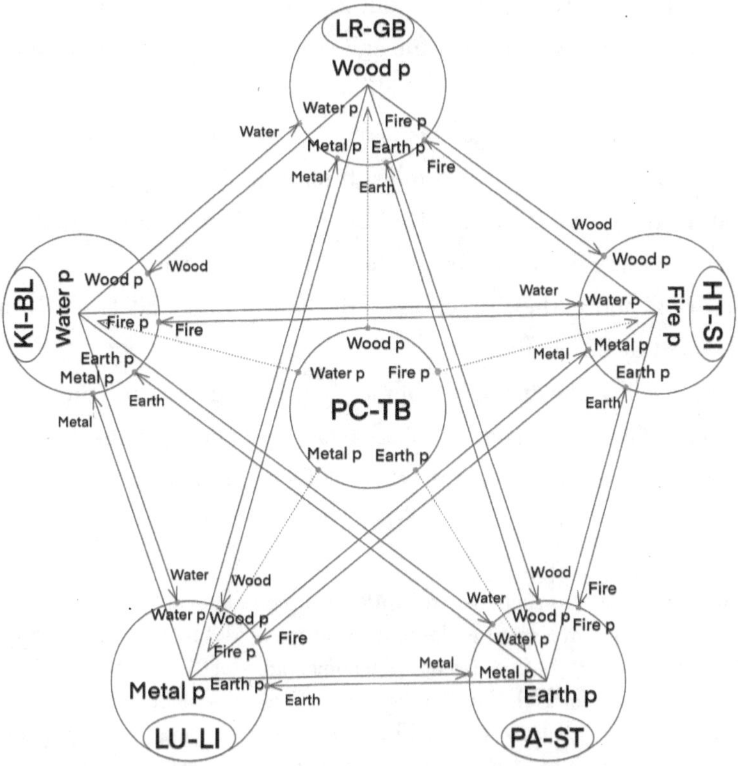

Figure 17. Flow chart of Qi between the Five Zangs and Five Fus

> This picture is a detailed view of Figure 8 earlier. The Synchronizing and Antagonizing relationship of the Five Phases is precisely depicted in the specific Qi flow generated from Five Zang-Fu organs. It is the definitive version of Oriental medicine's theory of Synchronizing and Antagonizing of the Five Phases.

Therefore, the Qi flow between the five pairs of Zang-Fu organs is depicted above as a perfectly symmetrical, geometric diagram of the so-called Synchronizing and Antagonizing relationship (see Figures 8 and 17). In this way, each Zang-Fu organ creates one of the Qis—Wood, Fire, Earth, Metal, or Water—and transmits it to the other four Zang-Fu organs through the transmitting acupoints to either activate or suppress their Qis.

While each of the Five Zangs and Five Fus exerts its own unique function by exchanging Qi with the other four Zang-Fu organs, as shown above, the Pericardium and Triple Burner integrate the individual actions of these Five Zangs and Five Fus from the overall perspective of the organism known as the human body. They regulate all the Zang-Fu organs in the body to ensure unified and optimally controlled functions. By doing so, the individual actions of the Five Zangs and Five Fus are coordinated, preventing any bias and maintaining harmony within the whole system, within a certain range. In Figure 17 above, these functions of the Pericardium and Triple Burner are represented by dotted lines.

I believe that the interaction of the Zang-Fu organs within the framework of the Five Phases, as I have described so far, represents the most sophisticated and accurate interpretation of the theory of Synchronizing and Antagonizing in the Five Phases of Oriental medicine.[36]

---

[36] This theory of the human body is reminiscent of the concept of "schéma corporel (body schema)," proposed by French philosopher Maurice Merleau-Ponty (1908-1961). In his book *Phénoménologie de la perception* (Phenomenology of Perception), Merleau-Ponty described body schema as the body's inherent ability to autonomously perform integrated movements at a pre-conscious level. This functions like an internal map, guiding the body in understanding and adjusting its movements and interactions with the environment. (*Phenomenology of Perception* by Maurice Merleau-Ponty, translated by Eui-geun Ryu, Seoul: Literature and Intelligence Publishing, 2023, pp. 165-171).

I think that the high degree of autonomy in the human body's living activities, as discussed in my theory of the dynamics of the Five Phases between the Zang-Fu organs, is the biological expression of the body schema that Merleau-Ponty mentioned. Strictly speaking, the body schema he refers to is a concept used to explain the unconscious spatial awareness and movement of the human body. In fact, it can be said that it only captures one aspect of the comprehensive view of the human body as presented by my theory of the Five Phases and Zang-Fu organs. However, I had a strong impression that his concept of body schema could serve as a useful framework for understanding my theory of the Five Phases and Zang-Fu organs. If Western medicine, which is based on anatomy, is constructed in terms of the "spatiality of position," the theory of the Five Phases and Zang-Fu organs is similar to one constructed in terms of the "spatiality of situation," much like the body schema.

In *Phenomenology of Perception*, Maurice Merleau-Ponty harshly criticizes the Cartesian dichotomy of mind and body, arguing that the human body is intricately intertwined with the mind and cannot be separated. His aim was to reveal the pre-objective and pre-scientific phenomenal field, the world as perceived by consciousness incarnated in such a body. He claimed that the mind and body, for him, are merely different layers (like two sides of the same coin) that make up a single existential situation. I believe this

Master Do-won Kuon also develops an elaborate theory of meridians in relation to these interactions between the Zang-Fu organs. He refers to the Five Qis of Wood, Fire, Earth, Metal, and Water generated in the Zang-Fu organs as "influential factors," explaining that they flow through the Zang-Fu acupoints when regulating the relationships between these Zang-Fu organs.

When these Five Qis are utilized as energy to operate the human body, they are synthesized separately in the Zang and Fu meridians and then form a complex that circulates throughout the body.[37] He explains that this complex, which runs across the entire body not between the Zang-Fu organs, enters and exits through the acupuncture points other than Zang-Fu acupoints which are directly connected to the Zang-Fu organs.

According to Do-won Kuon, the interaction of the Five Qis of Wood, Fire, Earth, Metal, and Water between the Zang-Fu organs is referred to as "mutual influence," while the effect of the complex of these Five Qis nourishing the entire body is called "vital influence." The functions of Zang-Fu acupuncture points and other acupuncture points are clearly distinguished according to him.

In this way, the complex that enables biological activities throughout the body originates from the Five Qis of the Five Phases, and these Five Qis, in turn, come from the Zang-Fu organs. Therefore, diseases that occur in the human body ultimately require the control of these Five Qis. It is revealed that

---

idea is closely related to Doh-ol Young-oak Kim's Ki (Qi) Philosophy or Mom (Body) Philosophy, which explains Heaven and Earth, and humans solely through the concept of Qi.

[37] "While meridians operate thus the mutual influence by the visceral points, they also synthesize the influential factors of all the organs according to the two separate systems of both Chang and Bhu." Do-won Kuon, *A Study Of Constitution-acupuncture*, 1965, p.18. I think this phrase is a bit ambiguous. This is because it sounds as if the meridians are combining the Five Qis of Wood, Fire, Earth, Metal, and Water. It would be more accurate to say that the Five Qis (influential factors) are generated in the Zang-Fu organs and are then utilized to synthesize a complex within the meridians of the Zang and Fu organs. Master Do-won Kuon referred to this complexes as "five influential factors."

the Five Qis are controlled by the Zang-Fu Points that regulate the Zang-Fu organs, and thus, fundamental treatment can only be achieved through these Zang-Fu Points.

So, regulating this Zang-Fu Points is called "radical regulation", and using the other acupoints is called "local regulation."[38] He is persuading us with the elaborate theories about the excellence of Eight-Constitution Medicine, which treats all diseases by regulating the Zang-Fu Points.[39] When treating an illness, be sure to grasp the root cause!

The body is imaging[40]

The above discussion of the Zang-Fu organs is all just a system of symbolic principles. It is not true that meridians exist as physical entities in the human body or that the Qi of the Five Phases physically moves through them. Meridians are virtual pathways that enable the exchange of Qis between the Zang-Fu organs. The Five Qis of Wood, Fire, Earth, Metal, and Water that circulate through the meridians are merely symbolic representations. A meridian, so to speak, is a signal transduction pathway[41] between Zang-Fu organs. The Five Zangs and Five Fus are anatomically real, but, at the same time, they are symbolic information centers that transmit the information of Qis associated with Wood, Fire, Earth, Metal, and Water.

---

[38] "Corporal acupuncture technique," commonly performed in general Oriental medicine clinics, can be considered similar to local regulation.

[39] Do-won Kuon, *A Study Of Constitution-acupuncture*, 1965, p.18. Local regulation refers to the acupuncture technique, such as corporal acupuncture, that does not use the principle of the Five Phases of the Zang-Fu organs, but usually performs inserting needles into the body and maintaining them for a certain period of time.

[40] Doh-ol Young-oak Kim's 9th lecture on *Donguisusebowon* (on May 21, 1994, at Doh-ol Academy): "Body is Imaging." All medical theories, no matter how elaborately they may be described in language, are ultimately nothing more than images drawn by humans on the human body. This idea is reminiscent of the "Proposition-Picture Theory" from *Tractatus Logico-Philosophicus* by Ludwig Wittgenstein (1889–1951), a leading figure in logical positivism, analytic philosophy, and linguistic philosophy in the 20th century.

[41] Vander, Sherman, and Luciano, *Human Physiology*, 9th edition, (McGraw-Hill, 2004), pp.136-150. In Western medicine, it refers to an information transmission system through chemical mediators such as neurotransmitters and hormones.

The method of conveying information in this symbolic system called the human body is surprisingly simple. It is the same as indicating whether something is plus (+) or minus (–), 1 or 0, positive or negative, on or off, and so on. It is merely a symbolic manipulation of two phases with equal magnitude in opposite directions. In other words, it is Yin and Yang.

The human body is dualistic. One aspect is a visible system of matter, composed of tissues made up of substances with mass, forming organs and carrying out the biological activities of the organism known as the human body through the flow of blood. The other aspect is an invisible system of symbols, consisting of the Zang-Fu, a symbolic system that cannot be quantified as material substances with mass, and that supports the biological activities of the human body through the flow of Qi, which represents symbolic information. This ongoing struggle between the visible world and the invisible world can be seen as the history of medicine and, by extension, the history of humanity.

What is important here in the theory of the Eight-Constitution Medicine is that it boldly hypothesized that the human body is a symbolic system of Five Zangs and Five Fus, based on the system of Five Phases, and discovered the deductive relational law between Five Zang-Fu organs under that hypothesis. We now face the task of integrating the visible and the invisible world. This will become the "Unified Field Theory of medical science" in the future.

CHAPTER 2

Definition of Constitution

CONSTITUTION IS A NEW ÉPISTÉMÈ THAT WILL OVERTURN THE WESTERN MECHANICAL VIEW OF HUMANITY. IT REPRESENTS A BIG PICTURE OF A NEW UNDERSTANDING ON THE HUMAN BEING.

CHAPTER 2

Definition of Constitution

The human body is a system of Zang-Fu. A system is defined as a unified structure in which each constituent part closely interacts with the others and functions together to achieve a common purpose. The human body is a system composed of the five pairs of Zang-Fu organs: the Liver and Gallbladder, the Heart and Small intestine, the Pancreas and Stomach, the Lungs and Large intestine, and the Kidneys and Bladder. These five pairs of Zang-Fu were referred earlier to as Five Zangs and Five Fus. In addition to these, there is an intangible system that regulates and coordinates the Five Zangs and Five Fus: the Pericardium and the Triple Burner. Unlike the others, they are not actual physical organs but invisible, virtual functional systems that coordinate the overall functioning of the human body.

Living creature is a world of discrimination

According to Western medicine, the human body is composed of cells. The cells are surrounded by extracellular fluid (ECF) bordering the cell membrane. Inside the cells, there is intracellular fluid (ICF). There is always a difference in electrolyte concentration between the intracellular and extracellular fluid. This is due to active transport, which intentionally pumps sodium ions that enter the cell back out, using biochemical energy, ATP (Adenosine Triphosphate). As a result, the sodium ion concentration inside the cell is consistently kept low, while the concentration outside the cell remains high.[42] However, the sodium ion continuously seeks an opportunity to enter the cell. Because of the concentration gradient between the inside and outside of the cell, the sodium ion, which is present in high concentration outside the cell, is at the higher energy level (higher potential) and can easily diffuse into the cell.

This non-equilibrium concentration difference between the inside and outside of the cell is maintained due to the active transport efforts to keep the cell in a non-equilibrium state. It is precisely this discrimination that makes the phenomenon of life possible. When the human body dies, the active transport ceases, allowing the extracellular sodium ion to freely enter the cells. Consequently, the electrolyte concentration inside and outside the cell reaches equilibrium, becoming indiscriminate.

The equilibrium of electrolyte concentration inside and outside the cell signifies death, as in this state of balance, there is no movement of matter or energy, leading to the cessation of metabolic activity. The world of indiscrimination is death.[43]

There is exchange of Qis between the Zang-Fu organs of the human body. The Liver-Gallbladder create Wood Qi and transmit it to the other four pairs of Zang-Fu organs; the Heart-Small intestine create Fire Qi and transmit it to the other four pairs of Zang-Fu; the Pancreas-Stomach create Earth Qi and transmit it to the other four pairs of Zang-Fu; the Lungs-Large intestine create Metal Qi and transmit it to the other four pairs of Zang-Fu; and the Kidneys-Bladder create Water Qi and transmit it to the other four pairs of Zang-Fu. The existence of Qi flow between Zang-Fu pairs implies that there is a difference in potential (Let me define this as

---

[42] This refers precisely to active transport by an enzyme called the sodium-potassium pump (Na-K pump). Thus, the electrolyte known as K+ also moves between the inside and outside of the cell, but for the sake of convenience in this discussion, it is omitted here. Meanwhile, the concentration of electrolytes (mainly sodium ion) in extracellular fluid is considered to be similar to that of seawater. This is said to be evidence that humans evolved from fish. It is also said that amniotic fluid during pregnancy has similar conditions. Our bodies still live in the sea!

[43] Doh-ol Young-oak Kim's 9th lecture on *Donguisusebowon* (on May 21, 1994, Doh-ol Academy): "Life was born from discrimination."

"Zang-Fu Potential") between the Zang-Fu pairs. Some Zang-Fu pairs have a high potential, and some have a low potential. If the potentials of the Zang-Fu pairs were equal, the Qi flow would cease.[44] When the flow of Qi stops, the physiological metabolic activities of the human body also cease, which essentially means death. The fact that the human body is alive and functioning means there is a potential difference that creates a greater or lesser influence among Zang-Fu pairs, maintaining a continuous flow of Qi between them. Just as the difference in the concentration of electrolytes must exist between the inside and outside the cell for metabolic activity to occur, there must be a difference in the potential of influence between Zang-Fu pairs for Qi flow to persist. This inequality or non-equilibrium is a prerequisite for life.[45] Life, therefore, is an existence of *Yi* (易), or constant change, which is continuously striving for equilibrium under the premise of non-equilibrium.

The second law of thermodynamics states: "Entropy increases."[46] An increase in entropy refers to an increase in disorder. The increase in disorder refers to moving from a state of unevenness to a state of uniformity. Heterogeneity means that there is a difference in concentration, that is, distinction within the system. Uniformity means that the difference in concentration has disappeared, and equilibrium or equality has been reached. The increase in entropy refers to the continuous tendency to progress from inequality to equality. When a living being dies, its body disperses. That

[44] In an electric circuit, current flows from high potential to low potential according to the potential difference. Similarly, in the human body, Qi flows from a higher Zang-Fu Potential to a lower Zang-Fu Potential according to the difference in Zang-Fu Potential.

[45] Doh-ol Young-oak Kim, *Ki Philosophy Sanjo or Impromptu* (Seoul: Tongnamu Publishing, 1992), p.33. "The beginning can be said to be an event in which the balance of Qi was changed to imbalance." This can be seen in the same context as the difference in electrolyte concentration inside and outside the cell discussed earlier.

[46] The laws of thermodynamics were discovered by German physicist and mathematician Rudolf Clausius (1822-1888). Entropy is expressed as the following state function: $dS = dQ/T$ (where S is entropy, Q is heat, and T is absolute temperature). Clausius mathematically derived the change in entropy (ΔS) for an isolated system and proved that the relation $\Delta S > 0$ always holds. This is the Second Law of Thermodynamics, known as the Law of Entropy Increase.

signifies an increase in entropy. The ultimate form of dispersion is uniformity. Scattering into pieces and entering a state of uniformity is death. An increase in entropy is the path to death.

But in the law of life, "entropy decreases."[47] Decreasing entropy means reverting from equality to inequality. It is a return from uniformity to distinction. It is a reversal from equilibrium to non-equilibrium. The second law of thermodynamics applies well to the inanimate material systems such as chemistry and physics. However, living creatures constantly strive to reduce entropy at every moment. That is why tens of trillions of cells can survive as one system for nearly 80 to 90 years or more, maintaining strong cohesion without dispersing. Living beings were created by defying the laws of physics and chemistry. By resisting the increase in entropy, life blossomed on Earth, the only planet in the universe. Until the day life ends, living organisms resist the increase in entropy. This resistance is the first prerequisite for the birth and existence of living beings. It is the initial condition for life to be life. The moment that life ceases to reduce entropy, it dies.[48]

[47] The law of entropy increase is a law that holds true in an isolated system. Living organisms, such as the human body, are not actually an isolated system. The human body is an open system in which input and output occur continuously. Therefore, it is difficult to say that it strictly undergoes entropy reduction. A phenomenon like entropy reduction occurs only temporarily. However, if we consider the external environment surrounding the human body, entropy increases as well. Strictly speaking, the human body continuously experiences both entropy decrease and entropy increase at every moment. However, if we look at the total lifespan, the decrease is less than the increase, so the overall trend is toward increasing entropy. So, even living beings ultimately cannot defy the law of increasing entropy. The cycle of birth, aging, illness, and death itself can be synonymous with the law of increasing entropy. The fact that we are born, grow old, get sick, and die is evidence of this law. Still, the fact that entropy decreases, even partially and temporarily, is truly remarkable. This is because, except for living beings, nothing else exhibits the phenomenon of entropy reduction.

[48] Doh-ol Young-oak Kim, *Ki (Qi) Philosophy Sanjo or Impromptu* (Seoul: Tongnamu Publishing, 1992), p.33. I believe that this phenomenon of entropy reduction in life is also in the same context as the transition from equilibrium to non-equilibrium in the primordial Qi.

Constitution is a prerequisite for life

The difference in potentials between the five Zang-Fu pairs is the first condition that must be met for the human body to be a living organism. It is the initial condition of the human body! There must be differences between the five Zang-Fu pairs from the very beginning. Due to this inequality, the biological activities known as the human body exists. The human body begins with these conditions of inequality. Some Zang-Fu pairs operate at a higher potential, while others function at a lower potential.

Je-ma Lee in Joseon Dynasty, the pioneer who initiated all discussions on the potential differences between the Zangs[49] in human history, conveys a subtle nuance suggesting that the formation of potential differences between the Zangs is an acquired result. Let's listen to what he himself has to say about Constitution.

> Taeyangin's Aixing (哀性, Nature of sorrow) radiates afar, while Nuqing (怒情, Sentiment of anger) erupts hastily. When the Aixing radiates afar, Qi flows into the Lungs, making them more active. On the other hand, when Nuqing erupts hastily, Qi agitates the Liver, causing further damage to it. This explains why the topography of the Zangs in Taeyangin features Large Lung and Small Liver.[50]

This is considered one of the most famous passages in Je-ma Lee's book of *Donguisusebowon*, the origin of Sasang-Consitution Medicine. Among the

---

[49] What is noteworthy here is that Je-ma Lee discussed Sasangin, or Four Constitutions, using only a combination of four "Zangs." The Fu organs are not included in his classification of Constitution.

[50] "太陽人哀性遠散，而怒情促急。哀性遠散，則氣注肺而肺益盛，怒情促急，則氣激肝而肝益削。太陽之臟局，所以成形於肺大肝小也。" Je-ma Lee, *Donguisusebowon* (Seoul: Haenglim Publishing, 1993), p.9. Here, "the Zang's dimensional difference" referred to by Lee Je-ma corresponds to "the potential difference between the Zangs" that I am referring to. What is notable here is that he addresses the concept of Constitution using only the two-Zang combination out of Four Zangs, rather than the Five Zang-Fu organs. In his classification of Constitutions, Fu-system is attributed to the Zang-system.

four Sasangins (Four Constitutional Types), only the case of Taeyangin is cited above for convenience. Here, Je-ma Lee presents his original theory on human nature and emotion.

Earlier, there have been debates on human nature for hundreds of years in Joseon Dynasty: Moral Nature of Four Beginnings of Benevolence, Righteousness, Propriety, and Wisdom, which have been regarded as human essence, and Human Emotion of Seven Sentiments of Joy, Anger, Sorrow, Fear, Love, Hatred, and Desire, which have been regarded as ever-changing phenomenon. All these dual distinctions of Nature and Emotion are integrated by Je-ma Lee into a single category of Nature-Emotion Continuum, that is, Joy, Anger, Sorrow, and Pleasure, and discussed in an extraordinary way in relation to the human Constitution.[51] A detailed discussion of this theory of Nature and Emotion is beyond the scope of this article, so I will refrain from further elaboration.

However, speaking only in relation to this article, for Je-ma Lee, the changing magnitude of Zangs for Taeyangin (太陽人), Soyangin (少陽人), Taeeumin (太陰人), and Soeumin (少陰人) is considered a progressive result of the excessive high or low of Joy, Anger, Sorrow, and Pleasure. For example, in

[51] For Je-ma Lee, Xing (性, Nature) and Qing (情, Emotion) belong to a single category, referred to as Joy, Anger, Sorrow, and Pleasure. There is no separate concept of Moral Nature such as Benevolence, Righteousness, Propriety, and Wisdom, nor separate Sentiments such as Joy, Anger, Sorrow, and Pleasure. Joy, Anger, Sorrow, and Pleasure. The two categories, for Je-ma Lee, can become either Nature or Emotion. The same Joy, Anger, Sorrow, and Pleasure can manifest as both Nature and Emotion depending on the circumstances of a person's life. Therefore, Je-ma Lee refers to the same Anger either as Anger in Nature (怒性) or Anger in Sentiment (怒情). Nature and Emotion is differentiated depending on how Joy, Anger, Sorrow, and Pleasure are expressed. He connects this concept to Constitution and develops a unique and creative theory of Nature and Emotion. For example, a Taeyangin is born with Nature of radiating-afar Sorrow and Sentiment of erupting-hastily Anger. From Je-ma Lee's theory of Nature and Emotion, I coined the term Nature-Emotion Continuum. It was inspired by the time-space continuum in Einstein's Theory of Relativity. Philosophically, Je-ma Lee sides with Dae-seung Ki (기대승, 奇大升, 1527-1572, philosopher in Joseon), not Hwang Yi (이황, 李滉, 1501-1570, philosopher in Joseon), in the long-standing debate over Theory of Li and Qi (이기론, 理氣論) in the Joseon history of thoughts. He thoroughly supported the Monism of Qi. Je-ma Lee's philosophy, I think, aligns with Ki (Qi) Philosophy of Doh-ol Young-oak Kim.

the case of Taeyangin, the Nature of Sorrow radiating afar and the Emotion of Anger erupting hastily, which have accumulated repeatedly over the course of life, gave rise to the terrain of Large Lung and Small Liver.

However, I do not believe that Je-ma Lee discussed the formation of Constitution with such a clear concept of innate or acquired nature. When viewed in the overall context of Je-ma Lee's *Donguisusebowon*, the innateness of Constitution is an undeniable fact. However, the logical context of the sentence here clearly indicates that Constitution is a progressive result of a life in which Joy, Anger, Sorrow, and Pleasure are not kept in moderation.

The fact that Je-ma Lee spoke of the formation of large and small Zangs, which leads to Constitutions with such an acquired nuance, is interpreted as emphasizing that, ultimately, the deepening of the large and small structures of the human Zangs results from the excessive expression of one's Nature and Emotion. For Je-ma Lee, Constitution is a fundamental prerequisite for advancing to the state of Middle Way and Harmony (中和, Zhonghe), which is the Confucian ideal, achieved through the cultivation of mind and body to regulate one's Nature and Emotion. Borrowing a term from Kantian philosophy, it can be seen as a postulate of practical reason (Postulate der praktischen Vernunft).

Therefore, he concludes the Chapter *Sadanlon* (Debate on Four Beginnings of Human Nature, 四端論), one of the most important chapters in *Donguisusebowon*, with the famous Theory on Middle Way and Harmony (中和論) from the Classic Bible of *Doctrine of the Mean*.[52] In *Sadanlon*, Je-ma Lee admits the inevitability of imbalanced human beings, that is, Sasangin (Four Constitutional Types), but, at the same time, declares the pursuit of the balanced, harmonious individual as the most important life attitude that all humans should strive for.

[52] "哀怒喜樂之未發, 謂之中, 發而皆中節, 謂之和. 哀怒喜樂未發, 而恒戒者, 此非漸近於中者乎? 哀怒喜樂已發, 而自反者, 此非漸近於節者乎?" Je-ma Lee, *Donguisusebowon* (Seoul: Haenglim Publishing, 1993), p.13.

Constitution is inequality of Zang-Fu

In Do-won Kuon's Eight-Constitution Medicine, the inequality of potential between the Zang-Fu pairs is firmly determined from birth. It is a fundamental human condition. That is the Constitution, the inequality of Zang-Fu pairs. Constitution is the starting point of biological phenomena. In the beginning of humans, there was inequality of Zang-Fu!

Among the Zang-Fu pairs in the human body, as mentioned earlier, there is a potential for each Zang-Fu pair ("Zang-Fu Potential") that causes the Qi flow of the Zang-Fu organ. This is a similar concept of the Large and Small Zangs that Je-ma Lee discusses. However, if we go into detail, there is a difference between my concept of "Zang-Fu Potential" and Je-ma Lee's concept of "Large and Small Zangs" (this will be explained in detail later). Since the difference in Zang-Fu Potential between the Zang-Fu pairs exists, there is a proportional difference in potential between the Five Qis of the Five Phases generated from the Zang-Fu pairs (let's call this the "Five Phases Potential" to distinguish it from the Zang-Fu Potential). Therefore, the pattern of dynamics or interactions between the pairs of Zang-Fu can be reduced to the pattern of dynamics or interactions between the Five Qis of the Five Phases. The interaction between the Five Zang-Fu pairs is replaced by the interactions between these Five Qis. Here, Zang-Fu is the Body (體), and Five Qis is the Function (用).[53]

Interactions constantly occur between the Five Qis of the Five Phases. There is a dynamic law that acts upon each Phase, which is referred to as Relationship of Synchronizing and Antagonizing as mentioned earlier. This can be considered a dynamic relationship theory, where each of the Five Qis

[53] It is called *Tiyonglun* (體用論). Ti (體) refers to the object itself, and Yong (用) refers to the function of the object. Although Ti and Yong are mentioned together, the emphasis is placed more on Yong than on Ti. This means that all objects perform their roles through their functions. The same applies to Zang-Fu theory here. While the Zang-Fu is discussed, there is not a single word about its ingredients or composition after analyzing it in terms of substance. There is almost no investigation of the Ti (substance). It only addresses its functions, the relationships between objects, and the laws of operation. I believe this is one of the representative characteristics of Eastern thought.

of the Five Phases exerts influence on the others. Now, let us arithmetically assume an arbitrary array based on the intensity of influence of these Five Qis, that is, the Five Phases Potential.

Just as the Zang-Fu Potentials in the human body differ between the pairs of Zang-Fu, the Five Phases Potentials in the human body are also proportionally different. These Phases or Qis (let's denote them as A, B, C, D, and E) can be arranged according to the differences in these Five Phases Potentials. This can be mathematically represented on a quadratic plane as follows.

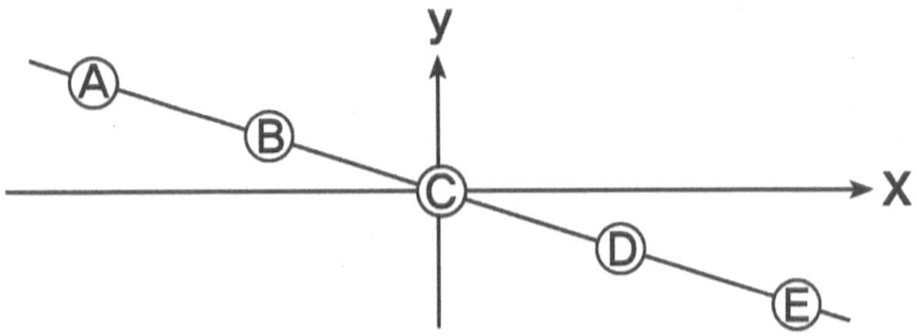

Figure 1. Five Phases Array Diagram

The x-axis represents the distance from the central Qi C at the origin, and the y-axis represents the Five Phases Potential.

The x-axis represents the distance from the central Qi of "C", and the farther this distance is, similar to the centrifugal force, the more dominant its influence becomes in the human body having the corresponding Array of Five Phases. Therefore, to the left of C, "A" has more influence than "B", and to the right of C, "E" has more influence than "D." This means that the influence of the Five Phases on the left side of C and on the right side of C are equivalent, with the only difference being that the signs are opposite to each other. In other words, A and B exert their influences in the positive direction, while D and E exert the same influences in the negative direction. I will refer to the operating areas of A and B, which have the influences in the positive direction of the y-axis, as "Yang Field," and the operating areas of D and E, which have the influences in the negative direction of the y-axis, as "Yin Field."

The y-axis represents the Five Phases Potential, which indicates the degree of dominance in the Array of Five Phases. The coordinates of A are symmetrical with the coordinates of E around the central point C at the origin, and the coordinates of B are also symmetrical with the coordinates of D around the central point C at the origin. From this, a relationship is established where the coordinate values of A and E have the same magnitudes but opposite signs, and the coordinate values of B and D, have the same magnitudes but opposite signs, too.

So, the coordinate of A is (Ax, Ay), the coordinate of B is (Bx, By), the coordinate of C is (0, 0), the coordinate of D is (Dx, Dy), and the coordinate of E is (Ex, Ey). Mathematically, the relationships Ex = -Ax, Ey = -Ay and Dx = -Bx, Dy = -By are established.

Constitutional Medicine has the following premise: "The human body is a system of Five Zangs and Five Fus that innately maintain a certain Array of their influences. From this, the array of the Qis of Five Phases generated in the Five Zangs and Five Fus follows a specific pattern."

This pattern does not change throughout the life. It forms a characteristic tendency in the physiology and the pathology that occurs in the human body. This is the Constitution.

So, based on this premise, let's arrange the Five Phases in order according to the rules of the Five Phases Array Diagram above. This can be considered a random array of the Five Qis—Wood, Fire, Earth, Metal, and Water—that do not overlap with each other. Therefore, it is the same as the permutation of arranging five different objects.

A·B·C·D·E (sometimes abbreviated as ABCDE) …… (1)

Constitution refers to the array of the Five Phases according to their influences, as mentioned earlier. This is because the array order of these Five Qis is the same as that of the Zang-Fu pairs.[54] Again, Constitution is the array of

[54] "The comparison of the mutual strength and weakness of the influential factors of the complex agrees with that of the organ functions of the same temperament." Do-won Kuon, *A Study Of Constitution-acupuncture*, 1965, p.18

the Five Zang-Fu pairs that exist in the human body.[55] As mentioned earlier, it is the same as the inequality structure of the Five Phases created from the Zang-Fu organs. Let's call this structure "Five Phases Structure Formula." And let's call the array of the Five Zang-Fu pairs "Zang-Fu Structure Formula."[56]

As mentioned earlier, the Five Phases Structure Formula is centered on the central Qi C, with A on the left and E on the right forming a symmetrical structure, and B on the left and D on the right also forming a symmetrical structure. Here, A and B belong to the positive potential (positive y-coordinate values) of the Five Phases, while D and E belong to the negative potential (negative y-coordinate values) of the Five Phases. If A and B have N-pole properties, then D and E have S-pole properties. If A and B are in clockwise motion, then D and E are in counterclockwise motion. I defined these symmetrical ambivalent aspects as Yang Field and Yin Field earlier.

A and B are the members of the Yang Field, and D and E are the members of the Yin Field. Centered on C, A and E form a pair with the same magnitude but opposite directions, and B and D also form a pair with the same magnitude but opposite directions (refer to Figure 1, Five Phases Array shown in the coordinates earlier).

The structure of Constitution is a dipolar system. A, B, D, and E may converge toward the horizontal x-axis to pursue the dynamic balance of the

---

[55] In his paper in 1965, Do-won Kuon, discussing *Donguisusebowon*, referred to this array as an innate imbalance. Here, we see the prototype of the concept of the Eight Constitutions. See the following: "And the Constitutions of the four types mean the four congenital imbalanced structures of the internal organ functions, and the names for them are respectively called Tae-yang-in (Hespera), So-yang-in (Saturna), Tae-um-in (Jupita) and So-um-in (Mercuria)." Do-won Kuon, *A Study Of Constitution-acupuncture*, 1965, p.4.

[56] Until recently, I expressed the Zang-Fu Structure Formula of the Constitution as "A>B>C>D>E." This expression indicates a one-sided superiority-inferiority relationship between the Qis, such as A being stronger than B, B being stronger than C, C being stronger than D, and D being stronger than E. This can lead to a misunderstanding of Constitution. From the perspective of influence on the human body, centering on C, the Zang-Fu organs A·B on the left and the Zang-Fu organs E·D on the right have equal influence. It is an Antagonistic Relationship in which both sides hold a equal status. Therefore, I clearly revealed the symmetry between left and right by introducing the concepts of Yang Field and Yin Field.

system (physiological condition),[57] or they may diverge in opposite directions, disrupting the dynamic balance (pathological condition). The closer the line connecting A, B, C, D, and E is to the x-axis, the closer the system is to the dynamic equilibrium. The further away it is, the farther it is from the dynamic equilibrium.

According to this dynamic equilibrium perspective, the Five Phases Potentials shown in the coordinates earlier follow the following inequality.

The absolute value of A potential > The absolute value of B potential
The absolute value of D potential < The absolute value of E potential

This means that in the Yang Field, "A" usually has a more dominant influence than "B", and in the Yin Field, "E" usually has a more dominant influence than "D." (Sometimes, there are exceptions where "B" can be more dominant than "A," and "D" can be more dominant than "E," indicating that the concept of "dominance" is not absolute but rather a relative tendency depending on one's physical condition.) What is important here is that the Yang and Yin Fields are symmetrical fields with equal influence. Therefore, it is not correct to say that the Qi of the Five Phases in the Yang Field is stronger or more dominant than the Qi of the Five Phases in the Yin Field (for example, A is not stronger than E. It is just that in the Yang Field, A tends to be more dominant than B, and in the Yin Field, E tends to be more dominant than D). Furthermore, even within the same Constitution, there are cases where either the influence of the Yang Field Qi (A or B) is dominant or the influence of the Yin Field Qi (E or D) is dominant. In other words, the influence of a Field may become more apparent depending on the physiological or pathological situation. However,

---

[57] Dynamic equilibrium is originally a concept from chemical reactions, meaning a state in which the rates of the forward and reverse reactions are equal. This implies that, although it is in an equilibrium state, it remains dynamic, with reactions constantly occurring in both directions. Slightly differently, I refers to the body's tendency, as dynamic balance, to constantly move toward the state of equilibrium from the state of non-equilibrium in the unequal Zang-Fu structures called Constitution. Strictly speaking, this is not the dynamic equilibrium. It would be more accurate to say that it is aimed at the dynamic equilibrium.

there is no definite rule as to which side is more proactive. It is a matter of chance, like rolling a dice.

For example, in the same Geumyang Constitution (with the array of Lungs Pancreas Heart Kidneys Liver), in some people, the Lungs, part of the Yang Field, cause a dominant physiological or pathological condition, while in others, the Liver, part of the Yin Field, causes a dominant physiological or pathological condition. The former tends to frequently cause symptoms in respiratory functions including the lungs, while the latter tends to frequently cause symptoms in detoxification functions including the liver.

Types of Constitution

Now, let's look at the types of arrays of the Five Phases, such as (1) above. The number of possible arrays will indicate the types of Constitution. Mathematically, the number of ways to arrange the Five Phases—Wood, Fire, Earth, Metal, and Water—as shown in (1) is 5! (factorial) = $5 \times 4 \times 3 \times 2 \times 1 = 120$. In other words, there are 120 possible arrays. So, do these 120 numbers represent the different types of Constitution?

The human body is an organism with the finite dimension. Therefore, the condition of "life called an organism" is definitely required. Not all of the 120 types above can be types of Constitution. This is only possible in a lifeless physical world. Therefore, among these 120, only those that meet the prerequisites for being the living beings are meaningful as Constitutions.

Living creatures pursue homeostasis

What is the first condition for life? It is homeostasis. So, how is the homeostasis maintained? It is through the dynamic equilibrium. Therefore, the array of the Five Phases cannot be random. Only the arrays that satisfy the first prerequisite for life, which is maintaining homeostasis in the human body, are meaningful as types of Constitution. In other words, only the arrays that can bring the equilibrium to the system become the correct Constitutional Structure. The arrays that disrupt the equilibrium cannot survive because they are not suitable for the conditions of living organisms. They are also naturally at an evolutionary disadvantage.

How can we bring the equilibrium to the system of the Five Phases Formula? "A" and "B" must converge toward the x-axis to decrease the potential of A and B. Similarly, "E" and "D" must also converge toward the x-axis to increase the potential of D and E. Here, the x-axis represents the ideal state in which the system has reached the perfect equilibrium. However, the human body can never fully reach this x-axis under any circumstances. It simply continues to move (converge) toward the x-axis endlessly.

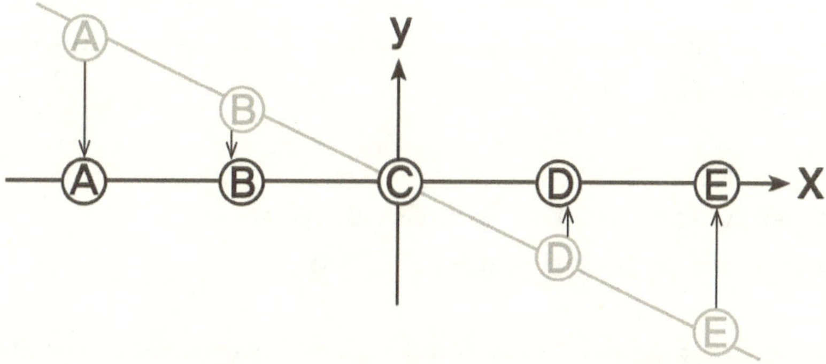

Figure 2. Model of the human body in the perfect equilibrium

> The human body is constantly striving to reach the state of equilibrium.

The word "convergence" is very important here. It means approaching closer forever. This implies that there is only the process of trying to get infinitely closer to the x-axis without ever actually reaching it. This can be seen as the reason why we constantly oscillate between health and illness. (There is no perfection of equilibrium.) Another important point derived from the word "convergence" is that the line representing the array of the Five Phases (A-B-C-D-E) can never cross the x-axis. The Yang Field remains only in the positive area, and the Yin Field remains only in the negative area. In other words, there is never a situation where the Yang Field becomes the Yin Field, or the Yin Field becomes the Yang Field. This is similar to how nothing in the universe, no matter how fast, can exceed the speed of light of 300,000 kilometers per second (absolute speed). In other words, Constitution is the "absolute structure" of human body that can never be changed. Therefore, from an academic perspective, the phrase "converting one's Constitution" is an impossible expression.

The human body presupposes a Constitution—a structure of inequality characterized by a potential difference between the Zang-Fu pairs, or a state of non-equilibrium. The activities of life is that this state of non-equilibrium constantly strives for the equilibrium (dynamic equilibrium). From non-equilibrium to equilibrium, from non-equilibrium to equilibrium![58] We live in the state of constant contradiction, where the state of non-equilibrium must always be assumed in order to aim for the state of equilibrium.

Constitution and the Relationship of Synchronizing and Antagonizing

The system of the Five Phases is regulated by the dynamic relationship of Synchronizing and Antagonizing. Let's consider the Five Phases Array like (1) defined earlier. The Qis of the Five Phases operate within a network of dynamic relationships involving Synchronizing and Antagonizing. Under these dynamic relationships, what are the conditions that allow a system with an array like (1) to maintain equilibrium? Naturally, there must be a relationship of tension in which the left side and the right side maintain a physiological balance of potential centered on C. In other words, they must oppose each other. In the Five Phases, an opposing relationship refers to the Antagonizing Relationship (a two-way Intersuppressing Relationship) between two Qis. Therefore, there must be an Antagonizing Relationship between A and E, as well as between B and D. To maximize this left-right relationship of tension,

[58] Returning from non-equilibrium to equilibrium is rest. The most important act of rest is sleep. Through sleep, we dramatically reduce entropy.

a Synchronizing Relationship (a two-way Interpromoting Relationship) is required between A and B, and between D and E (see Figure 3).[59] Only then can both sides maintain the strongest tension around C. This is the dynamic equilibrium of the human body.

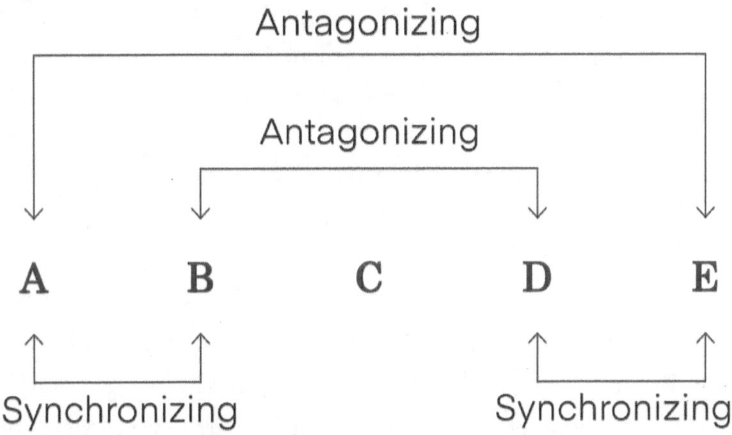

Figure 3. Conditions for Five Phases Array appropriate for Constitution

Antagonizing Relationship between A and E, and that between B and D must be established, and Synchronizing Relationship between A and B, and that between D and E must be established. Only then can the human body maintain the dynamic balance.

[59] Without these relationships, the system would not be able to maintain the equilibrium and would collapse. For example, if A and E are in Synchronizing Relationship, they will always be in sync with each other, so the tilted imbalance cannot be corrected. Let's suppose that the potential of E is too low and the potential of A is too high. Then when the potential of E is raised to correct this, A also will rise due to the synchronizing effect. The imbalance is never resolved because the same effect keeps happening. Additionally, what if A and B are Antagonizing? When the potential of A becomes too low, B, which is in an Antagonistic Relationship with A, will rise due to the antagonistic effect. Since B also belongs to an organ with second high potential in the Zang-Fu Structure Formula, if it rises further, the imbalance in the system worsens. To correct this, if B is lowered, A, in its Antagonistic Relationship, rises again. There is absolutely no way to correct the imbalance of the system.

How to find out the types of Constitution

Now, let's specifically identify the arrays that satisfy the conditions shown in Figure 3. They can be easily understood by considering the Synchronizing and Antagonizing Relationships of the Five Phases and the conditions of the Five Phases Array in Figure 3. First, let's consider the case where Earth is assigned to A. If Earth is assigned to A, then Water and Wood, which are in Antagonizing Relationship with Earth, can be assigned to E, as shown below.

Earth B C D Water ...... ①
Earth B C D Wood ...... ②

Let's look at case ① first. In ①, since Earth is located in the position of A, it is possible for Fire or Metal, which are Synchronizing with Earth, to be placed in B. First, if Fire is placed in B (Earth Fire C D Water), only Metal, which is Antagonizing Fire, can be placed in D (Earth Fire C Metal Water). This is because if Wood is placed in D (Earth Fire C Wood Water), it would form a Synchronizing relation with Fire and would not meet the conditions in Figure 3. If Metal is placed in D, the remaining Qi, Wood, is automatically placed in C. Therefore, one array is determined as follows: Earth Fire Wood Metal Water.

Next, let's look at the case where Metal is placed in position B (Earth Metal C D Water). In this case, Wood and Fire can be placed in D. If Fire is placed in D (Earth Metal C Fire Water), it does not meet the conditions of Figure 3 because it creates an Antagonizing relation with the Water in E. On the other hand, if Wood is placed in D (Earth Metal C Wood Water), it forms a Synchronizing relation with the Water in E, thus meeting the requirements of Figure 3. Then, the remaining element, Fire, is automatically placed in C. Accordingly, another array is determined: Earth Metal Fire Wood Water.

Now let's look at case ②. First, assuming that Fire is placed in B (Earth Fire C D Wood), either Water or Metal, which are Antagonizing Fire, can be placed in D. If Metal is placed in D (Earth Fire C Metal Wood), it does not meet the conditions of Figure 3 because it forms an Antagonizing relation with the Wood in E. Therefore, Metal cannot be placed in D. On the other hand, if Water is placed in D (Earth Fire C Water Wood), it forms a Synchronizing relation with the Wood in E, so it conforms to Figure 3. Then, the remaining Qi, Metal, is placed in C, and another array is determined: Earth Fire Metal Water Wood.

Finally, if Metal is placed in B (Earth Metal C D Wood), Wood and Fire, which are Antagonizing Metal, can be placed in D. Since Wood already exists in E, only Fire can be placed in D (Earth Metal C Fire Wood). Therefore, the remaining Qi, Water, is placed in C, and another array is determined: Earth Metal Water Fire Wood.

We have reviewed all the cases in which Earth is placed in A. If Earth is placed in A, the possible Five Phases Structure Formulas are as follows:

Earth Fire Wood Metal Water ... ①
Earth Metal Fire Wood Water ... ②
Earth Fire Metal Water Wood ... ③
Earth Metal Water Fire Wood ... ④

When Earth is placed in A, there are four possible Five Phases Structure Formulas as shown above. Similarly, if A assigns any of the remaining four Qis—Wood, Fire, Metal, or Water—it can be inferred that four Five Phases Structure Formulas are established for each. Therefore, mathematically, there are 4 × 5 = 20, meaning there are 20 types of Five Phases Structure Formulas that meet the conditions in Figure 3. To summarize everything, it is as follows.

(1) When Wood is placed in A

Wood Fire Earth Water Metal ... ①
Wood Fire Water Metal Earth ... ②
Wood Water Metal Fire Earth ... ③
Wood Water Fire Earth Metal ... ④

(2) When Fire is placed in A

Fire Wood Earth Metal Water … ①
Fire Wood Water Earth Metal … ②
Fire Earth Metal Wood Water … ③
Fire Earth Wood Water Metal … ④

(3) When Earth is placed in A

Earth Fire Wood Metal Water … ①
Earth Metal Fire Wood Water … ②
Earth Fire Metal Water Wood … ③
Earth Metal Water Fire Wood … ④

(4) When Metal is placed in A

Metal Water Earth Fire Wood … ①
Metal Water Wood Earth Fire … ②
Metal Earth Water Wood Fire … ③
Metal Earth Fire Water Wood … ④

(5) When Water is placed in A

Water Metal Earth Wood Fire … ①
Water Metal Wood Fire Earth … ②
Water Wood Fire Metal Earth … ③
Water Wood Metal Earth Fire … ④

The Birth of Eight Constitutions

The 20 Structure Formulae listed above represent the number of all Constitutions that can be theoretically deduced. I cannot say for certain whether all 20 Constitutions actually exist. The 20 Constitutions shown above are merely the result of mathematical deduction. Therefore, the existence of individual Constitutions can only be confirmed empirically through sufficient clinical experience. However, at least the following claim can be made: "The number of possible Constitutions in the human body is equal to or less than 20 (The number of possible Constitutions ≤ 20)."

Among these 20, if you select only those with Wood and Metal at both ends of the array, as well as those with Fire and Water at both ends, you will arrive at Master Do-won Kuon's Eight Constitutions, which I think are originally derived from Je-ma Lee's Sasang Constitutions. The Eight Constitutions are as follows (This selection is related to Je-ma Lee's Sasang Medicine. It will be detailed later):

① Metal Earth Fire Water Wood (Geumyang, 金陽)
② Metal Water Earth Fire Wood (Geumeum, 金陰)
③ Earth Fire Wood Metal Water (Soyang, 土陽)
④ Earth Metal Fire Wood Water (Soeum, 土陰)
⑤ Wood Water Fire Earth Metal (Mogyang, 木陽)
⑥ Wood Fire Earth Water Metal (Mogeum, 木陰)
⑦ Water Metal Wood Fire Earth (Suyang, 水陽)
⑧ Water Wood Fire Metal Earth (Sueum, 水陰)

In his book *Donguisusebowon*, Je-ma Lee states that the Heart (心, which corresponds to Fire in the Five Phases) is "The Supreme Ultimate in the Center" (中央之太極), meaning it is located at the center and holds the same position as the Supreme Ultimate, which presides over everything. Therefore, this Heart was excluded when discussing Sasangin's large and small Zang. The Heart is a Zang of neutrality that cannot be biased toward one side. Therefore, Sasangin was born with Four Constitutions: Taeyangin and Taeeumin as of the pair of Lungs and Liver, and Soyangin and Soeumin as of the pair of Pancreas and Kidneys.[60] Je-ma Lee's Four Constitutions are as follows.

[60] Je-ma Lee, *Donguisusebowon* (Seoul: Haenglim Publishing, 1993), p.7. "There are four differences in human innate Zangs theory. People with large Lungs and small Liver are called Taeyangin; Those with large Liver and small Lungs are called Taeeumin; Those with large Pancreas and small Kidneys are called Soyangin; Those with large Kidneys and small Pancreas are called Soeumin. ...... The Heart of the Five Zangs is The Supreme

Taeyangin: person with large Lungs and small Liver
Soyangin: person with large Pancreas and small Kidneys
Taeeumin: person with large Liver and small Lungs
Soeumin: person with large Kidneys and small Pancreas

Here, the large Zangs belong to Yang Field and the small Zangs belong to Yin Field if I assign the same idea as Eight Constitutions to Sasangins. My reference to the Yang and Yin Fields of Sasangin, as mentioned above, can be found as a clue in Je-ma Lee's book *Donguisusebowon*.

From the beginning when Master Do-won Kuon launched Constitutional Medicine, he developed a theory based on the Four Constitutions of Sasangin, that is, Taeyangin, Soyangin, Taeeumin, and Soeumin. What differs from Je-ma Lee is that, rather than discussing the Constitutions using only two pairs of Zang-Fu (more accurately, Je-ma Lee adopted only two Zangs), he discussed the Constitutions using five pairs of Zang-Fu by including three additional pairs beyond Je-ma Lee's two pairs. (This simple change became the decisive variable that made Eight Constitution Medicine so different from Sasang Constitutional Medicine.) Therefore, naturally, it was a structure in which the Heart could not come to both ends of the Constitution from the start. From Je-ma Lee's Four Constitutions, I infer that the Eight Constitutions were derived by defining two arrays for each Sasang Constitution: one for the Zang-system and the other for the Fu-system (2 × 4 = 8).

What I want to point out here is regarding the Yin and Yang classification of the Zang-Fu. Traditionally, it is said that Zang belongs to Yin and Fu to Yang, but Master Do-won Kuon, on the contrary, assigns the Zang to Yang and the Fu to Yin. Therefore, the Yang Constitutions (Geumyang, Toyang, Mogyang, and Suyang) are defined by the array of the Five Zangs, and the Yin Constitutions (Geumeum, Toeum, Mogeum, and Sueum) are defined by the array of the Five Fus.

Ultimate (Taiji) in the center. The Lungs, Pancreas, Liver, and Kidneys out of Five Zangs are the Sasang (Four Symbols) on the four supports."

There is no clear explanation for this, but in my opinion, in terms of physiological characteristics or pathological symptoms, the Geumyang, Toyang, Mogyang, and Suyang Constitutions, defined by the array of Zangs, are clinically closer to Yang attributes, while the Geumeum, Toeum, Mogeum, and Sueum Constitutions, defined by the array of Fus, are clinically closer to Yin attributes. While there are exceptions, I often observe this tendency in clinical practice.

Meanwhile, the current stance of Eight-Constitution Medicine does not actually place much significance on these distinctions between Yang and Yin. Instead, because the traditional concept of Yin and Yang is likely to distort the understanding of Constitution, an attempt was made to revise the Constitution names—previously divided into Yin and Yang—to names that reflect the magnitude of Zang-Fu influence, thereby aligning them with the definition of Constitution.[61] Therefore, the issue of Yin-Yang classification in relation to Zang-Fu will not be discussed here. The array of the Eight Constitutions as indicated by Master Do-won Kuon in the array of Zang-Fu is as follows.

---

[61] The Yin-Yang classification of the Zang and Fu has little practical significance in Eight-Constitution Medicine at the present. Since the names of the Constitutions are based on Yin and Yang, they often lead to unnecessary misunderstandings, as they are confused with the Yin and Yang Constitutions of traditional Oriental medicine. For this reason, Master Do-won Kuon once attempted to change the Constitution names based on the Zang-Fu. For example, the Geumyang Constitution could be called the "Lung-tonic Constitution" (肺强體質), and the Toeum Constitution could be called the "Stomach-tonic Constitution" (胃强體質). However, due to convention, the current Constitution names are widely used and are considered to have their own significance, so they remain in use today.

On the other hand, the English notation of Constitutions is based on the Zang-Fu. For example:

Pulmotonia (Geumyang Constitution = Strong Lung)
Colonotonia (Geumeum Constitution = Strong Large intestine)
Pancreotonia (Toyang Constitution = Strong Pancreas)
Gastrotonia (Toeum Constitution = Strong Stomach)
Hepatonia (Mogyang Constitution = Strong Liver)
Cholecystonia (Mogeum Constitution = Strong Gallbladder)
Renotonia (Suyang Constitution = Strong Kidney)
Vesicotonia (Sueum Constitution = Strong Bladder)

These names are based on the strongest Zang or Fu in each Constitution.

① Lungs Pancreas Heart Kidneys Liver (Geumyang)
② Large-intestine Bladder Stomach Small-intestine Gallbladder (Geumeum)
③ Pancreas Heart Liver Lung Kidney (Toyang)
④ Stomach Large-intestine Small-intestine Gallbladder (Toeum)
⑤ Liver Kidneys Heart Pancreas Lungs (Mogyang)
⑥ Gallbladder Small-intestine Stomach Bladder Large-intestine (Mogeum)
⑦ Kidneys Lungs Liver Heart Pancreas (Suyang)
⑧ Bladder Gallbladder Small-intestine Large-intestine Stomach (Sueum)

Master Do-won Kuon states that Yang Constitution is associated with the Zangs (Liver, Heart, Pancreas, Lungs, Kidneys), and Yin Constitution is associated with the Fus (Gallbladder, Small intestine, Stomach, Large intestine, Bladder).

Proposing new Zang-Fu arrays for Constitutions

In this way, the Zang array was applied to the Yang Constitutions of Geumyang, Toyang, Mogyang, and Suyang, and the Fu array was applied to the Yin Constitutions of Geumeum, Toeum, Mogeum, and Sueum. However, as mentioned earlier, this does not have much significance in actual clinical practice. This is because Yin and Yang do not exist completely apart from each other. From the perspective of Yin-Yang Interweaving,[62] the Lungs include the Large intestine, and the Large intestine includes the Lungs, making them a pair of Zang-Fu organs. To encapsulate the meaning of Master Do-won Kuon, I suggest the arrays of the Eight Constitutions as follows.

① LU-LI PA-ST HT-SI KI-BL LR-GB (Geumyang)
② LI-LU BL-KI ST-PA SI-HT GB-LR (Geumeum)
③ PA-ST HT-SI LR-GB LU-LI KI-BL (Toyang)
④ ST-PA LU-LI SI-HT GB-LR BL-KI (Toeum)
⑤ LR-GB KI-BL HT-SI PA-ST LU-LI (Mogyang)

[62] It is a term that expresses the process of Yin and Yang intertwining and mixing together to achieve various forms of harmony.

⑥ GB-LR SI-HT ST-PA BL-KI LU-LI (Mogeum)
⑦ KI-BL LU-LI LR-GB HT-SI PA-ST (Suyang)
⑧ BL-KI GB-LR SI-HT LU-LI ST-PA (Sueum)

[Legend]

LU = Lungs, LI = Large intestine, PA = Pancreas, ST = Stomach, HT = Heart, SI = Small intestine, KI = Kidneys, BL = Bladder, LR = Liver, GB = Gallbladder.

For the Yang Constitution, Zangs are listed first, and for the Yin Constitution, Fus are listed first. This means that the Zang or Fu listed in the front play a dominant role in the Constitution, while the Zang or Fu listed in the back play a secondary role. However, this is not necessarily absolute. This is because in physiology and pathology, the Zang and Fu are closely related and function simultaneously.

Sometimes a disease is treated by regulating only the dominant Zang-Fu organs of the Constitution, sometimes by regulating only the secondary Zang-Fu organs, and in some cases, by regulating them in combination. Therefore, I simply prefer to denote the front as the Zang-system and the back as the Fu-system, as follows[63]:

① LU-LI PA-ST HT-SI KI-BL LR-GB (Geumyang)
② LU-LI KI-BL PA-ST HT-SI LR-GB (Geumeum)
③ PA-ST HT-SI LR-GB LU-LI KI-BL (Toyang)
④ PA-ST LU-LI HT-SI LR-GB KI-BL (Toeum)
⑤ LR-GB KI-BL HT-SI PA-ST LU-LI (Mogyang)
⑥ LR-GB HT-SI PA-ST KI-BL LU-LI (Mogeum)
⑦ KI-BL LU-LI LR-GB HT-SI PA-ST (Suyang)
⑧ KI-BL LR-GB HT-SI LU-LI PA-ST (Sueum)

[63] Regarding the next array, keep in mind that, despite some exceptions, in Yang Constitutions, the Zang organs usually take the lead in physiology and pathology, while in Yin Constitutions, the Fu organs typically take the lead.

How many Constitutions are there?

I do not believe that all of the 20 theoretically derived Constitutions mentioned above actually exist. For example, if the Heart is located at either end of each Constitutional array, I conjecture that it would not be considered appropriate as a Constitution, considering the stability of the human body. According to the Zang-Fu structure, if there were a Constitution in which the Heart—the core engine of the human body—was the largest, that Constitution would likely be prone to collapse due to the Heart being too easily excited. Conversely, if the Heart was the smallest in the Zang-Fu structure, the human body would not function properly and would be prone to shutting down. This indicates that it would be difficult to maintain homeostasis within the human body system. In the end, I believe the eight cases in which Fire is located at either end should be excluded from the types of Constitutions.

Among the 20 arrays of Five Phases Structure Formulae logically derived earlier, the following eight arrays, in which Fire is positioned at either end of the Five Phases Structure Formula, are as follows: Fire Wood Earth Metal Water; Fire Water Earth Metal Wood; Fire Earth Metal Water Wood; Fire Wood Metal Earth Water; Metal Water Earth Wood Fire; Metal Wood Water Earth Fire; Water Metal Earth Fire Wood; and Wood Metal Earth Fire Water. I suppose that these arrays should be excluded from the types of Constitutions.

So if you subtract this 8 arrays from the 20 array, you are left with 12 arrays. Since only the 8 Constitutions are currently known as the types of Constitution, it must also be proven that the remaining four arrays do not exist. However, do the remaining four arrays—that is, the four arrays left after excluding the Eight Constitutions with Fire at either end of the 20 Constitutions—truly not exist? Or do they exist but are so rare that they are not easily discovered? It is not clear. Only when it is proven that these four arrays do not exist will the equation 20 − 8 − 4 = 8 confirm that only eight Constitutions exist. The four arrays whose existence remains unclear are as follows:

Wood Fire Water Metal Earth
Wood Water Metal Fire Earth
Earth Fire Metal Water Wood
Earth Metal Water Fire Wood

During the long course of my countless clinical treatments, most patients are experiencing good healing within the Eight Constitutions. Among the Eight Constitutions, the probability of the following six Constitutions—Geumyang, Geumeum, Toyang, Mogyang, Mogeum, and Suyang—is more than 90%.[64] People with the Sueum Constitution rarely visit my clinic, and people with the Toeum Constitution also seldom come to my clinic.

There are many ways to analyze the reasons for this. The Toeum Constitution is relatively rare in terms of absolute numbers, while the Sueum Constitution is not as rare, but it seems to maintain good health on one's own. In addition to the Suyang Constitution, the Sueum Constitution aligns well with the Korean diet, particularly its spicy food culture. Herbal medicines such as ginseng or red ginseng, as well as general health supplements, also have a positive effect on individuals with this Constitution. Therefore, the likelihood of falling ill is lower compared to other Constitutions, and it

---

[64] These statistics are based on the patients visiting my clinic, so rates in the general population may vary. This is because those with Constitution that is unfavorable to the current dietary culture or environment may have a higher frequency of clinic visits, while those with Constitution that is advantageous may have a lower frequency of visits. It is in the same context that Je-ma Lee, who lived at the end of the Joseon Dynasty, mentioned in his book of *Donguisusebowon* that Taeyangin (Geumyang and Geumeum Constitutions) were extremely rare. There would inevitably have been a bias in the statistic sample since it was conducted on the patients who visited Bowonguk, the clinic he founded.

From the perspective of the people of the late Joseon Dynasty, who had predominantly vegetarian diet, Taeyangin, many of whom were inherently vegetarians, must have been the healthiest, which is why the number of Taeyangin patients visiting his clinic was very small. Taeyangin, who are now exposed to the modern dietary culture centered on meat and processed foods—completely different from the Joseon era—are now frequently visiting clinics specializing in the Eight Constitutions. Taeyangin, who enjoyed the best health under the protection of the world's best vegetarian culture that lasted for half a millennium, are now coming out of the closet in large numbers because they cannot tolerate the greasy Western diet culture now in Korea.

seems that individuals with these Constitutions manage their health effectively through self-care. As a result, there is relatively less need to visit my clinic compared to other Constitutions. Thus, even though there are Eight Constitutions, approximately six Constitutions account for the majority of all patients.

In theory, we can speculate that there may be more than just the eight types of Constitutions. Theoretically, it is possible to have up to 20 Constitutions as derived earlier. Of course, whether they actually exist or not is a different matter. This is because there are countless cases where something is predictable in theory but does not exist in reality.[65] However, science logically develops theories and establishes laws through hypotheses. And the truth value of that law is measured through experiment. Only when it is proven through the experimentation is the theory accepted as truth.

Some may ask whether it is contradictory that there are theoretically 20 Constitutions, but only 8 Constitutions exist. However, this is a misunderstanding where the subject is reversed. There is no justification for assuming that the order of humans, nature, or even the universe should align with human theories. We simply investigate and develop theories using scientific methods to understand the order in which nature operates.

The same applies to the types of Constitutions discussed so far. In theory, 20 types are possible, but the types of Constitutions that are actually possible may vary under the conditions of the Earth's environment. However, what is clear is the undeniable fact that the condition of dynamic equilibrium between the Zang-Fu organs, inherent in the actual Constitutions, is an inevitable law.

---

[65] An example is the fact that an enormous number of species that once existed on Earth are now extinct. In particular, with the rise of human civilization, the extinction of species accelerated rapidly. Now, we are faced with a biodiversity problem that threatens the survival of humanity. The number of types of Constitutions may have approached 20 in the early days of mankind, but during the evolutionary process, many Constitutions that failed to adapt were eliminated, and those that successfully adapted remained, settling down to the current 8 Constitutions.

Distribution of Constitutions

The distribution of Constitutions varies depending on the region and the geopolitical conditions of a country and ethnic group. It is said that the Korean population is composed of two groups: northern peoples who migrated from the continent and primarily eat meat, and marine peoples who mainly farm and fish. This results in a diverse distribution of Constitutions, including the Mogyang Constitution, which is suited for eating meat; the Geumyang and Geumeum Constitutions, which are suited for vegetables, fish, and seafood; and the Toyang Constitution, which is generally suited for meat, vegetables, fish, and seafood.

On the other hand, in the case of Japan, being a maritime nation with islands surrounded by the sea, there are likely many Constitutions such as Geumyang or Geumeum, which are suited for eating fish and seafood, while Constitutions such as Mogyang or Mogeum, which are suited for eating meat, are relatively uncommon.

In countries like Germany or Mongolia, which are primarily inland, there are likely many Constitutions such as Toyang and Mogyang, which are well-suited for consuming meat and dairy products. However, there are likely fewer Geumyang or Geumeum Constitutions, which are better suited for vegetables, fish, and seafood.

Therefore, even though there are theoretically Eight Constitutions, their distribution is not uniform. Depending on the country or region, some Constitutions are more prevalent while others are relatively rare. Based on the patients who visited my clinic, I previously noted that in Korea, six Constitutions are particularly common: Geumyang, Geumeum, Toyang, Mogyang, Mogeum, and Suyang. This can be seen as more diverse distribution of Constitutions compared to other countries. The characteristics of Korea as a peninsula, influenced by both the continent and the ocean, are reflected in this varied distribution of Constitutions.

So far, we have examined the definition of Constitution and the types of Constitution theoretically derived from that definition.

CHAPTER 3

The Theory of Unit Formulae

MATHEMATICS IS THE KING OF THE BIG OTHER. FROM THE SHOULDERS OF THE KING, BEHOLD AND FEEL THE AWE-INSPIRING LAWS OF LIFE WOVEN INTO THE HUMAN BODY.

CHAPTER 3

The Theory of Unit Formulae

In Eight-Constitution Medicine, there are two main types of prescriptions. One is "Unit Formulae," and the other is "Compound Formulae," which consists of an appropriate combination of Unit Formulae.[66] If the Unit Formula is like a word, the Compound Formula is like a sentence formed by combining words. Here, we will learn about the principles of Unit Formulae, which correspond to words.

Unit Formulae in Constitutional Medicine are derived from the specific Zang-Fu Structure of each Constitution. Since every Constitution has a unique Zang-Fu array, even if treating the same disease, the acupoints that make up the Formulae differ for each Constitution. This is because, in Constitutional Medicine, treatment varies according to the inherent Zang-Fu Structure unique to each Constitution. While the specific acupoints differ across the Constitutions, the underlying principles that create the Formulae remain consistent for all Constitutions. This is where the logical coherence of Constitutional Medicine resides.

---

[66] Unit Formulae and Compound Formulae are the terms coined by me. A Compound Formula refers to a treatment that combines two or more Unit Formulae to address a disease. The more chronic or difficult the disease is, the more Compound the combination of Unit Formulae required. Typically, two-level Formula, consisting of a basic Unit Formula and another Unit Formula (sub-prescription), are used for simple diseases, while more serious chronic diseases, immune system disorders, viral infections, and benign or malignant tumors generally require three or more Unit Formulae, i.e., three-stage or higher Formulae.

Constitution is Congenital Imbalance

Here is a Constitution. Let's say the Zang-Fu structure of this Constitution is "A B C D E." In Constitutional Medicine, this inherent inequality in the human body is referred to as "Congenital Imbalance." Let's hear the meaning of these words directly in the words of Master Do-won Kuon.

> "The congenital unbalance (imbalance) of the organs of the 8 temperaments means that among the organs there are mutually controlling actions, so that the furthermore severe unbalance can not be made. Therefore, it appears as a characteristic individuality, and involves only a predisposition, being thus a healthy state."[67]

It can be seen that this concept of Congenital Imbalance originates from Je-ma Lee's Sasang Medicine. Master Do-won Kuon says:

> "And the constitutions of the four types mean the four congenital unbalanced structures of the internal organ functions, and the names for them are respectively called Tae-yang-in (Hespera), So-yang-in (Saturna), Tae-um-in (Jupita) and So-um-in (Mercuria)."[68]

This Congenital Imbalance is the non-equilibrium that serves as a prerequisite for life, as discussed in Chapter 2, "Definition of Constitution", and represents "the will to life" that constantly strives to reduce entropy. It is the initial condition of existence that is unconditionally bestowed upon humans from the moment they are born.

---

[67] Do-won Kuon, *A Study Of Constitution-acupuncture*, 1965, p.12. Here, the 8 temperaments correspond to the concept that represents the stage before the differentiation of the 8 constitutions. In Sasangin, each person was divided into Zang-temperament and Fu-temperament, resulting in eight temperaments. The unbalance he mentions, in fact, means imbalance.

[68] Do-won Kuon, *A Study Of Constitution-acupuncture*, 1965, p.4. The terms in parentheses are the names of the Sasang types as determined by Do-won Kuon.

Pathological Imbalance and Unit Formulae

If this tendency toward imbalance remains within certain limits and does not deepen further, it is not considered a disease. Therefore, the Congenital Imbalance refers to a Physiological Imbalance—a normal state of the body. This imbalance is not severe but represents a fundamental, slight imbalance inherent in the body.[69]

If a factor goes beyond this Congenital Imbalance and leads to a state of deeper imbalance, only then does a disease occur. This deeper imbalance is called Pathological Imbalance. It refers to the cause of disease manifesting in the human body and is the core of Constitutional pathology. Let's hear what Master Do-won Kuon has to say about this.

> "The more such constitutions get pretexts[70] mentally or physically, the stronger their strong organs have only the tendencies to become. And they cannot be weakened below their congenital functions. On the contrary, the weak organs have only the tendencies to be the more weakened, and cannot be strengthened above their own congenital functions. Hence, constitution cannot be changed a posteriori. Moreover, just as in the two poles of a balance there is a interrelation between the strong and the weak organs. Hence, when the strong part becomes stronger, the weak one weaker; when the weak one becomes weaker, the strong one stronger. Both the over-strengthenedness of this strong organ and the over-weakenedness of the weak one, namely

---

69 "The word 'congenital unbalance', used in the present thesis, means the unbalance of a narrow margin." Do-won Kuon, *A Study Of Constitution- acupuncture*, 1965, p.6.

70 Master Kuon comments that the term "pretext" has a similar meaning to the word "stressor," a stimulating factor mentioned by Professor Hans Selye (1907-1982). Professor Selye was a Hungarian-Canadian endocrinologist and physiologist known for his pioneering research on stress and the theory of General Adaptation Syndrome (GAS). General adaptation syndrome refers to the physical and pathological symptoms that occur when a person is subjected to continuous stress. Symptoms of general adaptation syndrome may include fatigue, headaches, insomnia, depression, anger, and anxiety.

> the state of over-unbalance, is the very disease; and it is the very cure of it to make the state of the over-unbalance return again to that of the congenital."[71]

If we synthesize Do-won Kuon's theories, we can establish the following important laws of Constitutional pathology. When the Zang-Fu Structure Array of a Constitution is ABCDE, in a pathological state, the Zang-Fu Potentials of A and B always tend to increase in the positive direction, and the Zang-Fu Potentials of D and E always tend to increase in the negative direction. (This means that the absolute value of the Zang-Fu Potentials of A, B, D, and E increases, while C, as the central Zang-Fu Potential, remains stable and does not make any changes in its potential.)

This is similar to the image of a seesaw. In a normal physiological state, the Zang-Fu Structure of a human body is constructed as follows: the Zang-Fu Potentials of A and B are slightly shifted in the positive direction, and the Zang-Fu Potentials of D and E are slightly shifted in the negative direction, while C being centered. This represents a state of Physiological Imbalance, which reflects the person's Constitutional structure and is considered a healthy state.

If this transitions into a diseased condition due to a factor, the imbalance among the Zang-Fu pairs can become so severe that A turns into A', B into B', D into D', and E into E'. This can be seen as the increase in entropy that occurs in a pathological state of the human body. In other words, one or more of A, B, D, and E cause excessive imbalance in the pathological state. This excessive imbalance leads to the state of disease. C remains as the central Zang-Fu and does not undergo any changes, similar to the central pivot of a seesaw. See the following picture.

---

[71] Do-won Kuon, *A Study Of Constitution-acupuncture*, 1965, p.5.

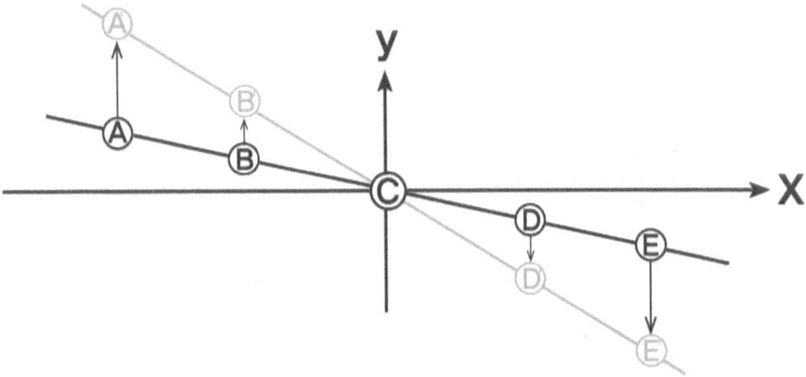

Figure 1. Schematic Diagram of Constitutional Pathology

This illustration is a typical diagram concisely depicting the Constitutional pathology of Eight-Constitution Medicine. For example, A', B', D', and E' represent a transient imbalanced Zang-Fu structure, where A, B, D, and E have shifted from their physiological state to a pathological state. Therefore, in order to cure this condition, it is necessary to correct the state of pathological imbalance and restore it to the original physiological state of Congenital Imbalance. This means that A' and B' must have their Zang-Fu Potentials lowered, while D' and E' must have their Znag-Fu Potentials raised. The prescriptions designed to return each of A', B', D', and E' to their original states are referred to as Unit Formulae.

Here we can derive the general principle for obtaining Unit Formulae. In other words, if the Zang-Fu in the Yang Field causes an excessive imbalance, the excessively raised Zang-Fu Potential must be lowered, so the "sedation method" is used. Conversely, if the Zang-Fu in the Yin Field causes an excessive imbalance, the excessively lowered Zang-Fu Potential must be raised, so the "tonification method" is applied (detailed information on the Eight-Constitution tonification and sedation methods will be provided shortly).

When the human body enters a state of disease, the Zang-Fu organs become excessively imbalanced. In this case, if the number of Zang-Fu organs in excessive imbalance is small, it is considered a mild disease, and if the number of Zang-Fu organs in excessive imbalance is large, it is considered a serious disease. Therefore, simple Formulae are used for mild diseases, while complex Formulae are used for serious diseases. In Eight-Constitution Medicine, the disease treatment is achieved through a combination of these Unit Formulae.

If a disease is caused by excessive imbalance in A and D, which deepens into A' and D', the treatment in this case involves using a Unit Formula to bring A' back to A and another Unit Formula to bring D' back to D, thus combining these two Formulae. If a disease is caused by excessive imbalance in A, D, and E, transitioning into A', D', and E', then three Unit Formulae are needed to return A', D', and E' to their original states A, D, and E. (Strictly speaking, it must also include the Unit Formula that regulates C, the central Zang-Fu, so four Unit Formulae are required, which will be detailed later.) Therefore, Unit Formulae are the foundational element of all prescriptions.

Unit Formulae of Toyang Constitution

Now, let's find Unit Formulae using an example of Toyang Constitution. The Zang-Fu Structure Array of the Toyang Constitution is "Pancreas-Stomach Heart-Small intestine Liver-Gallbladder Lungs-Large intestine Kidneys-Bladder." Therefore, centered around the Liver and Gallbladder, which are the central Zang-Fu organs, the Zang-Fu Potentials of the Pancreas and Stomach, and Heart and Small intestine on the left always tend to increase in the positive direction, while the Potentials of the Lungs and Large intestine, and Kidneys and Bladder on the right tend to increase in the negative direction.

Thus, the Unit Formulae for the Toyang Constitution consist of four formulae to tonify the Kidneys, Bladder, Lungs, and Large Intestine in the Yin field, and four formulae to sedate the Pancreas, Stomach, Heart, and Small Intestine in the Yang field, resulting in a total of eight Unit Formulae.

Since the central Zang-Fu organs, the Liver and Gallbladder, does not change the Zang-Fu Potentials, there are no Unit Formulae for them. Instead, there are two Unit Formulae each for the Pericardium and Triple Burner[72], which act on behalf of the central Zang-Fu organs and regulate the overall system of the human body. Therefore, a total of 12 Unit Formulae are required per Constitution. Let's begin finding each of them.

Unit Formulae for Kidneys and Bladder

First, let's examine the process of tonifying the Kidneys and Bladder. There are various methods for tonifying or sedating the Zang-Fu organs,[73] but Do-won Kuon adopted the methods for tonifying or sedating the Zang-Fu Points using the principles of Synchronizing and Antagonizing of the Five Phases. The method of tonifying or sedating, which utilizes the relationship of Synchronizing and Antagonizing within the Five Phases, originated from Saam Acupuncture[74], developed during the Joseon Dynasty. Initially, Master

[72] There are a total of four Unit Formulae for the Pericardium and Triple Burner. My view on the Pericardium and Triple Burner differs significantly from that of Master Do-won Kuon, which will be discussed in detail later.

[73] Tonifying and sedating techniques of acupuncture include the *Twisting-Based Tonifying and Sedating Method* (捻轉補瀉) according to the needle's rotational direction (clockwise rotation for tonigying and counterclockwise for sedating); the *Breath-Based Tonifying and Sedating Method* (呼吸補瀉), where inserting the needle during exhalation and removing it during inhalation serves as tonifying, while the reverse order serves as sedating; and the *Rotation Count-Based Tonifying and Sedating Method* (九六補瀉), where rotating the needle clockwise nine times is tonifying, and counterclockwise six times is sedating. However, I believe that the *Yinsuibuxie Method* mentioned above is the most reasonable and effective approach in Eight-Constitution Medicine.

[74] The Saam Acupuncture method, known to have been created by a Buddhist monk Saamdoin during the mid-Joseon Dynasty, is a unique Korean acupuncture theory, which is the first Zang-Fu tonifying/sedating method combining both the relationships of Interpromoting and Intersuppressing in the history of acupuncture. Master Do-won Kuon found significant clues regarding Zang-Fu tonifying/sedating method of the Eight Constitutions from this Saam acupuncture method.

The Saam acupuncture method builds on the theories of past Chinese medical doctors. The earliest clue appears in the *69th Nan* (phrase) of the Chinese classic of *Nanjing* (難經), which states, "For deficiency, replenish the mother; for excess, drain the child. Start with tonifying, and then apply sedating (虛者補其母, 實者瀉其子. 當先補之, 然後瀉之)." Gao Wu (高武) of the Ming Dynasty expanded on this with the method of tonifying and sedating within the self-meridian (自經補瀉法) in *Acupuncture Collection* (鍼灸聚英), applying

Do-won Kuon actively applied this Saam acupuncture method to tonify or sedate the Zang-Fu organs in Constitutions. However, after numerous clinical experiences and through trial and error, he developed a unique tonifying and sedating method for Eight Constitution Acupuncture. Nowadays, only a few Formulae mentioned in Saam Acupuncture are used for certain Constitutions, while most have been replaced with Formulae specifically tailored for the Eight Constitutions.

In Eight-Constitution Medicine, the *Yingsuibuxie Method* (迎隨補瀉法) is employed as a tonifying and sedating technique. This method, a form of acupuncture, combines the "Following Method," which places needles in alignment with the meridian flow, and the "Meeting Method," which places needles against the meridian flow. When using the Following Method, it acts as a tonifying approach by promoting Qi flow in the same direction as the meridian flow. Conversely, the Meeting Method acts as a sedating approach, controlling Qi flow in the opposite direction of the meridian flow. For details on meridian flow directions, please refer to the meridian theory introduced in Chapter 1.

The Kidneys and Bladder are Zang-Fu organs that receive Qis from other Zang-Fu organs and regulate the production of Water Qi. In the Toyang Constitution, the Kidneys and Bladder belong to the Yin Field, so if they cause excessive imbalance, Unit Formulae to restore the balance can be achieved through tonification.

---

the theory of Interpromoting relations within the same meridian. Zhang Shixian (張世賢) further extended tonifying/sedating techniques based on Interpromoting relations to other meridians in his book of *Nan Jing with Notes* (校圖注難經).

However, these earlier theories focused only on Interpromoting relations, without applying the concept of Intersuppressing relations. Saam developed his acupuncture method by incorporating both Interpromoting and Intersuppressing relations in meridian treatments, a novel approach at the time. Later, based on Saam's method, Do-won Kuon applied these principles to the Eight Constitutions, creating a distinctive acupuncture treatment for Eight-Constitution Medicine. (Presented by Director Seong-cheol Moon, a Korean Medicine practitioner, at the seminar of "Research Group for the Future of Eight-Constitution Medicine").

The essence of the restoration method utilizing the Synchronizing and Antagonizing relationships of the Five Phases is that, when tonifying or sedating a particular Zang-Fu organ, you should not treat that Zang-Fu organ directly. Instead, you should always engage other Zang-Fu organs that share a Synchronizing or Antagonizing relationship with the target organ, providing the tonifying or sedating technique indirectly through these dynamic interactions. This approach is based on the principle that all things exist in interdependence on one another.

Now, let's proceed with the discussion on Unit Formulae for Toyang Constitution. Since the Kidneys and Bladder are the Zang-Fu organs responsible for creating and regulating Water Qi, tonifying them corresponds to the method of tonifying Water Qi when interpreted within the framework of the Five Phases. See the diagram below for convenience.

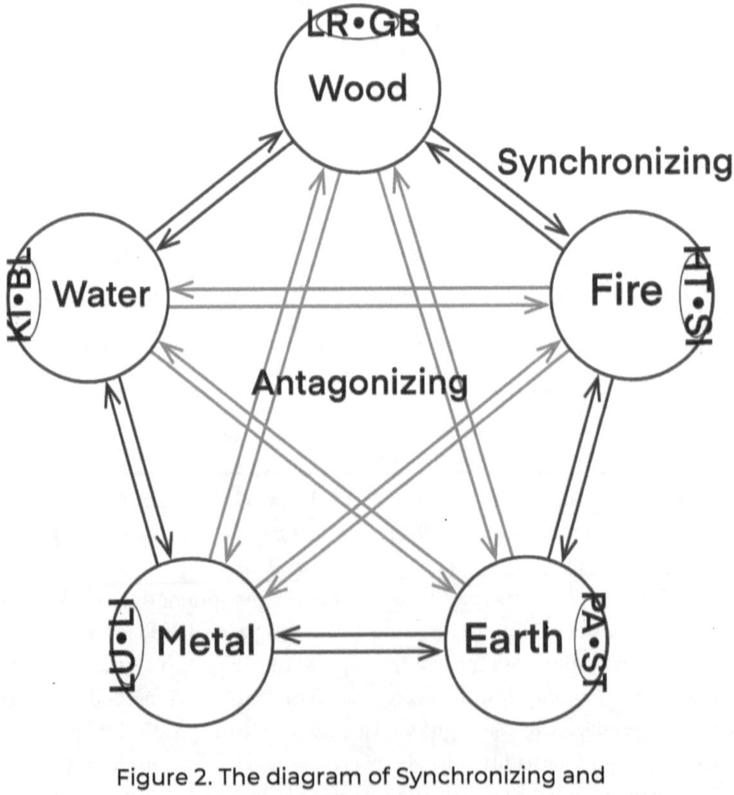

Figure 2. The diagram of Synchronizing and Antagonizing Relationships of Five Phases

First, let's explore how to tonify Water Qi by focusing solely on the Five Phases. Refer to the Synchronizing and Antagonizing relationships among the Five Phases illustrated in Figure 2 above. Within this system of the Five Phases, there are four possible ways to tonify Water by simultaneously adopting both Synchronizing and Antagonizing Relationships.

① sedating Earth and tonifying Metal
② sedating Earth and tonifying Wood
③ sedating Fire and tonifying Wood
④ sedating Fire and tonifying Metal

Proposal of Five Phases Arithmetic Method

Among the four methods above, if you select the one that best aligns with the Toyang Constitution—that is, the approach most suitable for the Zang-Fu structure of the Toyang Constitution—it becomes a Unit Formula for tonifying the Kidneys and Bladder specific to the Toyang Constitution. Here, I propose the "Five Phases Arithmetic Method" as a calculation technique to objectively determine which of the four methods above aligns most accurately with the Toyang Constitution.

The Five Phases Arithmetic Method is a straightforward calculation technique for analyzing relationships within the Five Phases, which I developed, inspired by Do-won Kuon's concept of the two-way relationships of Synchronizing and Antagonizing. By employing this method, one can accurately and quantitatively assess the impact on the entire system of the Five Zangs and Fus when a particular Zang or Fu is treated using the tonifying and sedating method utilizing Zang-Fu Points.

The fundamental principle of the Five Phases Arithmetic Method, as proposed by me, is that within the Synchronizing and Antagonizing relationships of the Five Phases, applying a tonifying method to one Qi also conveys tonifying effects to the two adjacent Qis in Synchronizing relationships due to the Synchronizing influence, while the two Qis in Antagonizing relationships receive sedating effects due to the Antagonizing influence.

On the other hand, when a sedating effect is applied to one Qi, the two adjacent Qis in Synchronizing relationships with that Qi receive sedating effects, while the two other Qis in Antagonizing relationships with that Qi receive tonifying effects.

These effects can be calculated quantitatively by assigning arbitrary values, such as +1 for the tonifying effect and -1 for the sedating effect. By assigning quantitative change values to the overall Qis each time a single tonifying or sedating operation is performed, and then summing these values for each Qi, the impact of multiple tonifying or sedating operations on the entire system can be comprehensively and accurately predicted. Although this is a very simple calculation method, it is an innovative way to quantitatively understand how the whole Five Phases system shifts.[75] Let's consider an example.

For example, what happens if you tonify Wood within the Five Phases? When you tonify Wood, Water and Fire, which share the Synchronizing relationships with Wood, will also receive tonifying effects, while Metal and Earth, which share the Antagonizing relationships with Wood, will receive sedating effects. Let's express this quantitatively.

$$\text{Tonifying Wood: } \Delta\text{Wood}=+1,\ \Delta\text{Water}=+1,\ \Delta\text{Fire}=+1,$$
$$\Delta\text{Metal}=-1,\ \Delta\text{Earth}=-1 \ \ldots\ldots \text{ⓐ}$$

[75] Due to the lack of such principles, most theories in the field of Oriental medicine risk falling into an unprincipled approach, selecting only the paths that suit individual preferences within the conventional Interpromoting and Intersuppressing relationship of the Five Phases. This issue is present even in China, which is considered the origin of Oriental medicine. When the concepts of Yin and Yang are added, it becomes almost chaotic—moving from Yin and Yang to the Five Phases back and forth, and then freely following any desired path, making it possible to support almost any theory. Based on our observations of Chinese medical masters, many of them also fall into this error without realizing it. This calculation method is developed with the hope of avoiding such unprincipled errors.

If ⓐ is represented in an illustration, it appears as follows.

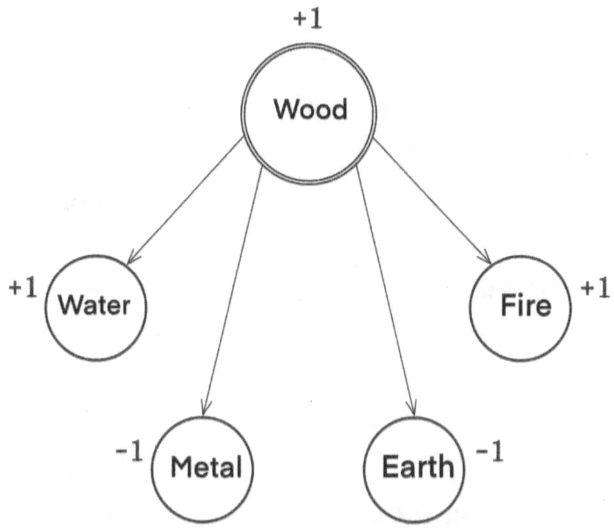

Figure 3. System-wide changes in the Five Phases when Wood is tonified

These numbers are relative values, not absolute values. Since any value can be assigned, we simply assigned the value of ±1. Additionally, it is assumed that the system has reached a steady state with respect to these values. The steady state refers to a stable condition achieved after a manipulation is applied to the system and it has settled over time without further changes. The time to reach this steady state is relatively short; it can be assumed that the steady state is achieved soon after the manipulation. Clinically, if you perform Constitution-acupuncture, you can observe an immediate response to the patient.

Then, this time, let's consider the case of sedating Earth. When you sedate Earth, Fire and Metal, which share the Synchronizing relationships with Earth, receive sedating effects, while Water and Wood, which have the Antagonizing relationships with Earth, receive tonifying effects. Therefore, if you sedate Earth, you obtain the following result.

Sedating Earth: ΔEarth=-1, ΔFire=-1, ΔMetal=-1,
ΔWater=+1, ΔWood=+1 …… ⓑ

If ⓑ is represented in an illustration, it appears as follows.

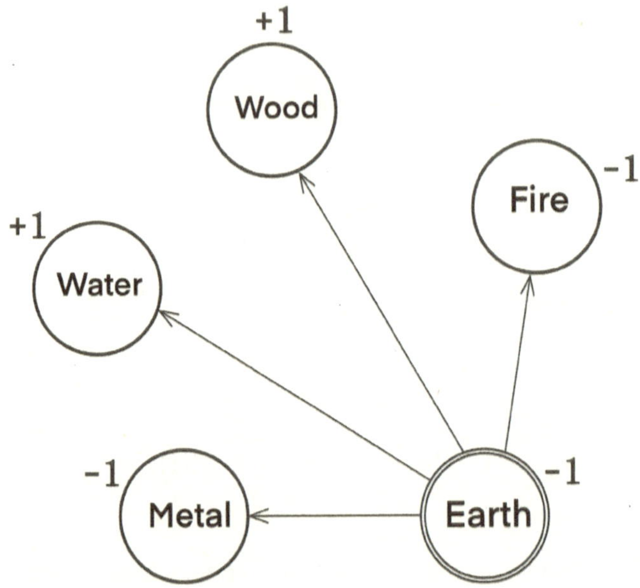

Figure 4. System-wide changes in the Five Phases when Earth is sedated

Then, if you tonify Wood and then sedate Earth, what will happen to the overall change in the Five Phases system? It's simple. Just add ⓐ and ⓑ above by matching the values of the corresponding Qis. This is because the effects of tonifying Wood and sedating Earth are independent. This is similar to calculating the amplitude of superimposed waves. In fact, the dynamic movement of Synchronizing and Antagonizing within the Five Phases is closer to the wave than the particle. Five Phases Theory is akin to the wave mechanics. The result is as follows:

Result: ΔWood=+2, ΔFire=0, ΔEarth=-2,
ΔMetal=-2, ΔWater=+2 …… ⓒ

In other words, within the entire Five Phases system, Wood was strengthened by 2, Fire remained unchanged, Earth and Metal were each weakened by 2, and Water was strengthened by 2. This represents the total change in the system when you tonify Wood and then sedate Earth in succession (the order doesn't matter—sedating Earth first and then tonifying Wood yields the same result). As previously mentioned, this phenomenon is similar to the reinforcement or cancellation of amplitudes that occurs when two waves interfere.

What would happen if you tonify Wood, sedate Earth, and then sedate Fire again? This too is simple. Using the above Five Phases Arithmetic Method, determine the change that occurs when sedating Fire and then add it to the result in © above.

Sedating Fire: ΔFire=-1, ΔWood=-1, ΔEarth=-1,
ΔMetal=+1, ΔWater=+1 ...... ⓓ

If ⓓ is represented as an illustration, it appears as follows.

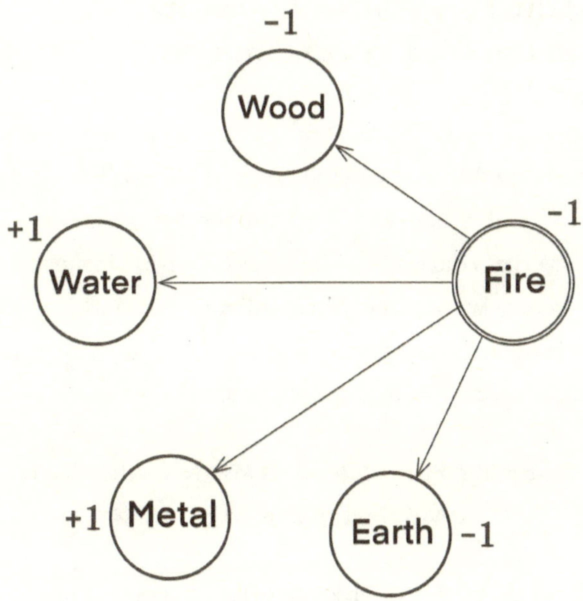

Figure 5. System-wide changes in the Five Phases when Fire is sedated

If you add the results of ⓒ and ⓓ, you will get the result as follows.

Result: ΔWood=+1, ΔFire=-1, ΔEarth=-3,
ΔMetal=-1, ΔWater=+3 …… ⓔ

Wood is strengthened by 1, Fire and Metal are weakened by 1, Earth is weakened by 3, and Water is strengthened by 3. In the end, it can be observed that, as a result of the three manipulations, Water was strengthened the most, while Earth was weakened the most. By calculating in this manner, you can easily and accurately understand the changes in the entire system, no matter how many times the manipulation is repeated! Now, let's take a closer look at how this Five Phases Arithmetic Method can be applied to the formation of Unit Formulae.

Applying the Five Phases Arithmetic Method to the Toyang Constitution

First, let's apply the Five Phases Arithmetic Method starting with sedating Fire and tonifying Metal (瀉火補金) method in example ④. When Fire is sedated, the Qis of Wood and Earth in the Synchronizing Relationships decrease due to the reduction in Fire's synchronizing influence. Meanwhile, Metal and Water, within the Antagonizing relationships, experience an anti-antagonizing influence from the sedated Fire, leading to an increase in their Qis. Let's express this in the operation.

Sedating Fire: ΔFire=-1, ΔWood=-1, ΔEarth=-1,
ΔMetal=+1, ΔWater=+1 …… (a)

As mentioned earlier, the absolute value of these numbers is not particularly important here. These values are assigned merely for convenience to observe the trend of change. What matters is the relative shift in whether each Qi's quantity increases or decreases after performing tonification and sedation. Therefore, from (a), it can be seen that the quantity of Fire, Wood, and Earth has decreased, while the quantity of Metal and Water has increased.

This time, let's examine the case of tonifying Metal. When Metal is tonified, the Qis of Earth and Water, which are in Synchronizing relationships with Metal, are strengthened due to the increased influence of Metal. Meanwhile, the Qis of Wood and Fire, which are in Antagonizing relationships with Metal, experience the antagonizing effect of Metal, resulting in their weakened Qis. This can be represented as follows:

$$\text{Tonifying Metal: } \Delta\text{Metal}=+1,\ \Delta\text{Earth}=+1,\ \Delta\text{Water}=+1,$$
$$\Delta\text{Wood}=-1,\ \Delta\text{Fire}=-1\ \ldots\ \text{(b)}$$

(a) represents the changes caused by sedating Fire, and (b) represents the changes caused by tonifying Metal. Since the changes in (a) and (b) are independent of each other, the overall change in the system resulting from sedating Fire and tonifying Metal can be determined by adding the results of (a) and (b) for each Phase. Let's sum the effects in (a) and (b) for each respective Qi.

$$\text{Result: } \Delta\text{Wood}=-2,\ \Delta\text{Fire}=-2,\ \Delta\text{Earth}=0,$$
$$\Delta\text{Metal}=+2,\ \Delta\text{Water}=+2\ \ldots\ \text{(c)}$$

Let's analyze this result. The Five Phases Structure Formula of Toyang Constitution is "Earth Fire Wood Metal Water." Therefore, Earth and Fire in the Yang Field always tend to increase their Qis, while Water and Metal in the Yin Field tend to decrease their Qis. If this tendency exceeds the normal range and progresses into a state of excessive imbalance, the body enters a pathological state, or disease. Thus, The Unit Formulae that further deepen this imbalance are not suitable. Conversely, The Formulae that alleviate this imbalance is the correct Unit Formulae. For Toyang Constitution, the correct Unit Formulae would require Earth and Fire values to be negative (or zero), Metal and Water values to be positive (or zero), and Wood, as the central Qi, should remain neutral, with a value of zero.

In the result of (c), the values of Fire and Earth are negative and zero respectively, and the values of Metal and Water are positive. According to the Five Phases Structure Formula, this result decreases Earth and Fire, which tend to increase, while it increases Metal and Water, which tend to decrease. Thus, it corrects the trend of probable Pathological Imbalance, meeting the requirements for an appropriate Unit Formula. However, the central Wood, which should have a value of zero, shows a negative value of −2, indicating a violation of Unit Formula Criteria here. Therefore, method ④ does not qualify for the correct Unit Formulae.

Next, let's examine the validity of method ③. Applying the Five Phases Arithmetic Method to ③ is as follows.

Sedating Fire: ΔFire=-1, ΔWood=-1, ΔEarth=-1,
ΔMetal=+1, ΔWater=+1 … (a)
Tonifying Wood: ΔWood=+1, ΔWater=+1, ΔFire=+1,
ΔEarth=-1, ΔMetal=-1 … (b)

From the results of (a) and (b), if you add up the values for the same Qis, you can get the result as follows:

Result: ΔFire=0, ΔEarth=-2, ΔMetal=0,
ΔWater=+2, ΔWood=0 … (c)

In the results of (c), Earth and Fire, which belong to the Yang Field, have a value of negative and zero, Water and Metal, which belong to the Yin Field, have a value of positive and zero, and Wood, the central Qi, has a value of zero. Thus, all requirements for the Unit Formula are met. Therefore, method ③ can be considered the correct Unit Formula.

Next, let's review method ② of sedating Earth and tonifying Wood. Applying the Five Phases Arithmetic Method is as follows.

Sedating Earth: ΔEarth=-1, ΔFire=-1, ΔMetal=-1,
ΔWater=+1, ΔWood=+1 … (a)
Tonifying Wood: ΔWood=+1, ΔWater=+1, ΔFire=+1,
ΔEarth=-1, ΔMetal=-1 … (b)

Adding the values of (a) and (b) together, we get the following result.

Result: ΔEarth=-2, ΔMetal=-2, ΔWater=+2,
ΔWood=+2, ΔFire=0 … (c)

In (c), the values of Earth, Water, and Fire meet the requirements of the Unit Formula. However, Metal, which should have a positive value, has a negative value of −2, and Wood, which should have a value of 0, has a positive value of +2. This violates the requirements for the Unit Formula. Therefore, method ② does not qualify for the correct Unit Formula.

Finally, let's examine method ① of sedating Earth and tonifying Metal. Applying the Five Phases Arithmetic Method yields the following:

Sedating Earth: ΔEarth=-1, ΔFire=-1, ΔMetal=-1,
ΔWater=+1, ΔWood=+1 … (a)
Tonifying Metal: ΔMetal=+1, ΔEarth=+1, ΔWater=+1,
ΔWood=-1, ΔFire=-1 … (b)

If you add up the results of (a) and (b),

Result: ΔEarth=0, ΔFire=-2, ΔMetal=0,
ΔWater=+2, ΔWood=0 … (c)

Looking at (c), Earth and Fire, which belong to the Yang Field, have 0 and a Yin value respectively; Metal and Water, which belong to the Yin field, have 0 and a Yang value respectively; and Wood, as the central Qi, has a value of 0. This meets all requirements for the Unit Formula. Therefore, it can be considered a correct Unit Formula.

In summary, methods ①sedating Earth and tonifying Metal and ③sedating Fire and tonifying Wood are the correct approaches for obtaining the Unit Formulae for replenishing Kidneys and Bladder of Toyang Constitution. Now, let's specifically determine the Zang-Fu acupoints that comprise the Unit Formulae according to methods ① and ③.

First, let's find the Unit Formula for replenishing Kidneys using method

①. Method ① involves sedating Earth and tonifying Metal, which ultimately enhances the Water production of Kidneys. Sedating Earth leads to reducing the amount of Earth Qi which is supplied to the Kidneys. Therefore, the Pancreas' Earth point, which plays a role in regulating Earth Qi, must be sedated. The acupuncture point responsible for creating and regulating Pancreas' Earth Qi is Taibai (太白, SP3), the transmitting point of the Pancreas meridian. The symbol of this acupuncture point is V5. Therefore, applying the Meeting Method to SP3 (Taibai) will reduce Pancreas' Earth Qi production.

It is helpful to think of the flow of Qi between Zang-Fu organs as similar to the movement of a particular substance within our cognitive system. However, in reality, there is no actual physical entity called "Qi" that exists and moves from one Zang-Fu organ to another. A more accurate understanding of the flow of Qi between Zang-Fu organs would be to view it as an intangible information transmission system or signal transduction pathway. For example, applying the Meeting Method to SP3 (Taibai), the Earth point for Pancreas, is essentially conveying an information or signal to reduce Pancreas' Earth Qi production to other Zang-Fu organs.

Now, the signal for the decrease in Pancreas' Earth Qi production is aimed at increasing the Water Qi production of the Kidneys. Therefore, the signal from needling Taebaek, the Earth point of Pancreas meridian, is received by Taixi (太谿, KI3), the Earth point of Kidneys meridian, as it needs to receive the signal to increase Water production by reducing Earth Qi. So, we apply the Meeting Method to this KI3 (Taixi) point (see Figure 6 below).

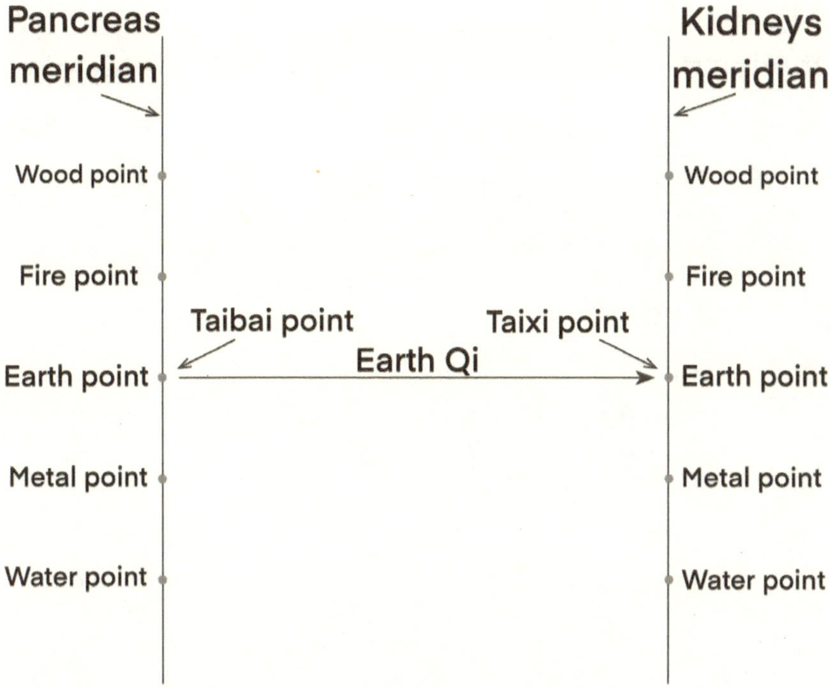

Figure 6. Transmission of Earth Qi from the Pancreas to the Kidneys[76]

Next, let's look at how to tonify Metal Qi. Since Metal Qi is produced in the Lungs, it needs to receive signals from the Metal point of the Lung meridian, which is the transmitting point of the Lungs. Therefore, the Following Method is applied to the Jingqu point (經渠, LU8), which is the Metal point of the Lungs meridian, and by subsequently applying the Following Method to the Fuliu point (復溜, KI7), which is the receiving Metal point of the Kidneys meridian, the signal is transmitted and accepted to the Kidneys.

[76] This picture is a modified version of an illustration from Do-won Kuon's treatise. The same applies to Figure 7 below. Do-won Kuon, *A Study of Constitution-Acupuncture*, 1965, p.17.

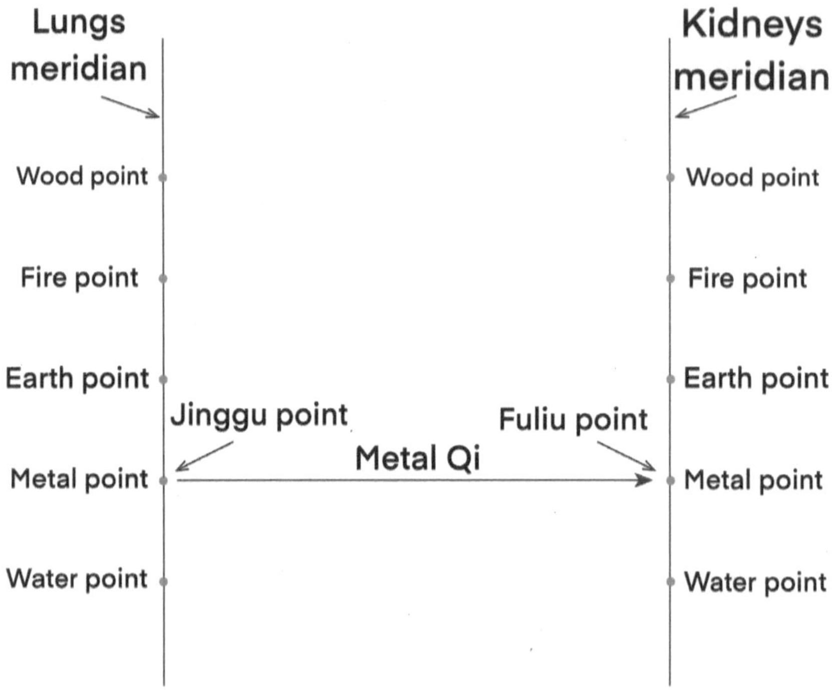

Figure 7. Transmission of Metal Qi from the Lungs to the Kidneys

Summarizing the above results, the Unit Formula for tonifying Kidney is as follows: Taibai(太白, SP3) c, Taixi(太谿, KI3) c, Jingqu(經渠, LU8) p, Fuliu(復溜, KI7) p. Here, "c" stands for "con-puncturing" (against the flow of the meridian) and corresponds to the "Meeting Method" in *Yingsuibuxie* (迎隨補瀉) Method, while "p" stands for "pro-puncturing" (following the flow of the meridian) and corresponds to the "Following Method" in *Yingsuibuxie* Method.

Now let's look at the Unit Formula to replenish the Bladder. The Bladder also manages the production of Water Qi, and it can be supported through sedating Earth and tonifying Metal. Therefore, by needling the Earth point of the Stomach using the Meeting Method, you can receive the signal through the Bladder's Earth point also using the Meeting Method. Similarly, by needling the Metal point of the Large Intestine meridian using the Following Method, the signal is received at the Bladder's Metal point using the Following Method.

The names of these acupoints obtained are as follows: Zusanli(足三里, ST36) c, Weizhong(委中, BL40) c, Shangyang(商陽, LI1) p, Zhiyin(至陰, BL67) p.

In conclusion, the method for replenishing the Kidneys and Bladder in Toyang Constitution using method ① is as follows.

Replenishing the Kidneys: SP3 (Taibai) c, KI3 (Taixi) c, LU8 (Jingqu) p, KI7 (Fuliu) p

Replenishing the Bladder: ST36 (Zusanli) c, Weizhong c, LI1 (Shangyang) p, Zhiyin p.

Now, let's find Unit Formulae to replenish the Kidneys and Bladder using the method ③. Method ③ is an approach to sedate Fire and tonify Wood.

First, to replenish the Kidneys, needle the Fire point of Shaofu (少府, HT8), the Heart's transmitting point, using the Meeting Method, and receive the signal through the Fire point of Rangu (然谷, KI2), the Kidney's receiving point, using the Meeting Method, and needle the Wood point of Dadun (大敦, LR1), the Liver's transmitting point, using Following Method, and receive the signal through the Wood point of Yongquan (湧泉, KI1), the Kidney's receiving point, using the Following Method.

Next, to replenish the Bladder, needle the Fire point (陽谷, Yanggu, SI5), the transmitting point of the Small intestine, using the Meeting Method, and receive the signal through the Fire point (崑崙, Kunlun, BL60), the receiving point of the Bladder, using the Meeting Method, and then needle the Wood point (足臨泣, Zulinqi, GB41), the transmitting point, using the Following Method, and receive the signal through the Wood point (束骨, Shugu, BL64), the receiving point of the Bladder, using the Following Method. Thus, the Unit Formula to replenish the Kidneys and Bladder for the Toyang Constitution is as follows.

Replenishing the Kidneys: HT8 (Shaofu) c, KI2 (Rangu) c, LR1 (Dadun) p, KI1 (Yongquan) p

Replenishing the Bladder: SI5 (Yanggu) c, BL60 (Kunlun) c, GB41 (Zulinqi) p, BL65 (Shugu) p

So far, we have obtained specific Unit Formulae for the Kidneys and Bladder of the Toyang Constitution through the methods ① and ③. This result was derived deductively based on the Structure Formula of the Toyang Constitution, using the Five Phases Arithmetic Method designed by me. Currently, in Master Do-won Kuon's Eight-Constitution Medicine, out of the two methods ① and ③, method ③ is not used, and only the Unit Formula according to the method ① is adopted.

In my opinion, the key difference between methods ① and ③ is that in method ③, the acupuncture points of the Liver and Gallbladder, which are the central Zang-Fu organs of the Toyang Constitution—namely, the LR1 (Dadun) and GB41 (Zulinqi) acupuncture points—are used. In Eight-Constitution Medicine, the central Zang-Fu organs' acupoints in the Constitutional Zang-Fu Arrays are not used directly. Instead, the Pericardium and Triple Burner serve as the central Zang-Fu organs and take on the function of coordinating all systems within the human body. Acupuncture points in the central Zang-Fu organs should not be used to regulate the specific Zang-Fu organs. Therefore, from now on, we will not adopt the method of using the central Zang-Fu organs' acupoints at all.[77] Accordingly, only the Unit Formulae for the method ① that replenish the Kidneys and Bladder, as discussed above, will be adopted. If displayed according to the symbol convention established earlier, the Unit Formulae are as follows.

Replenishing the Kidneys: V_5c, IX_5c, VII_7p, IX_7p
Replenishing the Bladder: VI_6c, X_6c, VIII_8p, X_8p

If we generalize the above results, we can obtain Unit Formulae for the Toyang Constitution. In other words, since the Five Phases Structure Formula of the Toyang Constitution is "Earth Fire Wood Metal Water," in general, in addition to the Kidneys and Bladder, Unit Formulae for the Pancreas and Stomach, Heart and Small intestine, Lungs and Large intestine, and Pericardium and Triple Burner can also be obtained.

[77] I have also applied method ③ in clinical practice. The results were not good. Discussions related to the Pericardium and Triple Burner will be covered in detail later.

Obtaining Unit Formulae for the Pancreas and Stomach

Let's obtain Unit Formulae for the Pancreas and Stomach. Since the Pancreas and Stomach correspond to Earth in terms of the Five Phases, the method for sedating Earth, based on the Synchronizing and Antagonizing relationships shown in Figure 2, is as follows.

① sedating Fire and tonifying Wood
② sedating Metal and tonifying Water
③ sedating Fire and tonifying Water
④ sedating Metal and tonifying Wood

Among these, you can find the one that matches the Five Phases Structure Formula of the Toyang Constitution by applying the Five Phases Arithmetic Method. Before applying the method, ① and ④ can be excluded from the Unit Formulae, as they induce changes in the central Zang-Fu organs—Liver and Gallbladder—which belong to Wood. Therefore, only ② and ③ need to be reviewed.

Let's first examine the case ②. Applying the Five Phases Arithmetic Method, the result is as follows:

Sedating Metal: ΔMetal=-1, ΔEarth=-1, ΔWater=-1,
ΔWood=+1, ΔFire=+1 … (a)
Tonifying Water: ΔWater=+1, ΔMetal=+1, ΔWater=+1,
ΔEarth=-1, ΔFire=-1 … (b)

If you add up the values of (a) and (b), you can get the result:

Result: ΔMetal=0, ΔEarth=-2, ΔWater=0,
ΔWood=+2, ΔFire=0 … (c)

This does not meet the requirements of the Unit Formula because the result shows a positive value where Wood should be zero, and a positive value where Fire should be negative.

Next, let's examine the case ③. Apply the Five Phases Arithmetic Method as follows.

Sedaing Fire: ΔFire=-1, ΔWood=-1, ΔEarth=-1,
ΔMetal=+1, ΔWater=+1 … (a)
Tonifyiong Water: ΔWater=+1, ΔMetal=+1, ΔWater=+1,
ΔEarth=-1, ΔFire=-1 … (b)

If you add up the values of (a) and (b), you can get the result:

Result: ΔFire=-2, ΔWood=0, ΔEarth=-2,
ΔMetal=+2, ΔWater=+2 … (c)

The values for Earth and Fire are negative, the values for Metal and Water are positive, and Wood has a value of zero, so it fully meets the requirements for the Unit Formula of Toyang Constitution. Therefore, it can be considered a correct Unit Formula. As a result, the Unit Formulae to drain Pancreas and Stomach can be obtained by using method ③sedating Fire and tonifying Water. Now, let's identify the specific acupuncture points that make up this Unit Formulae.

The Unit Formula according to the method ③ involves sedating Fire and tonifying Water, thereby draining the Pancreas and Stomach.

First, the Unit Formula for draining the Pancreas involves needling the Fire point, the transmitting acupoint of the Heart, using the Meeting Method and receiving the signal through the Fire point, the receiving acupoint of the Pancreas, also using the Meeting Method. Next, needle the Water point, the transmitting acupoint of the Kidney, using the Following Method, and receive the signal through the Water point, the receiving acupoint of the Pancreas, also using the Following Method. If expressed in terms of acupoint names, they are HT8 (Shaofu) c, SP2 (Dadu) c, KI10 (Yingu) p, and SP9 (Yinlingquan) p.

Next, the Unit Formula for draining the Stomach involves needling the Fire point, the transmitting acupoint of the Small intestine, using the Meeting Method, and receiving it through the Fire point, the receiving acupoint of the Stomach, also using the Meeting Method. Then, needle the Water point, the transmitting acupoint of the Bladder, using the Following Method, and receive it through the Water point, the receiving acupoint of the Stomach. Expressed in terms of the acupoint names, they are SI5 (Yanggu) c, ST41 (Jiexi) c, BL66 (Zutonggu) p, and ST44 (Neiting) p.

Draining Pancreas: HT8 (Shaofu) c, SP2 (Dadu) c, KI10 (Yingu) p, and SP9 (Yinlingquan) p

Draining Stomach: SI5 (Yanggu) c, ST41 (Jiexi) c, BL66 (Zutonggu) p, and ST44 (Neiting) p

Summary of the Unit Formulae for Toyang Constitution

So far, we have examined Unit Formulae for the Kidneys, Bladder, Pancreas and Stomach. All the other Unit Formulae for the Toyang Constitution can also be obtained in the same way. In other words, for the Heart and Small intestine, it is obtained through the Sedating Earth and Tonifying Metal method, and for the Lungs and Large intestine, it is obtained through the Sedating Fire and Tonifying Water method. Since the process is the same, only the results are summarized as follows.

Replenishing Kidneys: SP3 (Taibai) c, KI3 (Taixi) c, LU8 (Jingqu) p, KI7 (Fuliu) p

Replenishing Bladder: ST36 (Zusanli) c, BL40 (Weizhong) c, LI1 (Shangyang) p, BL67 (Zhiyin) p

Draining Heart: SP3 (Taibai) c, HT7 (Shenmen) c, LU8 (Jingqu) p, HT4 (Lingtao) p

Draining Small Intestine: ST36 (Zusanli) c, SI8 (Xiaohai) c, LI1 (Shangyang) p, SI1 (Shaoze) p

Draining Pancreas: HT8 (Shaofu) c, SP2 (Dadu) c, KI10 (Yingu) p, SP9 (Yinlingquan) p

Draining Stomach: SI5 (Yanggu) c, ST41 (Jiexi) c, BL66 (Zutonggu) p, ST44 (Neiting) p

Replenishing Lungs: HT8 (Shaofu) c, LU10 (Yuji) c, KI10 (Yingu) p, LU5 (Chize) p

Replenishing Large Intestine: SI5 (Yanggu) c, LI5 (Yangxi) c, BL66 (Zutonggu) p, LI2 (Erjian) p

Examining the above results, it can be seen that the methods for obtaining Unit Formulae for the Toyang Constitution can be reduced to the following two methods: sedating Earth and tonifying Metal method, and sedating Fire and tonifying Water method. In other words, Unit Formulae for the Kidneys, Bladder, Heart, and Small intestine can be obtained through sedating Earth and tonifying Metal method, and Unit Formulae for the Pancreas, Stomach, Lungs, and Large intestine can be obtained through sedating Fire and tonifying Water method.

Unit Formulae for Pericardium and Triple Burner

So far, we have discussed Unit Formulae for the Toyang Constitution for the Zang-Fu organs, except for the central Zang-Fu organs. From now on, we will discuss the Unit Formulae for Pericardium and Triple Burner, the system that exists solely as an intangible function unique to Oriental medicine, which differ somewhat from tangible Zang-Fu organs having specific forms. The Unit Formulae for Pericardium and Triple Burner are the so-called Mental Sub-formula.[78]

Unlike the Zang-Fu organs, such as the Liver, Heart, Pancreas, Lungs, Kidneys, Gallbladder, Small intestine, Stomach, Large intestine, and Bladder,

[78] It is commonly called Mental Formula, but strictly speaking, Mental Formula refers to a two-step Formula used in combination with a Basic Formula. In other words, "Mental Formula = Basic Formula + Mental Sub-formula." Since this is an additional prescription to the Basic Formula, I named it Mental Sub-formula. The detail will be discussed later in Chapter 4.

that perform unique, localized functions, the Pericardium and Triple Burner are the controlling organs that coordinate the entire body. They function as the central Zang-Fu. Therefore, it can be said that the Pericardium and Triple Burner perform the functions equivalent to the central Zang-Fu within the Constitutional Zang-Fu Structure Formula. In other words, the Qi controlled by the Pericardium and Triple Burner is the same as the Qi of the central Zang-Fu. Therefore, the Unit Formulae for the Pericardium and Triple Burner should naturally avoid causing changes to the central Zang-Fu's Qi.

In conclusion, the Unit Formulae that do not alter the central Zang-Fu can be achieved through the Sedating Earth and Tonifying Metal Method, and Sedating Fire and Tonifying Water Method, which are the two primary methods for obtaining Unit Formulae for the Toyang Constitution. As revealed earlier through the application of the Five Phases Arithmetic Method, these two methods are the only ones that align with the Five Phases Structure Formula without causing changes in the central Qi, Wood.

Also, since the Pericardium and Triple Burner do not receive Qis from other Zang-Fu organs, the Unit Formulae consist only of the acupoints from the Pericardium and Triple Burner meridians. This is because they function solely as the coordinators that transmit the Qi signals to the other Zang-Fu organs and facilitate the communication of Qi information between them. Now, let's obtain the Unit Formulae for the Pericardium and Triple Burner.

First, let's obtain Unit Formulae using the Sedating Earth and Tonifying Metal method. The Unit Formula for the Pericardium can be achieved by applying the Meeting Method to Daling (PC7), which is the Earth point of the Pericardium, and the Following method to Jianshi (PC5), which is the Metal point. For the Triple Burner, the Unit Formula can be obtained by applying the Meeting Method to Tianjing (TB10), which is the Earth point, and the Following method to Guanchong (TB1), which is the Metal point.

Pericardium: PC7 (Daling) c, PC5 (Jianshi) p
Triple Burner: TB10 (Tianjing) c, PC9 (Guanchong) p

Next, let's find the Unit Formulae using the Sedating Fire and Tonifying Water method. For the Pericardium, you can apply the Meeting Method to Laogong (PC8), which is the Fire point, and the Following method to Quze (PC3), which is the Water point. For the Triple Burner, you can apply the Meeting Method to Zhigou (TB6), Fire point, and then apply the Following method to Yemen (TB2), the Water point.

Pericardium: PC8 (Laogong) c, PC3 (Quze) p
Triple Burner: TB10 (Tianjing) c, TB2 (Yemen) p

Here, if we apply the Five Phases Arithmetic Method to the two methods above and examine only the final results, we obtain the following outcome in the case of Sedating Earth and Tonifying Metal:

ΔEarth=0, ΔFire=-2, ΔWood=0, ΔMetal=0, ΔWater=+2.

And in the case of Sedating Fire and Tonifying Water, we obtain the result:

ΔEarth=-2, ΔWater=-2, ΔWood=0, ΔMetal=+2, ΔWater=+2.

Considering that the Five Phases Structure Formula for the Toyang Constitution is "Earth Fire Wood Metal Water," both the methods above are suitable for Toyang Constitution, but it can be seen that the Sedating Fire and Tonifying Water Method, in particular, yields more appropriate results. This is because the Qis belonging to the Yang Field—Earth and Fire—were reduced, the Qis belonging to the Yin Field—Metal and Water—were increased, and the central Qi, Wood, showed the result with no change. Therefore, in my case, I more frequently use the Sedating Fire and Tonifying Water Method as Unit Formulae for the Pericardium and Triple Burner. However, in some cases, the Sedating Earth and Tonifying Metal Method may be used, or the Sedating Fire and Tonifying Water Method, and the Sedating Earth and Tonifying Metal Method may be combined and used simultaneously.

So far, we have examined the Unit Formulae for the Toyang Constitution. The general ways for obtaining the Unit Formulae for the Toyang Constitution were the Sedating Earth and Tonifying Metal Method, and Sedating Fire and Tonifying Water Method. In other words, the appropriate Unit Formulas can be obtained by using the Sedating Earth and Tonifying Metal Method for the Kidneys, Bladder, Heart, and Small Intestine; the Sedating Fire and Tonifying Water Method for the Pancreas, Stomach, Lungs, and Large Intestine; and by applying both methods for the Pericardium and Triple Burner.

General Equations for the Unit Formulae

If you expand this principle further, it can be equally applied to all the other Constitutions, not just Toyang Constitution. Now, let's define all the Constitution's Zang-Fu Structure Formula and Five Phases Structure Formula as follows.

A B C D E (Zang-Fu Structure Formula)
a b c d e (Five Phases Structure Formula)

Let's simply transpose the two Structure Formulae above into the case of the Toyang Constitution. For convenience, let me define Zang-Fu organs as: PA=Pancreas, ST=Stomach, HT=Heart, SI=Small intestine, LR=Liver, GB=Gallbladder, LU=Lungs, LI=Large intestine, KI=Kidneys, BL=Bladder. The Structure Formulae of the Zang-Fu and Five Phases for Toyang Constitution are as follows.

PA-ST(Earth) HT-SI(Fire) LR-GB(Wood) LU-LI(Metal) KI-BL(Water)

Therefore, it can be inferred that the method of obtaining the Unit Formulae for "A" and "D" here is the same as that for obtaining the Unit Formulae for the Pancreas-Stomach, Lungs-Large Intestine in the case of the Toyang Constitution. Thus, the second (B) and fifth (E) Zang-Fu organs should be used as the transmitting meridians, and in terms of the Five Phases, the method of sedating "b" and tonifying "e" can be applied. Similarly, the method of obtaining the Unit Formulae for "B" and "E" can be inferred to be the same as that for obtaining the Unit Formulae for the Heart-Small Intestine and Kidneys-Bladder in the case of the Toyang Constitution. Therefore, the first (A) and fourth (D) Zang-Fu organs should be used as the transmitting meridians, and in terms of the Five Phases, the method of sedating "a" and tonifying "d" can be applied.

In the case of Pericardium and Triple Burner, a pair of Unit Formulae can be obtained by applying both the methods above.

If this is expressed using the symbols introduced earlier, it is as follows. (Let's define Pericardium and Triple Burner as "S" here.) I refer to this as the "General Equation for Unit Formulae."

The Unit Formula for A (As): Bb(−) Ab(−) Ee(+) Ae(+)
The Unit Formula for D (Dt): Bb(−) Db(−) Ee(+) De(+)
The Unit Formula for B (Bs): Aa(−) Ba(−) Dd(+) Bd(+)
The Unit Formula for E (Et): Aa(−) Ea(−) Dd(+) Ed(+)
The Unit Formula for S (Sr): Sb(−) Se(+) or Sa(−) Sd(+)

Let me explain the meaning of the symbols above. For instance, in "As", the subscript "s" means "sedate," "t" means "tonify," and "r" means "regulate." Accordingly, "As" refers to the sedating of Zang-Fu "A", and "Dt" refers to the tonifying of Zang-Fu "D." "Sr" refers to the regulation by the Pericardium and Triple Burner.

"Bb" represents the acupoint "b" of the Zang-Fu "B", "De" represents the acupoint "e" of the Zang-Fu "D", and "Sa" represents the acupoint "a" of the Pericardium and Triple Burner. The symbol (+) indicates the direction aligned with the meridian's flow, known as the Following Method, while (−) denotes the direction against the meridian's flow, known as the Meeting Method. Therefore, Bb(−) means applying the Meeting Method to the point "b" of the Zang-Fu "B", and De(+) means applying the Following Method to the point "e" of the Zang-Fu "D."

As mentioned above, in the Unit Formulae for the Pericardium and Triple Burner, the former Sb(−) Se(+) is more suitable for achieving the balance within the Zang-Fu Structure than the latter Sa(−) Sd(+). I primarily use the former, Sb(−) Se(+).[79]

For example, let's find the Unit Formulae for the Geumeum Constitution using the General Equation for the Unit Formulae above. In the case of the Geumeum Constitution, the Zang-Fu Structure Formula and the Five Phases Structure Formula are as follows.

Zang-Fu Structure Formula: LU(A) KI(B) PA(C) HT(D) LR(E)
Five Phases Structure Formula: Metal(a) Water(b) Earth(c) Fire(d) Wood(e)

Here, as an example, let's derive the Unit Formula for the Heart. The Heart's Unit Formula corresponds to the Unit Formula "Dt." This formula can be easily obtained by directly substituting the parameters into the General Equation of Unit Formulae: Dt = Bb(−) Db(−) Ee(+) De(+). In this case, "Bb" represents the Water acupoint of the Kidneys, Yingu (KI10); "Db" represents the Water acupoint of the Heart, Shaohai (HT3); "Ee" represents the Wood acu-point of the Liver, Dadun (LR1); and "De" represents the Wood acupoint of the Heart, Shaochong (HT9). (Refer to the Zang-Fu acupoints in Chapter 1 for the specific acupoint names.) Thus, the Unit Formula is derived by applying the Meeting Method to KI10 (Yingu) and HT3 (Shaohai), and the Following Method to LR1 (Dadun) and HT9 (Shaochong).

Also, let's obtain the Unit Formula for Triple Burner, one of the Mental Sub-formula for the Geumeum Constitution. The Unit Formula for the Triple Burner can be obtained from Sb(−) Se(+) or Sa(−) Sd(+). Using the former, Sb represents the Water acupoint Yemen (TB2) of the Triple Burner, and Se represents the Wood acupoint Zhongzhu (TB3) of the Triple Burner. If we use the latter, Sa is the Metal acupoint, Guanchong (TB1) of the Triple Burner, and Sd is the Fire acupoint, Zhigou (TB6) of the Triple Burner. When applying the Five Phases Formula, I mainly uses the former as Mental

[79] I created this Mental Sub-formula and initially experimented with both the methods in various ways. I tried using the Sb(−) Se(+) method, I tried using the Sa(−) Sd(+) method, or I even tried using both the methods simultaneously. Each had certain effects, but the Sb(−) Se(+) method is preferred because it is most theoretically aligned with the structure of Constitution.

Sub-formula, as it yields the result more suited to the Five Phases Structure Formula. Therefore, the Unit Formulae for the Triple Burner can be derived by applying the Meeting Method to TB2 (Yemen) acupoint and the Following Method to the TB3 (Zhongzhu) acupoint. In this way, the Unit Formulae not only for Geumeum Constitution but also for all the other Constitutions can be derived from the General Equation above.

Shortcuts to the Unit Formulae

Another shortcut to obtaining the Unit Formulae can be easily identified by visually examining the balance conditions in the Constitutional Zang-Fu Structure Formula or the Five Phases Structure Formula introduced in Chapter 2, Definition of Constitution. This method intuitively utilizes the relationship of synchronizing and Antagonizing.[80] Refer to the picture below again.

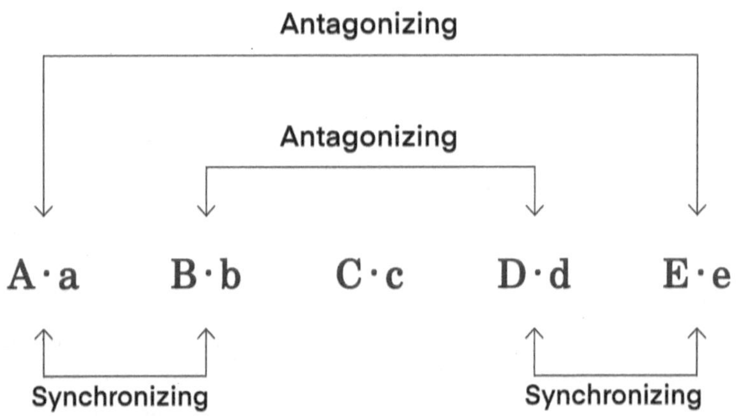

Figure 8. The Conditions for Zang-Fu or Five Phases Array of Constitution

A·B·C·D·E represent the symbols of the Zang-Fu, while a·b·c·d·e represent the symbols of the corresponding Five Phases.

Let's obtain the Unit Formula for "A" here. Obtaining Unit Formula for

[80] This method was presented by Professor Jong-wook Jeon of Chonbuk National University at the seminar of "Research Group for the Future of Eight-Constitution Medicine" (2006).

A means lowering the Zang-Fu potential of A, which belongs to Yang Field. Since A should be drained, in the diagram, B, which is in a Synchronizing relationship with A, should also be drained, and E, which is in an Antagonizing relationship with A, should be replenished. Therefore, the method of "sedating b and tonifying e" can be used.

If you look closely at the picture above, you will see that the answer lies right there. What are the Zang-Fu organs connected to A by an arrow? They are B and E. In other words, B is connected to A in the Synchronizing relationship, and E is connected to A in the Antagonizing relationship. When reduced to the Five Phases, "a" is connected to "b" as the Synchronizing relationship, and to "e" as the Antagonizing relationship. Therefore, to drain A, you simply need to suppress B and encourage E. Thus, it is immediately clear that the Unit Formula for draining A is represented by the equation: As = Bb(−) Ab(−) Ee(+) Ae(+).

Next, let's derive the Unit Formula for B. Since the Unit Formula for B is also to drain B, which belongs to the Yang field, in the figure, you can suppress A, which is in a Synchronizing relationship with B, and promote D, which is in an Antagonizing relationship. Therefore, the method of "sedating 'a' and tonifying 'd'" should be used. The Unit Formula is represented as the equation: Bs = Aa(−) Ba(−) Dd(+) Bd(+).

The Unit Formula for D is to replenish D, which is the Zang-Fu of the Yin field, so E, which is in the Synchronizing relationship with D, should be replenished, and B, which is in the Antagonizing relationship, must be drained. Therefore, the method of "sedating b and tonifying e" (=tonifying e and sedating b) is appropriate. In the same way, the Unit Formula is represented as the equation: Dt = Bb(−) Db(−) Ee(+) De(+).

Lastly, the Unit Formula for E is to replenish E, the Zang-Fu of the Yin Field, so you can replenish D, which is in the Synchronizing relationship with E, and to drain A, which is in the Antagonizing relationship with E. Therefore, it is obtained using the method of "sedating a and tonifying d" (=tonifying d and sedating a). The Unit Formula is represented as the equation: Et = Aa(−) Ea(−) Dd(+) Ed(+).

However, Unit Formulae for the Pericardium and Triple Burner cannot be obtained directly through this method. They can only be inferred from the other Unit Formulae. In other words, examining the above case, it can be seen that all the methods for obtaining Unit Formulae from the Five Phases relationship are either b(−) e(+) or a(−) d(+). Therefore, the Unit Formulae for the Pericardium and Triple Burner is Sb(−) Se(+) or Sa(−) Sd(+). I earlier noted that clinically, I used Sb(−) Se(+) more frequently. Although it is possible to obtain the Unit Formulae this simple way, the most accurate method is to derive the ones that align with the Zang-Fu Structure Formula through the Five Phases Arithmetic Method.

In the end, you can see that this simple method for obtaining the Unit Formulae and the method for obtaining them using the General Equation above are the same. This method is like a shortcut to easily obtain the Unit Formulae. However, it is confirmed to be correct only after undergoing a verification process through the Five Phases Arithmetic Method. Every insight must be confirmed by precise logic in the universal language that most people can understand. Therefore, the Five Phases Arithmetic Method must be assumed as the computational tool that makes this simple method possible. When calculated using the Five Phases Arithmetic Method, only those formulas that do not violate the Constitution's Zang-Fu Structure Formula or Five Phases Structure Formula can be considered valid Unit Formulas.

How to obtain the Unit Formulae for each Constitution

According to the previous General Equation, the method for obtaining the Unit Formulae for each Constitution is shown in the table below in Figure 9.

The Basic Formula, Fu (Fu-system) Inflammation Sub-formula, Zang (Zang-system) Inflammation Sub-formula, Mental Sub-formula, Vitality Sub-formula, Sterilization Sub-formula and Degeneration Sub-formula are the names given by Master Do-won Kuon.

Fu (Fu-system) Basic Formula, Fu (Fu-system) Mental Sub-Formula, and Fu (Fu-system) Degeneration Sub-formula are the names assigned by me based on Master Do-won Kuon's terminology. The term Sub-formula refers to an auxiliary Formula used in addition to the Basic Formula. The names of the Sub-formula here are relevant only for the two-stage Formulae in the Compound Formulae. A detailed explanation of the operation of Formulae is discussed in Chapter 4, Principles of Compound Formulae.

Let me explain Figure 9 on the next page with a few examples: In the Geumyang Constitution, the Basic Formula is a Unit Formula that replenishes the Liver, the outermost Zang of the Yin Field, and is obtained using the method of "sedating Metal and tonifying Water." Conversely, in the Mogyang Constitution, the Basic Formula is a Unit Formula that drains the Liver, the outermost Zang of the Yang Field, obtained using the method of "tonifying Metal and sedating Water." Additionally, in the Geumeum Constitution, the Zang Inflammation Sub-formula is a Unit Formula that replenishes the Liver, the outermost Zang of the Yin Field, and is obtained using the method of "sedating Metal and tonifying Fire." In the Sueum Constitution, the Sterilization Sub-formula is a Unit Formula that drains the Gallbladder, the second Fu in the Yang Field, and is obtained using the method of "tonifying Metal and sedating Water."

In other words, for the Geumyang, Geumeum, Toyang, and Toeum Constitutions, the method above is used from the two methods (above and below) in each cell of the table, while for the Mogyang, Mogeum, Suyang, and Sueum Constitutions, the method below is used.

Unit Formulae for Zang-system

Zang system Formulae	Geumyang/ Mogyang	Geumeum/ Mogeum	Toyang/ Suyang	Toeum/ Sueum
Basic	Metal- Water+ (Liver+)/ Metal+ Water- (Liver-)	Water- Wood+ (Lungs-)/ Water+ Wood- (Lungs+)	Earth- Metal+ (Kidneys+)/ Earth+ Metal- (Kidneys-)	Metal- Water+ (Pancreas-)/ Metal+ Water- (Pancreas+)
Fu Inflam.	Metal- Water+ (Pancreas-)/ Metal+ Water- (Pancreas+)	Water- Wood+ (Heart-)/ Water+ Wood- (Heart+)	Earth- Metal+ (Heart-)/ Earth+ Metal- (Heart+)	Metal- Water+ (Liver+)/ Metal+ Water- (Liver-)
Mental	Earth- Wood+ (Pericardium)/ Metal+ Water- (Pericardium)	Water- Wood+ (Pericardium)/ Metal+ Fire- (Pericardium)	Fire- Water+ (Pericardium)/ Earth+ Metal- (Pericardium)	Metal- Water+ (Pericardium)/ Earth+ Wood- (Pericardium)
Zang Inflam.	Earth- Wood+ (Lungs-)/ Earth+ Wood- (Lungs+)	Metal- Fire+ (Liver+)/ Metal+ Fire- (Liver-)	Fire- Water+ (Pancreas-)/ Fire+ Water- (Pancreas+)	Earth- Wood+ (Kidneys+)/ Earth+ Wood- (Kidneys-)
Degen.	Earth- Wood+ (Kidneys+)/ Earth+ Wood- (Kidneys-)	Metal- Fire+ (Kidneys-)/ Metal+ Fire- (Kidneys+)	Fire- Water+ (Lungs+)/ Fire+ Water- (Lungs-)	Earth- Wood+ (Lungs-)/ Earth+ Wood- (Lungs+)

Unit Formulae for Fu-system

Fu system Formulae	Geumyang/ Mogyang	Geumeum/ Mogeum	Toyang/ Suyang	Toeum/ Sueum
Fu Basic	Metal- Water+ (Gallbladder+)/ Metal+ Water- (Gallbladder-)	Water- Wood+ (L. intestine-)/ Water+ Wood- (L. intestine+)	Earth- Metal+ (Bladder+)/ Earth+ Metal- (Bladder-)	Metal- Water+ (Stomach-)/ Metal+ Water- (Stomach+)
Steril.	Metal- Water+ (Stomach-)/ Metal+ Water- (Stomach+)	Water- Wood+ (S. intestine-)/ Water+ Wood- (S. intestine+)	Earth- Metal+ (S. intestine-)/ Earth+ Metal- (S. intestine+)	Metal- Water+ (Gallbladder+)/ Metal+ Water- (Gallbladder-)
Fu Mental	Earth- Wood+ (Triple Burner)/ Metal+ Water- (Triple Burner)	Water- Wood+ (Triple Burner)/ Metal+ Fire- (Triple Burner)	Fire- Water+ (Triple Burner)/ Earth+ Metal- (Triple Burner)	Metal- Water+ (Triple Burner)/ Earth+ Wood- (Triple Burner)
Vital.	Earth- Wood+ (L. intestine-)/ Earth+ Wood- (L. intestine+)	Metal- Fire+ (Gallbladder+)/ Metal+ Fire- Gallbladder-)	Fire- Water+ (Stomach-)/ Fire+ Water- (Stomach+)	Earth- Wood+ (Bladder+)/ Earth+ Wood- (Bladder-)
Fu Degen.	Earth- Wood+ (Bladder+)/ Earth+ Wood- (Bladder-)	Metal- Fire+ (Bladder-)/ Metal+ Fire- (Bladder+)	Fire- Water+ (L. intestine+)/ Fire+ Water- (L. intestine-)	Earth- Wood+ (L. intestine-)/ Earth+ Wood- (L. intestine+)

Figure 9. How to derive Unit Formulae for each Constitution

The abbreviation rules in the table are as follows:

1) Unit Formulae for Zang-system

Basic = Basic Formula, Fu Inflam. = Fu-system Inflammation, Sub-formula, Mental = Mental Sub-formula, Zang Inflam. = Zang-system Inflammation Sub-formula, Degen. = Degeneration Sub-formula

2) Unit Formulae for Fu-system

Fu Basic = Fu-system Basic Formula, Steril. = Sterilization Sub-formula, Fu Mental = Fu-system Mental Sub-formula, Vital. = Vitality Sub-formula, Fu Degen. = Fu-system Degeneration Sub-formula

3) Method for acupuncture

Let me show you an example in the first cell "Basic (Basic Formula)" of Zang-system Formulae which reads Metal- Water+ (Liver+) / Metal+ Water- (Liver-). The method above, that is, "Metal- Water+ (Liver+)" means the method of "sedating Metal and tonifying Water" to replenish the Liver of Geumyang Constitution, and that below, that is, "Metal+ Water- (Liver-)" means the method of "tonifying Metal and sedating Water" to drain the Liver of Mogyang Constitution.

For another example, "Fu Mental (Fu-system Mental Sub-formula)" for Geumyang/Mogyang reads "Earth- Wood+ (Triple Burner) / Metal+ Water- (Triple Burner)." The method for Geumyang is sedating Earth and tonifying Wood to regulate Triple Burner, and that for Mogyang is tonifying Metal and sedating Water to regulate Triple Burner.

4) Zang-Fu organs

L. intestine = Large intestine, S. intestine = Small intestine

Let's verify it using the Five Phases Arithmetic Method!

It is necessary to check whether the methods in the table align with the Zang-Fu Structure of each Constitution through the Five Phases Arithmetic Method. First, let's look at the case of the Geumyang Constitution.

The Zang-Fu and Five Phases Structure Formula of the Geumyang Constitution is as follows:

LU-LI(Metal) PA-ST(Earth) HT-SI(Fire) KI-BL(Water) LR-GB(Wood)

where LU is Lungs, LI is Large intestine, PA is Pancreas, ST is Stomach, HT is Heart, SI is Small intestine, KI is Kidneys, BL is Bladder, LR is Liver, and GB is Gallbladder as mentioned before.

The Unit Formulae for the Geumyang Constitution are divided into the two categories: "sedating Metal and tonifying Water", and "sedating Earth and tonifying Wood." Therefore, you can apply the Five Phases Arithmetic Method to check whether they fit the Constitutional structure of the Geumyang Constitution. Let's first examine the method of sedating Metal and tonifying Water. Applying the Five Phases Arithmetic Method, you can get the following.

Sedating Metal: ΔMetal=-1, ΔEarth=-1, ΔWater=-1, ΔWood=+1, ΔFire=+1
Tonifying Water: ΔWater=+1, ΔMetal=+1, ΔFire=+1, ΔFire=-1, ΔEarth=-1

If you add these according to the same Qi, you can get the following.

Result: ΔMetal=0, ΔEarth=-2, ΔWater=0, ΔFire=0, ΔWood=+2

It can be seen that it fits the Structure Formula of the Geumyang Constitution (Metal Earth Fire Water Wood). Next, let's examine the method of sedating Earth and tonifying Wood.

Sedating Earth: ΔEarth=-1, ΔFire=-1, ΔMetal=-1, ΔWater=+1, ΔWood=+1
Tonifying Wood: ΔWood=+1, ΔWater=+1, ΔFire=+1, ΔEarth=-1, ΔMetal=-1

If you add these two rows together according to the same Qi, you can get the following.

Result: ΔMetal=-2, ΔEarth=-2, ΔWater=0, ΔFire=+2, ΔWood=+2

It also fits the Constitutional Structure of the Geumyang Constitution.

Next, let's examine the case of the Mogyang Constitution, which is the opposite of the Geumyang Constitution. The Structure Formula of the Mogyang Constitution is as follows:

LR-GB(Wood) KI-BL(Water) HT-SI(Fire) PA-ST(Earth) LU-LI(Metal)

The Unit Formula for the Mogyang Constitution is derived by "tonifying Metal and sedating Water", and "tonifying Earth and sedating Wood." First, let's look at tonifying Metal and sedating Water.

Tonifying Metal: ΔMetal=+1, ΔEarth=+1, ΔWater=+1, ΔWood=-1, ΔFire=-1
Sedating Water: ΔWater=-1, ΔMetal=-1, ΔWood=-1, ΔFire=+1, ΔEarth=+1
Result: ΔWood=-2, ΔWater=0, ΔFire=0, ΔEarth=+2, ΔMetal=0

Therefore, it fits the Structure of the Mogyang Constitution (Wood Water Fire Earth Metal). Next, let's examine the method of tonifying Earth and sedating Wood.

Tonifying Earth: ΔEarth=+1, ΔFire=+1, ΔMetal=+1, ΔWater=-1, ΔWood=-1
Sedating Wood: ΔWood=-1, ΔWater=-1, ΔFire=-1, ΔEarth=+1, ΔMetal=+1
Result: ΔWood=-2, ΔWater=-2, ΔFire=0, ΔEarth=+2, ΔMetal=+2

Therefore, it fits the Structure of the Mogyang Constitution. Through this, we can see that if the structure of the Constitution is reversed, the method of obtaining the Unit Formula is also reversed.

Next, let's examine the case of the Geumeum Constitution. The Structure of the Geumeum Constitution is as follows:

LU-LI(Metal) KI-BL(Water) PA-ST(Earth) HT-SI(Fire) LR-GB(Wood)

The Unit Formulae for the Geumeum Constitution is derived by "sedating Water and tonifying Wood", and "sedating Metal and tonifying Fire." First, let's look at the method of sedating Water and tonifying Wood.

Sedating Water: ΔWater=-1, ΔMetal=-1, ΔWood=-1, ΔFire=+1, ΔEarth=+1
Tonifying Wood: ΔWood=+1, ΔWater=+1, ΔFire=+1, ΔEarth=-1, ΔMetal=-1
Result: ΔMetal=-2, ΔWater=0, ΔEarth=0, ΔFire=+2, ΔWood=0

Therefore, it fits the Structure of the Geumeum Constitution. Next, let's look at the method of sedating Metal and tonifying Fire.

Sedating Metal: ΔMetal=-1, ΔEarth=-1, ΔWater=-1, ΔWood=+1, ΔFire=+1
Tonifying Fire: ΔFire=+1, ΔWood=+1, ΔEarth=+1, ΔMetal=-1, ΔWater=-1
Result: ΔMetal=-2, ΔWater=-2, ΔEarth=0, ΔFire=+2, ΔWood=+2

It also fits the Structure of the Geumeum Constitution. It can be inferred that for the Constitution opposite to the Geumeum Constitution—the Mogeum Constitution—the reverse method would align with the Constitutional structure, similar to the relationship between the Geumyang and Mogyang Constitutions. So, let me omit the examination of the Mogeum Constitution. The Toyang Constitution was also studied in detail in the Unit Formulae derivation process, so it will be omitted, too. The examination of the reverse Constitution, the Suyang Constitution, can also be omitted because it will align with the Constitutional structure. Lastly, let's examine the Toeum Constitution.

The Constitutional Structure of the Toeum Constitution is as follows:

PA-ST(Earth) LU-LI(Metal) HT-SI(Fire) LR-GB(Wood) KI-BL(Water)

The way to obtain the Unit Formulae is through "sedating Metal and tonifying Water", and "sedating Earth and tonifying Wood."

Sedating Metal: ΔMetal=-1, ΔEarth=-1, ΔWater=-1, ΔWood=+1, ΔFire=+1
Tonifying Water: ΔWater=+1, ΔMetal=+1, ΔWood=+1, ΔFire=-1, ΔEarth=-1
Result: ΔEarth=-2, ΔMetal=0, ΔFire=0, ΔWood=+2, ΔWater=0

Sedating Earth: ΔEarth=-1, ΔFire=-1, ΔMetal=-1, ΔWater=+1, ΔWood=+1
Tonifying Wood: ΔWood=+1, ΔWater=+1, ΔFire=+1, ΔEarth=-1, ΔMetal=-1
Result: ΔEarth=-2, ΔMetal=-2, ΔFire=0, ΔWood=+2, ΔWater=+2

Therefore, it can be seen that both "sedating Metal and tonifying Water", and "sedating Earth and tonifying Wood" fit the structure of the Toeum Constitution. Naturally, for the opposite Constitution, the Sueum

Constitution, it can also be predicted that it matches the Constitutional structure. Verification is omitted.

My opinion on Mental Sub-formulae

My Unit Formula theory was developed through studying Do-won Kwon's 1965 thesis and exploring its underlying principles. Most of it is consistent with Do-won Kuon's theory, but there is a significant difference between Do-won Kuon's and my theories regarding the Mental Sub-formulae. While I have unified all Mental Sub-formula into the Unit Formulae for the Pericardium and the Triple Burner Meridians, Master Do-won Kuon uses the Pericardium and Triple Burner Meridians for Geumyang, Mogyang, Toeum, and Sueum, and the Heart and Small Intestine Meridians for Geumyang, Mogeum, Toeum, and Suyang.

In his classification of Sasangin, Je-ma Lee excluded the Heart from Zang-Fu Structure Arrays of Constitutions because he referred to it as the Ultimate of the Center. Therefore, it was believed that the Heart (including the Small intestine) functions like the central axis that regulates the other Zang-Fu organs of the human body. In this way, Master Do-won Kuon assigned the Mental Sub-formula a function similar to the central axis of the Heart mentioned by Je-ma Lee.

We also refer to Heart as the mind or the organ heart. When referred to as the heart, it functions as a simple local organ, one of the organs that make up the human body. However, when referred to as the mind, it is an abstract entity, an intangible center that regulates the human body as a whole and coordinates the other organs, similar to the central nervous system. Problems arise from this duality—viewing the heart as both one of the five organs and as the center that controls the human body as a whole.

Traditionally, the Pericardium and Triple Burner are referred to as the Ministerial Fire. This originates from the statement in "*Chapter on Heavenly Foundations*" in the medical classic, *Neijing*: "The Sovereign Fire acts with brightness, while the Ministerial Fire acts with status." Although countless theories from various scholars have emerged throughout medical history to interpret this saying, I view it as a discussion of the relationship between the Heart and the Pericardium-Triple Burner, comparable to the relationship between a monarch and a prime minister, as clearly reflected in the terms Sovereign Fire and Ministerial Fire. In other words, the monarch governs through non-action, relying only on his own brilliant virtue, while the prime minister, as a subject to the monarch, supports and governs the country in practice. Here, Sovereign Fire refers to the Heart, while Ministerial Fire refers to the Pericardium and Triple Burner. The Pericardium and Triple Burner act on behalf of the Heart and directly govern the human body.

To say that the Pericardium and Triple Burner act on behalf of the Heart means that they take over the Heart's overall regulating function of the human body. In other words, the Pericardium and Triple Burner have the practical function of regulating the entire body. In this way, the Heart transfers its regulatory function for the whole body to the Pericardium and Triple Burner, leaving the Heart with only a local Zang organ role. The Heart now functions just as one of the Zang-Fu organs. On the other hand, the Pericardium and Triple Burner perform the comprehensive regulating function for the Five Zangs and Five Fus of the human body, taking on the role of the central Zang-Fu in each Constitution's Structure. Therefore, the Pericardium and Triple Burner occupy the central Zang-Fu position in the Constitution's Zang-Fu Arrays on behalf of all the Zang-Fu organs—the Liver and Gallbladder, Heart and Small Intestine, Pancreas and Stomach, Lungs and Large Intestine, and Kidneys and Bladder.

However, Master Do-won Kuon follows the traditional view and considers the Pericardium and Triple Burner only as the representatives of the Heart and Small Intestine. Therefore, in Constitutions where the Heart and Small Intestine occupy the central Zang-Fu organ position, the Mental Sub-formulae are derived from the Pericardium and Triple Burner. If the Heart and Small Intestine are not in the central Zang-Fu organ position, the Mental Sub-formulae are derived directly from the Heart and Small Intestine themselves. In other words, the Heart and Small Intestine function as local Zang-Fu organs, but at the same time, they serve as central Zang-Fu organs. It's as if they are both a director and an actor, directing and performing simultaneously. This is where a divergence emerges between Do-won Kwon's theory of Mental Sub-formulae and my own.

I believe that the Pericardium and Triple Burner, as representatives of the central Zang-Fu, are responsible for coordinating the functions of the entire body. Additionally, the Heart is strictly a local organ, constituting only one part of the Constitution's Zang-Fu Array, and it faithfully performs its limited role, namely, the creation and regulation of Fire Qi within the Five Phases. The duality of "The Part and The Whole" of the Heart must be completely dismantled.

For Master Do-won Kuon, the Mental Sub-formula is essentially to fulfill the role of the Heart and Small Intestine as the Ultimate of the Center. However, in the Geumyang, Mogyang, Toeum, and Sueum constitutions, the Heart and Small Intestine are positioned in the middle of the Zang-Fu array, which leads to the restriction of not being able to use the central Zang-Fu organs. Therefore, the Pericardium and Triple Burner were adopted as the Zang-Fu organs acting on behalf of the Heart and Small Intestine. On the other hand, in the Geumeum, Mogeum, Toyang, and Suyang Constitutions, where the Heart and Small Intestine are not positioned in the central Zang-Fu, they are used directly as Mental Sub-formulae.

However, when Do-won Kuon defined the Eight Constitutions, he included the Heart and Small Intestine as components in the Arrays of Zang-Fu organs that make up each Constitution, thereby already regarding the Heart and Small Intestine as local Zang-Fu organs, not as the overseeing authority that manages and coordinates all bodily functions. If there is a master that coordinates the human body as a whole, it cannot be the Heart and Small Intestine, as they are limited to specific local forms and functions among the Five Zang-Fu organs. Instead, it must be an intangible force that exists throughout the entire body and permeates every part. This role can only be fulfilled by the Pericardium and Triple Burner. Therefore, I formulated the Mental Sub-formulae solely with the Pericardium and Triple Burner.

Next, there is also a difference between him and me in the selection of acupuncture points for the Mental Sub-formulae. I believe it must be carried out in a way that does not disrupt the physiological balance of the Constitution's Zang-Fu array—that is, the Zang-Fu Structure Formula—or, in other words, does not cause pathological imbalance.

For the example of Toyang Constitution, I consider the method of "sedating Fire and tonifying Water" as the best way to obtain Mental Sub-formula based on the Five Phases Arithmetic Method, while Do-won Kuon adopts the method of "sedating Earth and tonifying Water" as the best approach.[81] However, when calculated using the Five Phases Arithmetic Method, Do-won Kuon's method results in breaking the Physiological Balance of the Toyang Constitution. Let's apply the Five Phases Arithmetic Method.

If we apply the case of draining Earth, through Master Do-won Kuon's method of "sedating Earth and tonifying Water," to the Five Phases Arithmetic Method, we get the following.

Draining Earth: ΔEarth=-1, ΔWood=+1, ΔFire=-1, ΔMetal=-1, ΔWater=+1
Replenishing Water: ΔWater=+1, ΔWood=+1, ΔFire=-1, ΔEarth=-1, ΔMetal=+1
Result: ΔWood=+2, ΔFire=-2, ΔEarth=-2, ΔMetal=0, ΔWater=+2

Here, the Wood, which represents the Central Qi, shows +2 increase, which means this method is inappropriate as it intensifies the Constitutional imbalance. If it is truly necessary to find a Mental Sub-formula that aligns with the Five Phases Structure of the Constitution in the Heart meridian, it would be suitable to choose "HT8 (Shaofu) c, HT3 (Shaohai) p" as the method of sedating Fire and tonifying Water. For the other Constitutions as well, his approach to the Mental Sub-formulae and mine do not align at all. It is evident that there are significant differences in the opinion between him and me. Below is a comparison table of the Mental Sub-formulae for the Eight Constitutions between Master Do-won Kuon and me.

[81] For Zang-system's Mental Sub-formula, I choose Laogong (PC8) as the sedating point and Quze (PC3) as the tonifying point of the Pericardium meridian, while Do-won Kuon uses Shenmen (HT7) as the sedating point and Shaohai (HT3) as the tonifying point of the Heart meridian.

	Kuon		Joowonjang			
Geum yang	Earth- Water+	PC7c, PC3p	Earth- Wood+	PC7c, PC9p	Metal- Water+	PC5c, PC3p
		TB10c, TB2p		TB10c, TB3p		TB1c, TB2p
Geum eum	Metal- Wood+	HT4c, HT9p	Water- Wood+	PC3c, PC9p	Metal- Fire+	PC5c, PC8p
		SI1c, SI3p		TB2c, TB3p		TB1c, TB6p
To yang	Earth- Water+	HT7c, HT3p	Fire- Water+	PC8c, PC3p	Earth- Metal+	PC7c, PC5p
		SI8c, SI2p		TB6c, TB2p		TB10c, TB1p
To eum	Metal- Wood+	PC5c, PC9p	Metal- Water+	PC5c, PC3p	Earth- Wood+	PC7c, PC9p
		TB1c, TB3p		TB1c, TB2p		TB10c, TB3p
Mog yang	Earth+ Water-	PC7p, PC3c	Metal+ Water-	PC5p, PC3c	Earth+ Wood-	PC7p, PC9c
		TB10p, TB2c		TB1p, TB2c		TB10p, TB3c
Mog eum	Metal+ Wood-	HT4p, HT9c	Metal+ Fire-	PC5p, PC8c	Water+ Wood-	PC3p, PC9c
		SI1p, SI3c		TB1p, TB6c		TB2p, TB3c
Su yang	Earth+ Water-	HT7p, HT3c	Earth+ Metal-	PC7p, PC5c	Fire+ Water-	PC8p, PC3c
		SI8p, SI2c		TB10p, TB1c		TB6p, TB2c
Su eum	Metal+ Wood-	PC5p, PC9c	Earth+ Wood-	PC7p, PC9c	Metal+ Water-	PC5p, PC3c
		TB1p, TB3c		TB10p, TB3c		TB1p, TB2c

Figure 10. Comparison of Kwon's Mental Sub-formulae and Mine

List of Unit Formulae for the Eight Constitutions

Apart from the Mental Sub-formulae, all other Unit Formulae for the Eight Constitutions—including Basic Formulae, Fu-system Inflammation Sub-formulae, Zang-system Inflammation Sub-formulae, Sterilization Sub-formulae, and Vitality Sub-formulae—are all consistent between Kwon and me.[82] Below are the Unit Formulae for the Eight Constitutions.

Zang-system Formulae	Geumyang/ Mogyang	Geumeum/ Mogeum	Toyang/ Suyang	Toeum/ Sueum
Basic	LU8, LR4 KI10, LR8	KI10, LU5 LR1, LU11	SP3, KI3 LU8, KI7	LU8, SP5 KI10, SP9
Fu-system Inflammation	LU8, SP5 KI10, SP9	KI10, HT3 LR1, HT9	SP3, HT7 LU8, HT4	LU8, LR4 KI10, LR8
Mental	PC7, PC9 (Geumyang)/ PC5, PC3 (Mogyang)	PC3, PC9 (Geumeum)/ PC5, PC8 (Mogeum)	PC8, PC3 (Toyang)/ PC7, PC5 (Suyang)	PC5, PC3 (Toeum)/ PC7, PC9 (Sueum)
Zang-system Inflammation	SP3, LU9 LR1, LU11	LU8, LR4 HT8, LR2	HT8, SP2 KI10, SP9	SP3, KI3 LR1, KI1
Degeneration	SP3, KI3 LR1, KI1	LU8, KI7 HT8, KI2	HT8, LU10 KI10, LU5	SP3, LU9 LR1, LU11

Figure 11a. Unit Formulae for Eight Constitutions (Zang-system)

[82] Sub-formulae are the prescriptions that combine with the Basic Formula to achieve the desired effect. For instance, the inflammation of the Zang-system is treated with the ratio of Basic formula vs Zang-system Inflammation Sub-formula = 5:1, and for almost all other treatments, the ratio of Basic formula vs other Sub-formulae is = 4:2. This is discussed in Chapter 4, Principles of Compound Formulae.

Fu-system Formulae	Geumyang/ Mogyang	Geumeum/ Mogeum	Toyang/ Suyang	Toeum/ Sueum
Fu-system's Basic	LI1, GB44 BL66, GB43	BL66, LI2 GB41, LI3	ST36, BL40 LI1, BL67	LI1, ST45 BL66, ST44
Sterilization	LI1, ST45 BL66, ST44	BL66, SI2 GB41, SI3	ST36, SI8 LI1, SI1	LI1, GB44 BL66, GB43
Fu-system Mental	TB10, TB3 (Geumyang)/ TB1, TB2 (Mogyang)	TB2, TB3 (Geumeum)/ TB1, TB6 (Mogeum)	TB6, TB2 (Toyang)/ TB10, TB1 (Suyang)	TB1, TB2 (Toeum)/ TB10, TB3 (Sueum)
Vitality	ST36, LI11 GB41, LI3	LI1, GB44 SI5, GB38	SI5, ST41 BL66, ST44	ST36, BL40 GB41, BL65
Fu-system Degeneration	ST36, BL40 GB41, BL65	LI1, BL67 SI5, BL60	SI5, LI5 BL66, LI2	ST36, LI11 GB41, LI3

Figure 11b. Unit Formulae for Eight Constitutions (Fu-system)

In the table of Unit Formulae for the Eight Constitutions above, the four Constitutions—Geumyang, Geumeum, Toyang, and Toeum—are needled in the order of "c → c → p → p" (for the Mental Sub-formulae, c → p), whereas the other four Constitutions—Mogyang, Mogeum, Suyang, and Sueum—are needled in the order of "p → p → c → c" (for the Mental Sub-formulae, p → c). For example, the Basic Formula for Geumyang is "LU8 (Jingqu) c, LR4 (Zhongfeng) c, KI10 (Yingu) p, LR8 (Ququan) p," and for Mogyang, it is "LU8 p, LR4 p, KI10 c, LR8 c." Additionally, Geumyang's Mental Sub-formula is "PC7 (Daling) c, PC9 (Zhongchong) p," and for Mogyang, it is "PC5 (Jianshi) p, PC3 (Quze) c."

The Mental Sub-formulae are described only for the case of the General Equation Sb(−) Se(+). To obtain another Mental Sub-formulae, refer to the list of Mental Sub-formulae above (Figure 10).

What is Disease-origin?

In the early days of Eight-Constitution Medicine, all diseases of each Constitution were treated with just one Basic Formula. Master Do-won Kuon mentioned that he was able to cure almost all diseases just with that. The Basic Formula is a prescription that targets the root cause of disease for each Constitution. The Disease-origin refers to the underlying cause of all diseases occurring in each Constitution.[83] As a vast amount of clinical experience accumulated and the Zang-Fu Structure of the Constitutions was gradually refined, the Basic Formulae were continuously revised accordingly. The current Basic Formulae are entirely different from those of the early days of Eight-Constitution Medicine, when his thesis was written in 1965. The Disease-origin currently targeted in the Basic Formulas for each Constitution is as follows: For Geumyang and Mogyang, it targets the Liver; for Geumeum and Mogeum, it targets the Lungs; for Toyang and Suyang, it targets the Kidneys; and for Toeum and Sueum, it targets the Pancreas. Let's hear directly from Master Do-won Kuon about the Basic Formulae.

> As mentioned in the above, constitutional pathology demands the recovery of the disease-origins of the 8 morbidities to their congenital states. In other words, it demands the over-strengthened disease-origins to be repressed and the over-weakened ones to be animated.[84]

Here, a morbidity refers to an excessive imbalance in the Zang-Fu organs of a Constitution that leads to pathology. Each Sasang Constitution causes

[83] The concept of Disease Root is explained in the paper in 1965 as follows. "However, when they are placed continuously under some bad conditions, the tendencies of each organs, mentioned (In his original text, it was written as "mentions," but it appears to be a typo, so it is corrected as this.) in the summary of *Donguisusebowon*, appear; and the structures of the 8 Chang- and Bhu-temperaments become the hotbeds for the 8 disease-orgins or etiologies. When both the Chang- and Bhu-temperaments have become the hotbeds of these disease-origins, the present writer pathologically designates the first or the second morbidity of each constitution." Do-won Kuon, *A Study Of Constitution-acupuncture*, 1965, p.9.

[84] Do-won Kuon, *A Study of Constitution-acupuncture*, 1965, p.13.

two types of morbidities—one from the Zang-system and the other from the Fu-system—making a total of eight morbidities. This was a transitional theory before the concept of the Eight Constitutions was fully established. The cause of these morbidities was considered the root of the disease, and the prescription for treating this disease later became the Basic Formulae. Listen to the following words from Do-won Kuon to sense the pride he had in his discovery of these Basic Formulae. Looking back, the Formulae were not yet perfect. It exudes the freshness of the embryonic period of Eight-Constitution Medicine.

> According to the clinical statistics, made by the present writer, these 8 treatment-formulas can cure almost all of the diseases, so that any other one can be regarded as unnecessary.[85]

At that time, was Korea, even in the modern era, not as advanced as it is now? And were people's diseases as simple and straightforward as they had been in ancient times? I find this somewhat difficult to believe.

Power of the Five Element Arithmetic Method

The eight treatment prescriptions for the diseases listed in the paper in 1965 are called the Basic Formulae now. At that time, the Saam acupuncture method was used to treat the disease origins, but it was not the standardized, well-planned, and perfected treatment using four acupuncture points as it is today. Instead, it appeared in an undeveloped form in its early stages, where three or four points were used depending on the condition of each Constitution, with some points being used repeatedly. This indicates that it was not yet the fully established methods.

For example, the current prescription for Disease-origin in Taeyangin Chang-temperament, which corresponds to the Geumyang Constitution, consists of "LR4 (Zhongfeng) c, KI10 (Yingu) p, LR8 (Ququan) p, KI10

[85] Do-won Kuon, *A Study of Constitution- acupuncture*, 1965, p.31.

(Yingu) p, LR8 (Ququan) p." If you compare this with the current Basic Formula for the Geumyang Constitution, "LU8 (Jingqu) c, LR4 (Zhongfeng) c, KI10 (Yingu) p, and LR8 (Ququan) p", you'll notice it is similar but a little different. The Formula in 1965 uses an incomplete method of "sedating Metal and tonifying Water" for replenishing the Liver. This shows that the current approach of using both the other meridian and the self-meridian simultaneously had not yet been established. Compared to the current Formula, the transmitting point "LU8 (Jingqu)" of the Lung meridian, which is needed to sedate Metal, is missing; instead, only the acupoint LR4 (Zhongfeng) from the Liver meridian, the self-meridian, is used to sedate Metal. In the case of tonifying Water, the current method of using both the other meridian and the self-meridian is adopted, but with a variation: the points for tonifying Water are repeated an additional time.

Let's look at another example. The formula for the Disease-origin of Soyangin Chang-temperament, which corresponds to the current Toyang Constitution, consists of "SP3 (Taibai) c, KI3 (Taixi) c, LU8 (Jingqu) p, KI7 (Fuliu) p, LU8 (Jingqu) p, KI7 (Fuliu) p." It also appears similar to the current Toyang Constitution's Basic Formula: "SP3 (Taibai) c, KI3 (Taixi) c, LU8 (Jingqu) p, KI7 (Fuliu) p." However, upon closer examination, it becomes clear that it is actually an incomplete formula. How can you verify this? With the Five Elements Arithmetic Method!

The Zang-Fu Array of Soyang's Chang-temperament is "Pancreas Heart Liver Lungs Kidneys," which corresponds to the current Toyang Constitution. Therefore, the Formula for replenishing the Kidneys becomes the Basic Formula for treating the Disease-origin of this Constitution. Considering the Zang-Fu Structure of this Constitution, the Formula for replenishing the Kidneys can be obtained using the method of "sedating Earth and tonifying Metal." However, if we analyze the Formula for Soyangin's Chang-temperament here, it appears that the method of "sedating Earth and tonifying Metal, followed by tonifying Metal" is applied—that is, Metal is repeatedly tonified. The sedating is done in the same way as the current Formula, but the tonifying is repeated one additional time. So, which one is correct between this and the current one? Checking this is not as straightforward as it might seem—it's a bit confusing. But now we can calculate it precisely. How? By applying the Five Phases Arithmetic Method! By applying the method, we can accurately see the impact this approach has on the Zang-Fu Structure of the Toyang Constitution. Let's apply the Five Phases Arithmetic Method.

If you first sedate Earth, it becomes as follows.

Sedating Earth: ΔEarth=-1, ΔMetal=-1, ΔFire=-1, ΔWater=+1, ΔWood=+1 … ①

Next, if you tonify Metal, it becomes as follows:

Tonifying Metal: ΔMetal=+1, ΔWater=+1, ΔEarth=+1, ΔWood=-1, ΔFire=-1 … ②

Next, Metal was added once more, so the result is the same as above.

Tonifying Metal: ΔMetal=+1, ΔWater=+1, ΔEarth=+1, ΔWood=-1, ΔFire=-1 … ③

Therefore, the total change in the system due to the operation above is as follows. If you combine the three results of ①, ②, and ③ together, you get the result as follows:

Result: ΔEarth=+1, ΔFire=-3, ΔWood=-1, ΔMetal=+1, ΔWater=+3

If you examine the Five Phases Structure Formula of this Constitution, "Earth Fire Wood Metal Water", you'll notice that the changes in Earth and Wood do not align with the Constitution. Earth should decrease, and Wood should remain stable with a value of 0, indicating no change. Therefore, the previous method of "SP3 (Taibai) c, KI3 (Taixi) c, LU8 (Jingqu) p, KI7 (Fuliu) p, LU8 (Jingqu) p, KI7 (Fuliu) p" is incorrect. Master Do-won Kuon later recognized this discrepancy and adjusted the Formula to form the Basic Formula for the Toyang Constitution that we use today. It appears that these insights were gained empirically, one by one, through clinical trials.

It seems that compiling all the established Unit Formulae for the Eight Constitutions as we know them today took well over a decade since the paper in 1965. Even in his Myongji University thesis in 1974, the Unit Formulae were still quite different from the current ones, with some consisting of just three acupuncture points rather than the usual four.[86] However, through extensive clinical experience, Master Do-won Kuon eventually arrived at the perfected Unit Formulae for each Constitution. Although the journey included many detours, the insight he gained through reasoning and clinical practice is truly remarkable. The reason it took so long was the absence of the straightforward tool like the Five Phases Arithmetic Method.

Contributions and limitations of Saam Acupuncture

This is the same reason why Saam acupuncture is not entirely compatible with Eight-Constitution Medicine. It does not take into account the unequal Zang-Fu structure of each Constitution but rather assumes an equal status

[86] Do-won Kuon, *Studies on Constitution-Acupuncture Therapy*, 1974. This paper introduces the two-stage Formulae system we commonly know today: Basic Formula coupled with Sub-formula, including their application techniques and clinical cases. It also presents a revised version of the pulse patterns essential for pulse diagnosis, the most critical diagnostic tool in Eight-Constitution Medicine. Notably, the names of the Eight Constitutions—Geumyang, Geumeum, Mogyang, Mogeum, Toyang, Toeum, Suyang, and Sueum—which are now widely recognized, were revised and introduced for the first time in this work. However, the Basic Formula and Sub-formulae introduced here are still in an incomplete state. For example, the Formulae for Geumyang and Toeum consist of only three acupoints instead of the four typically used today. Additionally, the Yang Constitutions use acupoints from the Zang-system, while the Yin Constitutions utilize acupoints from the Fu-system. Of these updated Formulae, only the Toyang Constitution remains identical to the present. At the end of this paper, the famous chart of the Eight-Constitutions Diet is provided, along with the most critical precautions and health maintenance tips for each Constitution. This Constitutional Diet chart was created by Do-won Kuon for the first time in human history and is considered invaluable wisdom for maintaining the health of the general public.

among the Five Zang-Fu organs. Under this assumption, Saam acupuncture considers only the tonification and sedation of each Zang or Fu individually. Additionally, it mechanically applies the principles of Interpromoting and Intersuppressing in the unilateral direction, as in traditional Oriental medicine, so each Zang-Fu organ has only one fixed approach for treatment. Consequently, when Saam acupuncture is applied to the field structure defined by Constitution, it generally does not align. Applying the Five Phases Arithmetic Method reveals that it often conflicts with the Five Phases Structure Formula of the Constitution. Occasionally, a few formulas may coincide by chance with the Constitutional structure, but without a precise understanding of one's Constitution, these isolated instances hold little practical significance.

Saam acupuncture is no longer sufficient to meet the diverse needs of Eight-Constitution Medicine. Consequently, Saam acupuncture was excluded from Eight-Constitution Medicine. However, it greatly contributed to the early development of this field. Thanks to the Saam acupuncture method, the creation of today's various Unit Formulae and Compound Formulae became possible. Saam acupuncture faithfully fulfilled its historical role during the transitional period in the evolution of Eight-Constitution Medicine. (I am saying this solely from the perspective of Eight-Constitution Medicine; I believe Saam acupuncture holds a solid position in the clinical practice in its own right.)

The importance of Unit Formulae

Master Do-won Kuon has conducted numerous clinical trials and developed a vast array of Formulae capable of treating most diseases people commonly experience. Each disease affects different Zang-Fu organs. Especially diseases with the most complex pathologies, like cancer and immune system disorders, involve multiple Zang-Fu organs. That is, four or five Zang-Fu organs combine to create an imbalance. As a result, Compound Formulae of four or more steps are necessary. Nowadays, Formulae have become even more intricate, with 6-, 7-, and even 10-stage Formulae being utilized.[87]

10-step Formula indicates that imbalances have arisen in all five Zangs and Fus. Regardless of how complex a Formula becomes, it is ultimately just a combination of Unit Formulae, which underscores the significance of Unit Formulae. Therefore, Master Do-won Kuon refers to the treatment of diseases by regulating the Zang-Fu organs through Unit Formulas composed of Zang-Fu Acupoints as "radical regulation." On the other hand, the treatment using the acupuncture points other than Zang-Fu Acupoints is termed "local regulation." This distinction is based on the fact that local regulation does not involve the Zang-Fu Acupoints directly. This terminology highlights his pride in the Eight-Constitution Medicine.

The intended effects of the Sub-formulae—such as reducing inflammation, enhancing vitality, or providing sterilization—are relevant only in the 2-stage treatment within the Compound Formulae.[88] In cases of more extensive treatment, that is, with Compound Formulae of three or more stages, the disease is treated by sequentially correcting the imbalanced Zang-Fu organs in the appropriate order. The principles of Compound Formulae will be discussed in the next chapter. Above, we have explored the principles of Unit Formulae.

[87] The specific application of Unit Formulae is covered in detail in the next chapter, "Principles of Compound Formulae."

[88] This is explained in detail in the next chapter, *Principles of Compound Prescription*. Please refer to Do-won Kuon's Myongji University thesis in 1974, Do-won Kuon, *Studies on Constitution-Acupuncture Therapy*, 1974.

CHAPTER 4

The Theory of Compound Formulae

TREATING A DISEASE IS LIKE A CHESS GAME. YOU CAN MOVE THE PIECES WHEREVER YOU WANT AND HOWEVER YOU LIKE, BUT ONLY UNDER THE STRICT RULE.

CHAPTER 4

The Theory of Compound Formulae

The pathology of Eight-Constitution Medicine is very simple. The saying that "all truths are simple and easy" is an unchanging truth. All theories of Eight-Constitution Medicine—namely, physiology, pathology, treatment, and regimen—are deductively derived from the definition of Constitution. The definition of Constitution is said to be the arrangement of the five Zang-Fu pairs in terms of their Zang-Fu potentials. This naturally can be inferred from this Zang-Fu Structure. So, what is Constitutional pathology? It is the "excessive imbalance of the Zang-Fu organs." Constitutional pathology refers to the state in which the Zang-Fu that form the Constitution deviate significantly from their Congenital Imbalance, resulting in Pathological Imbalance.

Constitutional pathology is an excessive imbalance of the Zang-Fu pairs

Let's consider a Constitution with the following Zang-Fu Structure: ABCDE. As mentioned repeatedly before, when a pathological condition arises, the Zang-Fu Potentials of A and B in the Yang Field tend to increase even further, while the Zang-Fu Potentials of D and E in the Yin Field tend to decrease even further. However, human body has an innate instinct to maintain homeostasis. Therefore, it attempts to preserve dynamic equilibrium by counteracting these pathological tendencies.

This dynamic equilibrium opposes the tendency for Zang-Fu Potentials in the Yang Field to increase and that for Zang-Fu Potentials in the Yin Field to decrease. This process is an example of negative feedback in system theory. If this negative feedback mechanism functions properly, the body remains in a healthy state. However, if you are overworked, exposed to low temperatures for prolonged periods, or consume excessive amounts of harmful food, and so on, the feedback mechanism may fail to operate effectively. In such cases, the Zang-Fu Potentials of A or B in the Yang Field rise even higher, and the Zang-Fu Potentials of D or E in the Yin Field drop even lower. When this surpasses the body's physiological control limits, a pathological condition develops, leading to the onset of disease and the associated symptoms.

What, then, constitutes the healing of a disease? The process of cure is naturally derived from the pathology theory of Eight-Constitution Medicine. It involves lowering the potentials of Zang-Fu organs that have risen excessively and raising the potentials of those that have fallen excessively, both in a corrective, reversed manner. By returning the body to its original physiological state, which is the state of Congenital Imbalance, the human body can regain its previous health. This is the process of healing in Eight-Constitution Medicine.

For this type of healing, the Unit Formulae discussed in detail earlier are employed. The Unit Formulae are the fundamental remedies designed to correct imbalances in an individual Zang-Fu organ. The number of imbalanced Zang-Fu organs varies depending on the severity of the disease. Generally, a mild disease involves a small number of imbalanced Zang-Fu organs, while a severe disease involves a larger number of imbalanced Zang-Fu organs. As a result, the prescriptions used to treat diseases can range from simple to complex. However, the underlying principle remains straightforward: the goal is to correct the Zang-Fu organs that have become excessively imbalanced.

The principles of natural numbers

The laws that govern all things in the natural world are surprisingly simple. Although humans use advanced mathematics and complex science to describe the intricate phenomena and the movement of objects, we often find that the underlying principles themselves are very simple. The same applies to chemistry, which represents the intrinsic laws of matter. The numerous biochemical reactions that take place inside and outside the human body typically occur based on straightforward principles, akin to the arithmetic skills of elementary school students. These reactions operate at the level of basic arithmetic operations. Most of them can be resolved with simple addition and subtraction, and in many cases, only addition is required. The calculations primarily involve natural numbers, such as one, two, three, and four, rather than fractions, rational numbers, irrational numbers, or real numbers.

It is easy to perceive the double-helix structure of DNA—often considered the catalyst for the development of molecular biology—as something deeply profound. However, in reality, it is merely a repetitive chemical structure composed of sugar, phosphate, and base. Within this structure, the four bases—A (adenine), G (guanine), C (cytosine), and T (thymine)—form complementary bonds, A-T and G-C, following extremely simple pairing rules of number "2." These pairing rules determine the genetic information encoded in DNA.

The atomic model of a Danish physicist, Niels Bohr (1885–1962), which laid the foundation for the advanced field of quantum mechanics, states that the energy levels of electrons around protons are integer multiples: 1, 2, 3, 4, and so on. This principle of natural numbers, which can be understood even at an elementary school level, forms the basis of Bohr's atomic model—a model developed by a Nobel Prize-winning physicist renowned for his exceptional achievements in the field.

Additionally, most people are likely aware that Mendeleev's (1834-1907) periodic table of the elements, which we memorize by rote in chemistry class, is based on the arithmetic of natural numbers representing the protons and electrons.

Master Do-won Kuon frequently discusses his unique numerology for explaining the Eight-Constitution Medicine. In an article he contributed to the May 1995 issue of the magazine *Light and Salt*, he made the following statement.

> There are strict laws that govern all things, observed in practice. The structure of everything is represented by the number 7, the movement of everything by the number 12, and the individuality of everything by the number 8.

For example, there are 7 musical notes, 7 colors of light, 12 months in a year, 24 hours (2×12) in a day, and the seasons are divided into initium spring (the beginning of spring), spring equinox, initium summer, summer solstice, initium autumn, autumn equinox, initium winter and winter solstice, forming the 8 seasonal terms. Similarly, the human body has 8 Constitutions. While these are just a few specific examples and cannot be generalized, it is evident—just as seen in the examples from Western science mentioned above—that the principle of natural numbers exists in the laws of nature. This numerical principle frequently appears in Eight-Constitution Medicine. With this perspective, let's examine the treatment principles of Eight-Constitution Medicine in detail.

A Zang-Fu is not the same as an organ

In Eight-Constitution Medicine, pathology refers to the state of excessive imbalance in the Zang-Fu organs of the human body. Therefore, it can be inferred that by examining the potential imbalances that may occur in the Zang-Fu organs, we can identify all possible pathologies that could arise in the human body. However, it is important to address the issue of distinguishing between the concepts of Zang-Fu organs and the Western medicine's organs here.

What I refer to as "Zang-Fu" is different from the organs as understood in Western medicine. As repeatedly mentioned in the previous chapters, these Zang-Fu organs are symbolic information centers that create and regulate the Qis of Wood, Fire, Earth, Metal, and Water, rather than physical visceral organs in Western medicine. While they may sometimes seem similar to the concept of western organs, this is purely coincidental. Therefore, the imbalance of Zang-Fu organs mentioned here does not imply the presence of a lesion in the corresponding physical organ.

This is a crucial concept for understanding Constitutional pathology. While Western medicine consistently focuses on the material pathological changes occurring in the physical organs, Eight-Constitution Medicine adheres to the concept of the "Zang-Fu" as the subject of communication of symbolic information until the end. Hence, it is important to remember that the pathology discussed in Eight-Constitution Medicine is unrelated to physical lesions of the organs. Occasionally, the Zang-Fu organs involved in Constitutional pathology may coincide with the affected organs of a lesion, but this is purely coincidental.

To understand this clearly, let's examine the difference between "physical organs" and "Zang-Fu organs" in detail using the example of the disease, gastritis. The term "gastritis" refers to an inflammation of the stomach. This is the most common way of naming diseases in modern Western medicine. In other words, the name consists of the organ or tissue where the lesion is located, combined with the histological findings of pathology in that area. That is why it is called "gastritis" in English. The disease name is formed by adding the suffix "itis", which means inflammation, to the root word "gastr" (stomach), resulting in gastritis (gastr + itis).

In Eight Constitutional Medicine, the gastritis can be treated in two-stage Formula if the condition is not severe. Since the organ stomach is associated with the Fu-system, the treatment involves combining the Basic Formula with the Fu-system Inflammation Sub-formula (Basic Formula : Fu-system Inflammation Sub-formula = 4:2 ratio)[89] as follows:

For the Geumyang Constitution, a combination of Unit Formulae that nourish the Liver and drain the Pancreas is used.

For the Mogyang Constitution, conversely, a combination of Unit Formulae that drain the Liver and nourish the Pancreas is applied.

For the Geumeum Constitution, a combination of Unit Formulae that drain the Lungs and nourish the Heart is used.

---

[89] Do-won, "*Studies on Constitution-Acupuncture Therapy,*" 1974. In this paper, the two-stage treatment Formulae of Constitution-acupuncture is presented along with clinical case studies.

For the Mogeum Constitution, on the other hand, a combination of Unit Formulae that nourish the Lungs and drain the Heart is employed.

For the Toyang Constitution, a combination of Unit Formulae that nourishes the Kidneys and drain the Heart is applied.

For the Suyang Constitution, the opposite approach is taken, using a combination of Unit Formulae that drain the Kidneys and nourishes the Heart.

For the Toeum Constitution, a combination of Unit Formulae that drain the Pancreas and nourish the Liver is used.

For the Sueum Constitution, the opposite method is employed, using a combination of Unit Formulae that nourish the Pancreas and drain the Liver.

This means that, in the case of the Geumyang Constitution, gastritis results from an excessively low Liver potential and an excessively high Pancreas potential. In the Mogyang Constitution, the opposite is true: gastritis results from an excessively high Liver potential and an excessively low Pancreas potential. In the Geumeum Constitution, gastritis occurs due to an excessively high Lung potential and an excessively low Heart potential, whereas in the Mogeum Constitution, it results from an excessively low Lung potential and an excessively high Heart potential.

Additionally, in the Toyang Constitution, gastritis arises from an excessively low Kidney potential and an excessively high Heart potential, whereas in the Suyang Constitution, it results from an excessively high Kidney potential and an excessively low Heart potential. In the Toeum Constitution, gastritis occurs due to an excessively high Pancreas potential and an excessively low Liver potential. Conversely, in the Sueum Constitution, gastritis results from an excessively low Pancreas potential and an excessively high Liver potential.

This illustrates the pathology of excessive imbalance as described in Eight-Constitution Medicine.

In other words, the Geumyang and Mogyang Constitutions cause gastritis due to the excessive imbalance of the Liver and Pancreas; the gastritis of the Geumeum and Mogeum Constitutions result from the excessive imbalances of the Lungs and Heart; the Toyang and Suyang Constitutions experience the gastritis due to the excessive imbalances of the Kidneys and Heart; and gastritis of the Toeum and Sueum Constitutions result from the excessive imbalance of the Pancreas and Liver.

What is noteworthy here is that the pathology of gastritis involves an imbalance in organs such as the Liver, Pancreas, Lungs, Heart, and Kidneys, which are entirely unrelated to the Stomach itself. Therefore, the treatment does not directly target the Stomach but instead focuses on regulating the excessively imbalanced Zang-Fu organs. In Western medicine, if there is a problem with the stomach, treatment is typically directed at the stomach itself. Treating the Liver and Pancreas for a stomach issue would be considered absurd in Western medicine. However, in Eight-Constitution Medicine, the local organ is not directly treated. (There may be cases where the affected organ and the lesion coincide by chance, however.) Instead, the approach aims to restore the excessive imbalance in the Zang-Fu organs caused by the disease to its original, physiological state.

In this way, the concept of organs in Western medicine and the concept of Zang-Fu organs in Oriental medicine differ significantly. With this distinction in mind, let's delve into the principles of the disease treatment.

Number of cases of excessive imbalance

Consider a Constitution with a Zang-Fu Structure labeled as "ABCDE." In this structure, there are only four possible types of pathology that can occur:

① When only one Zang-Fu experiences the excessive imbalance.
② When any two Zang-Fu experience the excessive imbalance.
③ When any three Zang-Fu experience the excessive imbalance.
④ When any four Zang-Fu experience the excessive imbalance.

Here, C is the central Zang-Fu organs and remains unchanged, so it is excluded from the calculation of the number of cases. The number of cases is determined using permutations, as the treatment varies depending on the order of the Zang-Fu organs that exhibit excessive imbalance. In other words, the prescription (Compound Formula) changes based on both the number and order of imbalances. Now, let's examine the number of possible cases in detail.

In case ①, it is straightforward. Since it involves selecting one out of the four Zang-Fu organs, the possibilities are A, B, D, or E causing excessive imbalance, resulting in a total of four cases.

In case ②, it is a bit more complex. It is equivalent to the number of permutations for selecting two out of the four Zang-Fu organs. The possible pairs are: AB (assuming A and B are experiencing excessive imbalance, and similarly for the others), AD, AE, BA, BD, BE, DA, DB, DE, EA, EB, and ED. This gives a total of 12 cases (4 × 3).

In case ③, it becomes even more complicated. It involves selecting three out of the four Zang-Fu organs, resulting in the following permutations: ABD, ABE, ADB, ADE, AEB, AED, BAD, BAE, BDA, BDE, BEA, BED, DAB, DAE, DBA, DBE, DEA, DEB, EAB, EAD, EBA, EBD, EDA, and EDB. This results in 24 cases (4 × 3 × 2).

In case ④, the scenario involves selecting all four Zang-Fu organs, resulting in the following permutations: ABDE, ABED, ADBE, ADEB, AEBD, AEDB, BADE, BAED, BDAE, BDEA, BEAD, BEDA, DABE, DAEB, DBAE, DBEA, DEAB, DEBA, EABD, EADB, EBAD, EBDA, EDAB, and EDBA. This gives a total of 24 cases (4 × 3 × 2 × 1).

One thing to consider here is the central Zang-Fu organs. The Pericardium and Triple Burner are said to function on behalf of the central Zang-Fu organs by harmoniously coordinating the other Zang-Fu organs without undergoing changes themselves. In cases ③ and ④, where the excessive imbalances occur in three or more Zang-Fu organs, the control function of the Pericardium or Triple Burner is necessary. However, in cases ① and ②, where the excessive imbalances involve two or fewer Zang-Fu organs, the control function of the Pericardium or Triple Burner is not necessary. (It is sometimes utilized, but usually, it is not.) We will discuss this further in relation to Mental Sub-formula later.

In case of excessive Imbalance in one Zang-Fu organ

Now, let's examine the principles of prescription formulation in detail. Assume that the Disease-origin of a Constitution with the structure ABCDE lies in A. In this case, the Unit Formula that regulates A becomes the Basic Formula. The Unit Formula for A aims to suppress an excessive increase of A, which means draining A. The Unit Formula for A (denoted as As) is derived from the General Equation for Unit Formulae in Chapter 3 as follows: Bb(−) Ab(−) Ee(+) Ae(+).

For the Mogyang Constitution, the Zang-Fu Structure is "Liver-Gallbladder Kidney-Bladder Heart-Small Intestine Pancreas-Stomach Lungs-Large Intestine." To find the Formula for the Zang-system, commonly known as the Basic Formula, draining the Liver is necessary. Therefore, it includes the acupuncture points: LU8 (Jingqu) p, LR4 (Zhongfeng) p, KI10 (Yingu) c, and LR8 (Ququan) c (If derived using the General Equation, the result is KI10 (Yingu) c, LR8 (Ququan) c, LU8 (Jingqu) p, and LR4 (Zhongfeng) p. Conventionally, the points are needled in the order of LU8 (Jingqu) p, LR4 (Zhongfeng) p, KI10 (Yingu) c, and LR8 (Ququan) c. I will continue following this conventional order).

Additionally, the Fu-system Basic Formula involves the acupoints such as LI1 (Shangyang) p, GB44 (Zuqiaoyin) p, BL66 (Zutonggu) c, and GB43 (Xiaxi) c.

The Basic Formula is used for the simplest diseases. Typically, illnesses in children under the age of 3 are treated using this Basic Formula. Generally, the standard method involves repeating the sequence LU8 (Jingqu) p, LR4 (Zhongfeng) p, KI10 (Yingu) c, LR8 (Ququan) c four times. However, in the case of a sprain, the sequence is repeated five times. Repeating this Basic Formula six times can treat hemostasis. It often has a dramatic hemostatic effect, even for relatively severe internal or external bleeding. This method can be applied to both children and adults. The rules for the number of repetitions will be discussed later.

The case of excessive imbalances in B, D, and E can also be addressed in the same manner. Since there is an excessive imbalance only in one Zang-Fu, the Unit Formula for each Zang and Fu for B, D, and E becomes the Unit Formula we want. For the Mogyang Constitution, the Unit Formula for B involves regulating the Kidneys and Bladder. The excessive increase of the Kidneys is controlled using SP3 (Taibai) p, KI3 (Taixi) p, LR1 (Dadun) c, and KI1 (Yongquan) c, while the excessive increase of the Bladder is managed with ST36 (Zusanli) p, BL40 (Weizhong) p, GB41 (Zulinqi) c, and BL65 (Shugu) c. The cases for D and E follow the same method and are thus omitted.

In clinical practice, the Basic Formula is primarily used in general. Therefore, for Mogyang, Geumeum, Suyang, or Toeum Constitution, which have the Disease-origin in A, the outermost Zang of the Yang Field, the Formulae that drain A are mainly applied. Conversely, for Geumyang, Geumeum, Soyang, or Sueum, which have the Disease-origin in E, the outermost Zang of the Yin Field, the Formulae that replenish E are mainly used.

In case of excessive Imbalance in Two Zang-Fu organs

Now, let's consider the case where two Zang-Fu organs in case ② have caused excessive imbalances. Specifically, let's look at the second case, AD, where "A" and "D" exhibit the excessive imbalances. In this situation, A has increased excessively, while D has decreased excessively. Therefore, the Unit Formulae that drain A and replenish D can be used together. We can derive "As" and "Dt" using the General Equation. As remains the same as previously derived, while Dt is derived from Bb(−) Db(−) Ee(+) De(+).

For the Mogyang Constitution, A corresponds to the Liver and Gallbladder, while D corresponds to the Pancreas and Stomach. This results in the four possible cases of excessive imbalance: Liver and Pancreas; Liver and Stomach; Gallbladder and Pancreas; and Gallbladder and Stomach. Let's take an example of the excessive imbalances of the Liver and Pancreas.

The Unit Formula for the Pancreas is LU8 (Jingqu) p, SP5 (Shangqiu) p, KI10 (Yingu) c, and SP9 (Yinlingquan) c, and that for the Stomach is LI1 (Shangyang) p, ST45 (Lidui) p, BL66 (Zutonggu) c, and ST44 (Neiting) c. Therefore, in cases of excessive imbalance in the Liver and Pancreas, LU8 (Jingqu) p, LR4 (Zhongfeng) p, KI10 (Yingu) c, LR8 (Ququan) c are applied, followed by LU8 (Jingqu) p, SP5 (Shangqiu) p, KI10 (Yingu) c, and SP9 (Yinlingquan) c. This is known as the Fu-system Inflammation Formula, a Formula used for treating inflammatory diseases of Fu-system organs and tissues.

This Formula can be applied to the inflammatory diseases of organs such as the stomach, small intestine, large intestine, or gallbladder, or to inflammatory conditions in Fu-system tissues (most organs and tissues except the Five Zang organs), including diseases of the eyes, nose, and skin. In other words, in the Mogyang Constitution, inflammatory diseases of Fu-system organs or tissues cause excessive imbalances in the Liver and Pancreas. Therefore, a combination of the Basic Formula (draining the Liver) and the Fu-system Inflammation Sub-formula (replenishing the Pancreas) is applied, as these two Unit Formulas are used to correct the excessive imbalances in the Liver and Pancreas.

The Formula composed of Unit Formulae for two or more Zang-Fu organs in this manner is known as Compound Formula. Depending on the number of Unit Formula that makes up the Compound Formula, it is referred to as a 2-stage, 3-stage, 4-stage, or 5-stage Compound Formula.

2-Stage Compound Formula

Additionally, the principle of Constitution-acupuncture treatment usually involves repeating the treatment sequence to enhance its therapeutic effect. A Formula used for addressing imbalances of two Zang-Fu organs is called two-stage Formula, which includes the formulae such as Fu-system Inflammation Formula, Zang-system Inflammation Formula, Sterilization Formula, and Vitality Formula. This is a Compound Formula that functions as a combination of Basic Formula and Sub-formula, and it can be broadly applied to general diseases before they become severe.

First, in the case of the Fu-system Inflammation Formula mentioned as an example earlier, it is applied as a combination of 4 times of Basic Formula treatment and 2 times of Fu-system Inflammation Sub-formula treatment. In other words, the **Fu-system Inflammation Formula** consists of four repetitions of the Basic Formula and two repetitions of the Fu-system Inflammation Sub-formula (4 x Basic Formula + 2 x Fu-system Inflammation Sub-formula).

For example, in the case of the Mogyang Constitution, the treatment involves applying the Basic Formula (draining the Liver) four times, followed by the Fu-system Inflammation Sub-formula (replenishing the Pancreas) twice in sequence. Thus, LU8 (Jingqu) p, LR4 (Zhongfeng) p, KI10 (Yingu) c, and LR8 (Ququan) c are repeated four times, followed by LU8 (Jingqu) p, SP5 (Shangqiu) p, KI10 (Yingu) c, and SP9 (Yinlingquan) c twice. In general, the basic structure of a 2-stage Formula is as follows: 2-stage Formula = ○ times Basic Formula + ○ times Sub-formula.[90]

In cases of imbalance in the Liver and Stomach in the Mogyang Constitution, a combination of 4 sessions of Basic Formula (draining the Liver) and 2 sessions of Sterilization Sub-formula (replenishing the Stomach) is applied. Thus, LU8 (Jingqu) p, LR4 (Zhongfeng) p, KI10 (Yingu) c, and LR8 (Ququan) c are repeated four times, followed by LI1 (Shangyang) p, ST45 (Lidui) p, BL66 (Zutonggu) c, and ST44 (Neiting) c repeated twice. This is known as the **Sterilization Formula**, and it is primarily used for bacterial infectious diseases. In the Mogyang Constitution, bacterial infections can cause the excessive imbalance of the Liver and Stomach. The basic structure of the Sterilization Formula is as follows: Sterilization Formula = 4 times Basic Formula + 2 times Sterilization Sub-formula.

The Sterilization Formula can be used for all bacterial diseases such as tuberculosis, typhoid fever, bacterial gastritis, bacterial cystitis, and so on. Since the bacterial diseases are often accompanied by inflammation, the Fu-system Inflammation Formula or the Zang-system Inflammation Formula can be used

---

[90] The technical details presented here, such as the number of repetitions for Formulae and the selection of left or right sides, are not absolute rules. They are primarily based on Master Do-won Kuon's unique acupuncture techniques and are the result of experience accumulated through clinical practice. Therefore, questioning the necessity of why it is applied this way is meaningless. Besides the method described here, various other approaches are also possible. However, this method has been validated over a long period in clinical practice and is widely used. Thus, if the first three chapters cover the theoretical principles of Eight-Constitution Medicine, the fourth chapter can be seen as the start of its practical clinical application.

as auxiliary treatments. In this case, the acupuncture is applied to both the left and right sides. The Sterilization Formula is applied to the Constitutional side,[91] while the auxiliary Formula is applied to the opposite side.

For example, in the case of gastritis caused by Helicobacter pylori bacteria, it is similar to using the Sterilization Formula on the Constitutional side and the Fu-system Inflammation Formula on the opposite side. For any disease where pus is present, the Sterilization Formula should be used first. For conditions such as hemorrhoids, the Sterilization Formula and the Fu-system Inflammation Formula can be used together.

Treatment with Constitution-acupuncture usually begins with the Basic Formula, because according to Do-won Kuon's theory, most disease originates from the Zang-Fu organ which are considered the root of the disease. This is why Basic Formula is referred to as a prescription for treating the Disease-origin.

The cases of the excessive imbalance in the Gallbladder and Pancreas or in the Gallbladder and Stomach are also theoretically possible, and the Compound Formulae can be formulated in the same way as in the previous examples. However, the frequency of use in these cases is much lower compared to cases that begin with the Basic Formula, as used in previous instances.

The number of repetitions is based on Do-won Kuon's unique numerology. The general rule is roughly divided into two cases: repeating 4 times (even number) and repeating 5 times (odd number). Specifically, in the two-stage Compound Formula, when a Sub-formula is added to the Basic Formula, the total number of repetitions becomes six. (This rule applies only to two-stage Compound Formulas.) Thus, if the Basic Formula is repeated 4 times, the Sub-formula is repeated 2 times. If the Basic Formula is repeated 5 times, the Sub-formula is repeated 1 time.

When the ratio of the Basic Formula to the Sub-formula is 5:1, it applies only to the Zang-system Inflammation Formula used for Zang-system

---

[91] The Constitutional side refers to the side where the major Formula for each Constitution is applied. This will be explained in detail later.

inflammatory diseases (Basic Formula: Zang-system Inflammation Sub-formula = 5:1). In all other cases, the ratio is usually Basic Formula: Sub-formula = 4:2.

In the case of the Mogyang Constitution, the Basic Formula for Zang-system inflammation consists of LU8 (Jingqu) p, LR4 (Zhongfeng) p, KI10 (Yingu) c, and LR8 (Ququan) c, repeated 5 times. The Zang-system Inflammation Sub-formula (replenishing the Lungs) consists of SP3 (Taibai) p, LU9 (Taiyuan) p, LR1 (Dadun) c, and LU11 (Shaoshang) c, applied once. The Zang-system Inflammation Formula is mainly used for the inflammatory diseases of the Zang-system. Thus, it can be applied to conditions such as pneumonia, emphysema, pancreatitis, hepatitis, fatty liver, nephritis, etc. It is particularly effective for treating hepatitis. In most cases, hepatitis is difficult to treat with medication due to the liver lesions, as the liver is the main organ for detoxification. Here, Constitution-acupuncture treatment offers the best solution for such issues. It can be effectively used for all types of hepatitis, including types A, B, and C.

Formula for treating the lethargic condition of organs, tissues, or the whole body are referred to as **Vitality Formula**. In the case of the Mogyang Constitution, the prescription consists of the Basic Formula—LU8 (Jingqu) p, LR4 (Zhongfeng) p, KI10 (Yingu) c, and LR8 (Ququan) c—repeated 4 times, along with the Vitality Sub-formula for replenishing the Large Intestine—ST36 (Zusanli) p, LI11 (Quchi) p, GB41 (Zulinqi) c, and LI3 (Sanjian) c—repeated 2 times.

This Formula can be used for conditions like gastric ptosis, where the stomach becomes weakened and sags downward; colonic ptosis, where the intestines lose tone and droop; hernia, where the intestines protrude into the inguinal canal or scrotum; or uterine prolapse, where the uterus descends. It can also be applied to anal prolapse, kidney or urethral stones, etc. If gallstones are not too large, they can be treated using this Vitality Formula without the need for surgery.

For colonic ptosis, hernia, uterine prolapse, anal prolapse, and urethral stones, the Lower Burner treatment can be used. For gastric ptosis and gallstones, the Middle Burner treatment is appropriate. (The acupuncture techniques for the Upper, Middle, and Lower Burner treatments will be explained shortly.) This Vitality Formula can also be applied to general muscle weakness, including in the arms, legs, or back.

For mild neurotic disorders such as insomnia, headaches, or anxiety, a Mental Formula is used. The **Mental Formula** involves 4 Basic Formula sessions and 2 Mental Sub-formula sessions. In the case of the Mogyang Constitution, the sequence LU8 (Jingqu) p, LR4 (Zhongfeng) p, KI10 (Yingu) c, and LR8 (Ququan) c is applied four times, followed by PC5 (Jianshi) p and PC3 (Quze) c twice. Strictly speaking, it is difficult to classify the Mental Formula as the Formula belonging to the case of imbalances of two Zagn-Fu organs. It is more appropriate to view it as an application for neurosis by adding the Mental Sub-formula to the Basic Formula that addresses the excessive imbalance of one Zang-Fu organ.

When the Zang-Fu Structure is 'ABCDE', the structure of the 2-stage Formula for Mogyang, Geumeum, Suyang, and Toeum Constitutions, where A is the Disease-origin, is as follows. For convenience, the Zang-Fu Array is represented as AA' BB' CC' DD' EE', distinguishing between the Zangs and the Fus. Here, A, B, C, D, and E refer to the Zangs (Zang-system), while A', B', C', D', and E' refer to the Fus (Fu-system). Additionally, Pericardium is denoted as S, and Triple Burner is denoted as S'. In the future, if necessary, we will continue to list the Zang-system and the Fu-system together in this manner.

As•A's	Bs•B's	Sr•S'r	Dt•D't	Et•E't
↑	↑	↑	↑	↑
Basic F. & Fu-system Basic F.	Degen. Sub-f. & Fu-system Degen. Sub-f.	Mental Sub-f. & Fu-system Mental Sub-f.	Fu-system Inflam. Sub-f. & Sterilization Sub-f.	Zang-system Inflam. Sub-f. & Vitality Sub-f.

Figure 1. 2-stage Compound Formulae for Constitutions with Disease-origin A

The abbreviation rule in Figure 1 is as follows:

As: Basic Formula (Basic F.)
A's: Fu-system Basic Formula (Fu-system Basic F.)
Bs: Degeneration Sub-formula (Degen. Sub-f.)
B's: Fu-system Degeneration Sub-formula (Fu-system Degen. Sub-f.)
Sr: Mental Sub-formula (Mental Sub-f.)
S'r: Fu-system Mental Sub-formula (Fu-system Mental Sub-f.)
Dt: Fu-system Inflammation Sub-formula (Fu-system Inflam. Sub-f.)
D't: Sterilization Sub-formula (Sterilization Sub-f.)
Et: Zang-system Inflammation Sub-formula (Zang-system Inflam. Sub-f.)
E't: Vitality Sub-formula (Vitality Sub-f.)

In other words, for a Constitution where A is the Disease-origin, the Unit Formula for A and A' become the Basic Formula (As) and the Fu-system Basic Formula (A's), respectively. The Unit Formulae for draining B and B' are called Degeneration Sub-formula (Bs) and Fu-system Degeneration Sub-formula (B's), respectively. The Unit Formulae that replenish D and D' are referred to as Sterilization Sub-formula (Dt) and Fu-system Sterilization Sub-formula (D't). The Unit Formulae that replenish E and E' are called Zang-system Inflammation Sub-formula (Et) and Vitality Sub-formula (E't), respectively. Lastly, the Unit Formulae that regulate S and S' are termed Mental Sub-formula (Sr) and Fu-system Mental Sub-formula (S'r), respectively.

In the case of Geumyang, Mogeum, Toyang, and Sueum Constitutions where E is the Disease-origin, conversely, Et and E't become the Basic Formula and the Fu-system Basic Formula, respectively; Dt and D't become the Degeneration Sub-formula and the Fu-system Degeneration Sub-formula, respectively. Meanwhile, Bs and B's become the Fu-system Inflammation Sub-formula and Sterilization Sub-formula, respectively, and As and A's become Zang-system Inflammation Sub-formula and Vitality Sub-formula, respectively. For more details, please refer to the Unit Formulae list in Chapter 3, *Principles of Unit Formulae.*

The Upper Burner treatment and the Lower Burner treatment

The two-stage Compound Formula enables targeted treatment for Upper or Lower Burner lesions when the disease is concentrated in these areas. For treating the Upper Burner of the body, the acupuncture points applied by the Meeting Method in the Sub-formula are needled twice, while for the Lower Burner of the body, the acupuncture points applied by the Following Method in the Sub-formula are needled twice. The former is referred to as ana-puncture, and the latter as cata-puncture. If the lesion is located in the Middle Burner or affects the entire body, the original Formula is used.

For example, in the case of Mogyang Constitution, when treating an inflammatory disease of the lungs, the Zang-system Inflammation Formula can be used with a focus on the Upper Burner of the body. Repeat the Basic Formula points, LU8 (Jingqu) p, LR4 (Zhongfeng) p, KI10 (Yingu) c, and LR8 (Ququan) c, five times in sequence (VII7p, I7p, IX9c, I9c—5 times in total), and apply Zang-system Inflammation Sub-formula points, SP3 (Taibai) p, LU9 (Taiyuan) p, LR1 (Dadun) c, and LU11 (Shaoshang) c, once in sequence, with LR1 (Dadun) and LU11 (Shaoshang) once again each using the Meeting Method (V5p, VII5p, I1c, I1c, VII1c, VII1c, once in total).

If there is inflammation in the bladder of Mogyang Constitution, the Fu-system Inflammation Formula can be used with a focus on the Lower Burner of the body. Repeat the Basic Formula four times (repeat the sequence— VII7p, I7p, IX9c, I9c—four times in total). Then, apply the Fu-system Inflammation Sub-formula points, LU8 (Jingqu) p, SP5 (Shangqiu) p, KI10 (Yingu) c, and SP9 (Yinlingquan) c, repeating twice in sequence each with LU8 (Jingqu) and SP5 (Shangqiu) once again using the Following Method (VII7p, VII7p, V7p, V7p, IX9c, V9c—twice in total). In Eight-Constitution Medicine, the body is divided into Upper, Middle, and Lower Burners as follows.

Upper Burner: the area above the diaphragm. It includes the lungs, heart, bronchi, head, eyes, ears, nose, throat, ribs, upper thoracic spine, and cervical spine.

Middle Burner: the area between the diaphragm and the navel. It includes the liver, gallbladder, pancreas, stomach, duodenum, and thoracic spine.

Lower Burner: the area below the navel. It includes the kidneys, bladder, large intestine, rectum, uterus, prostate, lumbar spine, and sacral spine.

Therefore, if the lesion is in the Upper Burner of the body, use the Upper Burner treatment; if it is in the Lower Burner, use the Lower Burner treatment. If the lesion is in the Middle Burner or spread throughout the body, the 2-stage Formula is applied without any additional repetition.

In stage 4 and above, the operation of the Upper and Lower treatment is differentiated.

In the 4-stage Formulae, the Upper Burner treatment is applied in ratios such as 4:4:2:4 or 5:5:1:5, while the Lower Burner treatment is administered in ratios such as 4:4:4:2 or 5:5:5:1.

In the 5-stage Formulae, the Upper Burner treatment follows ratios such as 4:4:4:2:4 or 5:5:5:1:5, and the Lower Burner treatment follows ratios such as 4:4:4:4:2 or 5:5:5:5:1.

For Middle Burner treatment or a whole body treatment, the ratios are 4:4:4:4:4 or 5:5:5:5:5. Specific usage examples will be introduced later.

As mentioned earlier, two-stage Formulae can yield better results when both the left and right prescriptions are used together. For example, in cases of bladder inflammation, the Fu-system Inflammation Formula can be applied on one side and the Sterilization Formula on the other.

In other words, for Fu-system Inflammation, the therapeutic effect can be enhanced by applying the Sterilization Formula in addition. This is because the Fu-system, like the gastrointestinal tract, is more susceptible to bacterial infections.

For example, Formula for the bladder Inflammation, if "A" is the Disease-origin, the prescription is as follows: L. As 4 times, Dt cata 2 times (Fu-system Inflammation Formula) / R. As 4 times, D't cata 2 times (Sterilization Formula), where L = left, R = right, cata = cata-puncture, and the slash '/' indicates separation between the left and right sides.

Usually, for Yang Constitutions such as Geumyang, Mogyang, Toyang, and Suyang, the Fu-system Inflammation Formula is applied to the left, and the Sterilization Formula is applied to the right. Conversely, for Yin Constitutions such as Geumeum, Mogeum, Toeum, and Sueum, the Fu-system Inflammation Formula is applied to the right, and the Sterilization Formula is applied to the left.

In other words, for Yang Constitution, the main Formula is applied to the left, and the auxiliary Formula is applied to the right. For Yin Constitution, the main Formula is applied to the right, and the auxiliary Formula is applied to the left. This is because the left corresponds to Yang and the right to Yin—the left being the positive side and the right the negative side. However, this is not necessarily absolute. In some cases, the rule can be reversed.

If there is a clear bacterial disease, such as tuberculosis, typhoid fever, leprosy, bacterial gastritis, etc., the Sterilization Formula becomes the primary prescription. In this case, the primary prescription (Sterilization Formula) is applied to the Constitutional side, while the auxiliary prescription is applied to the opposite side.

For instance, in cases of bacterial pneumonia or pulmonary tuberculosis, a Sterilization Formula is applied to the Constitutional side, and an Zang-system Inflammation Formula is applied to the opposite side.

You may recall pulmonary tuberculosis as a disease that was prevalent during times of poverty. Unfortunately, this disease is reportedly on the rise again due to significant declines in overall immunity caused by rapid environmental changes and the overuse of antibiotics. Tragically, some individuals succumb helplessly, unable to receive proper treatment due to the severe side effects of tuberculosis medications, which are potent antibiotics. This Formula approach can be effective in such situations. Since the lungs belong to the Upper Burner, the Upper Burner treatment is used. The prescription is as follows: L. As 5 times, D't ana once / R. As 5 times, Et ana once, where ana refers to ana-puncture.

Generally, when the Zang-system Inflammation Formula is used as the main formula, a Mental Formula is also used as an auxiliary Formula on the opposite side. For instance, in the case of hepatitis, as briefly mentioned earlier, the Zang-system Inflammation Formula and the Mental Formula are used together. The Formula for the Constitution where A is the Disease-origin, using General Equation, is as follows: L. As 5 times, Et 1 time / R. As 5 times, Sr 1 time.

Two-stage Formulae can be applied to a variety of other diseases. For example, in the case of gastric ptosis, the Vitality Formula can be used on the Constitutional side, and the Fu-system Inflammation Formula can be used on the opposite side. The Formula, using General Equation, is as follows: L. As 4 times, E't 2 times / R. As 4 times, Dt 2 times.

Special application of two-stage Compound Formulae

Next, there is a special example of applying the two-stage Compound Formulae. In the case of the Zang-system Inflammation Formula, the ratio of the Basic Formula to the Sub-formula is typically 5:1. However, for conditions like hiccups and diseases affecting tissues such as the heart valve, bronchus, glomeruli, and blood vessels of the heart and liver, the Zang-system Inflammation Formula is applied at a ratio of 4:2. This adjustment is made because, although these tissues belong to Zang organ, they also exhibit characteristics similar to Fu-system. Diseases affecting these areas are referred to as Zang-system Fu-symptom.

Conversely, there is the Fu-system Zang-symptom, which refers to inflammatory diseases affecting tissues such as the esophagus, nostrils, and ear canals. This term indicates that, although these tissues are part of a Fu-system, they exhibit properties characteristic of the Zang organs. The esophagus is a tissue connected to the stomach but classified as Zang, while the nostrils and ear canals are part of bone (cartilage tissue), making them also classified as Zang tissues. In such cases, the Fu-system Inflammation Formula is applied with the ratio of Basic Formula to Fu-system Inflammation Sub-formula = 5:1.

Additionally, the Sterilization Formula ratio is usually 4:2, but for diseases with severe pain, a ratio of 5:1 is used. For example, conditions like tennis elbow cause intense pain due to epicondylitis of the upper arm, and in such cases, a 5:1 ratio is applied to treating epicondylitis. While the Vitality Formula Ratio is typically set at 4:2, when it is used to activate muscles, it can be adjusted to 5:1.

The commonly used two-stage Compound Formulae are shown below in general form. There are two tables: The first table is for the Mogyang, Geumeum, Suyang, and Toeum Constitutions, where A is the Disease-origin. The second table is for the Geumyang, Mogeum, Toyang and Sueum Constitutions, where E is the Disease-origin. Of course, additional two-stage Compound Formulae not included in the table below can also be applied.[92]

Formula	Basic Formula	Sub-formula
Zang-system Inflammation	As x5	Et x1
Fu-system Inflammation	As x4	Dt x2
Sterilization	As x4	D't x2
Vitality	As x4	E't x2
Mental	As x4	Sr x2

(a) 2-stage Compound Formulae for Constitutions with Disease-origin A

[92] Figure 2 presents two-stage Compound Formulae published in Do-won Kuon's thesis at Myongji University. It is widely used for treating simple diseases. Two-stage Compound Formulae for combinations such as BA, BD, BE, DA, DB, DE, EA, EB, and ED, which are not included here, can also be formulated. The Compound Formulae for them can be BsAs, BsDt, BsEt, DtAs, DtBs, DtEt, EtAs, EtBs, and EtDt. The number of repetitions follows a 5:1 or 4:2 ratio, similar to other two-stage Compound Formulae.

Formula	Basic Formula	Sub-formula
Zang-system Inflammation	Et x5	As x1
Fu-system Inflammation	Et x4	Bs x2
Sterilization	Et x4	B's x2
Vitality	Et x4	A's x2
Mental	Et x4	Sr x2

(b) 2-stage Compound Formulae for Constitutions with Disease-origin E

Figure 2. Two-stage Compound Formulae Tables

The general scope of application for the two-stage Compound Formulae is as follows.

Basic Formula	Minor sprain (repeat 5 times), any trauma (repeat 5 times), bleeding from any internal or external injury (repeat 6 times), other common pediatric diseases (repeat 4 times), etc.
Fu-system Inflammation Formula	Infectious and inflammatory diseases of the Five-Fu organs: stomach, small intestine, large intestine, gallbladder, and bladder; diseases of other related tissues such as the duodenum, esophagus, uterus, blood vessels, and skin; diseases of the mucous membrane areas that secrete mucus; and conditions affecting the eyes, as well as ENT (ear, nose, and throat) diseases, oral diseases, etc.
Zang-system Inflammation Formula	Inflammatory diseases of Five Zangs such as the liver, heart, pancreas, lungs, and kidneys; diseases of Zang-system tissues such as bones; and musculoskeletal diseases including sprains.

Sterilization Formula	All bacterial diseases (treated in combination with the Fu-system Inflammation Formula), pulmonary tuberculosis (treated in combination with Zang-system Inflammation Formula), rhinitis, sinusitis, otitis media, purulent infections, hemorrhoids (treated in combination with the Fu-system Inflammation Formula), etc.
Vitality Formula	Diseases caused by organ or tissue dysfunction: gastric ptosis, colonic ptosis, stones, loss of appetite, frequent urination, enuresis, low blood pressure, lethargy, etc.
Mental Formula	Diseases classified as neurosis: dysautonomia, insomnia, headache, depression, etc.

3-Stage Compound Formulae

First, we need to examine the rules of using Mental Sub-formula. Mental Sub-formulae (denoted as Sr or S'r) must be applied when excessive imbalances occur in three or more Zang-Fu organs. This means that when the excessive imbalances affect three Zang-Fu organs and more, the regulatory functions of the Pericardium or Triple Burner are necessary. Since the central Zang-Fu organs are positioned third in the Zang-Fu Array of Constitution, this Mental Sub-formula is also utilized in the third position.

As a specific example of using the Mental Sub-formula, if there is an excessive imbalance in only one Zang-Fu organ, apply the Basic Formula four times, followed by the Mental Sub-formula twice, as mentioned earlier, to address mild neurosis. In cases of excessive imbalances in two Zang-Fu organs, use only the 2-stage Compound Formulae as previously described, or apply the 2-stage Compound Formulae along with an additional Mental Sub-formula (3-stage Compound Formula).

The most well-known 3-stage Compound Formula is the one consisting of "5 times Basic Formula, 5 times Zang-system Inflammation Sub-formula, and 1 time Mental Sub-formula." An example for Mogyang Constitution is:

"Is applied 5 times, VIIt applied 5 times, and III'r applied once." In other words, this includes the Basic Formula applied 5 times to address the Disease-origin (the Liver in the case of Mogyang Constitution), the Zang-system Inflammation Sub-formula applied 5 times to correct the excessive imbalance of the Zang organ (the Lungs in the case of Mogyang Constitution), which is in an Antagonizing relationship with the Disease-origin, and the Unit Formula for the Pericardium applied once.

Applications of Disc Formula

This Compound Formula is primarily applied to spine-related diseases. It is a key Formula that is always used for herniated cervical or lumbar discs, which is why it is often nicknamed the "Disc Formula." It is an essential treatment for inflammatory diseases in the spine. It is also highly effective for other joint diseases, such as sprains or inflammatory conditions of the neck, lower back, knees, ankles, wrists, etc. Even in cases where the ankle is so severely sprained that walking is nearly impossible, patients often experience rapid relief, sometimes being able to walk immediately after undergoing the Disc Formula treatment procedure.

This Formula is also well-suited for conditions like myalgia, numbness or pain in the limbs. In short, it is a Formula that can be broadly applied to most musculoskeletal diseases in the human body. It is frequently used for mild neuroses as well, including headaches, anxiety, and insomnia. (It is particularly effective in cases of spinal diseases-related conditions.) This Compound Formula is considered one of the most effective and frequently used Formula in Eight-Constitution Medicine.

Let's look at some specific applications of the Disc Formula. Here too, for convenience, the Zang-Fu Array is denoted as AA' BB' CC' DD' EE', distinguishing the Zang-system from the Fu-system. Pericardium is represented as S, and Triple Burner as S'. This is exemplified by the cases where the outermost Zang-Fu (A or A') of Yang Field serves as the Disease-origin.

First, let's look at disc disease, specifically herniation of nucleus pulposus (HNP). The Disc Formula is used for these disc diseases, regardless of whether it is cervical (neck) or lumbar (lower back). The Formula obtained from General Equation is AsEtSr (5:5:1), which represents a Constitution-acupuncture treatment consisting of five times As, five times Et, and one time Sr. This is used primarily for disc diseases that cause pain. If the main symptom is numbness or tingling, use AsEtSr 4:4:2. Although basic disc therapy alone can be effective, for greater efficacy, additional Formulae can be combined and applied to both the left or right sides. One example is using the Disc Formula (AsEtSr 5:5:1) on one side and Vitality Formula on the other side. The purpose of placing the Vitality Formula is to reduce pressure on the spine by strengthening the muscles surrounding the spine.

For conditions affecting the cervical spine and upper thoracic spine, use the Upper Burner treatment. For diseases involving the lumbar spine and symptoms in the lower extremities, use the Lower Burner treatment. For example:

For cervical disc disease, use AsEtSr 5:5:1 / AsE't ana 4:2 (abbreviated as AES 551 / AE'a 42, if necessary for convenience).

For lumbar disc disease that affects the lower extremities, use AsEtSr 5:5:1 / AsE't cata 4:2.

If the symptoms are confined to the lower back, Middle Burner treatment may be used. If the pain is severe, the Sterilization Formula can be substituted for the Vitality Formula. For example, in cases of severe leg pain due to lumbar disc disease, AES 551 / AD'c 51 can be used. The method remains the same.

It can also be used for humeral epicondylitis, commonly known as tennis elbow or golfer's elbow. Use AES 551 / AD'a 51 (for severe epicondyle pain), or AES 551 / AE'a 42 (for chronic pain). Using the same technique, you can also apply the "Disc Formula/Sterilization Formula for Upper Burner treatment" or "Disc Formula/Vitality Formula for Upper Burner treatment" to treat trigeminal neuralgia, facial muscle spasm, and temporomandibular joint (TMJ) disorder. It is also effective to use the Disc Formula and the Sterilization Formula together for conditions like gum disease and gingivitis.

This remedy can also be used for sciatic neuralgia and other types of back pain. In chronic cases, muscle vitality tends to decrease, so the Vitality Formula can be additionally used. The prescription is: AES 551 / AE'c 42.

If the symptoms of rheumatoid arthritis (RA) are mild, Disc Formula can be applied in the same way. In severe cases, a specialized Formula for rheumatoid arthritis (4-stage or 5-stage Formula) must be used. In such cases, the Disc Formula also can be applied to the opposite side.

Knee joint diseases, ligament injuries, muscle cramps, plantar pain, ankle pain, and any joint-related conditions—such as those affecting the shoulder joint and wrist—as well as simple muscle pain, neuralgia, joint pain, and intercostal neuralgia (joint stiffness) can all be treated using the Disc Formula. It is also effective for tenosynovitis and ankylosing spondylitis. In other words, the Disc Formula can be applied to most conditions affecting the muscles, bones, joints and nerves. Whenever there is pain anywhere in the body, the Disc Formula can always be used as a treatment option.

3-Stage Formulae Derived from 2-Stage Formulae

A two-stage Formula can effectively treat a variety of diseases on its own, but more importantly, it serves as a basis for progressing to a higher-stage Compound Formulae. For example:

The Disc Formula evolved from the Zang-system Inflammation Formula (AsEt) into AsEtSr.

There is an ulcer treatment for conditions like stomach, duodenal, and colon ulcers, which evolved from the Fu-system Inflammatory Formula (AsDt) into AsDtSr (4:4:2).

The Virus Formula developed from the Sterilization Formula (AsD't) into AsD'tSr (5:5:1).

The Virus Formula is literally used for viral diseases. It is typically effective for conditions like the common cold and shingles. The viral diseases are among the most challenging to treat in modern medicine. This is because viruses differ from bacteria, making it difficult to develop effective drugs like antibiotics. Although there are several antiviral agents available, their effectiveness is much lower compared to antibiotics. This is due to the nature of viruses, which constantly mutate, unlike bacteria that have relatively stable cell structures, making it extremely difficult to develop specific drugs.

For viral diseases that are hard to treat with medication, this Virus Formula is highly effective. In some cases, the common cold can develop into more serious conditions, and in such instances, the Virus Formula can be used. It is a very useful formula for colds that linger for an extended period, chronic colds in both children and adults who suffer from them year-round, and for colds in pregnant women, who may have difficulty using medication.

Herpes zoster, commonly known as shingles, is a challenging neurological condition often seen in individuals with weakened immune systems due to overwork or stress. The disease is named because the shingles virus invades the nervous system, causing band-shaped lesions along the nerve pathways. If the virus affects the trigeminal nerve, it can lead to herpes zoster ophthalmicus, which may result in complications such as keratitis, conjunctivitis, retinitis, uveitis, exophthalmos, glaucoma, and in severe cases, even blindness.

Ramsay-Hunt Syndrome occurs when the virus invades the facial nerve and acoustic nerve, leading to facial nerve paralysis and nystagmus, along with ear pain.

When the intercostal nerves are affected, band-shaped lesions appear along the ribs. Since the virus directly invades the nervous system, the most common and painful complication of these diseases is postherpetic neuralgia, which is characterized by blistering lesions and severe pain.

Because these conditions are viral, there is not much definitive cure. While antiviral medications are used, there is much debate regarding their effectiveness. In addition, auxiliary treatment usually relies on symptomatic relief, using oral steroids, painkillers, and anti-inflammatory medications, while waiting for the immune system to strengthen through adequate rest.[93] However, if you apply this Virus Formula specifically designed for shingles, it can yield excellent results without any lasting aftereffects.

However, even though hepatitis is also a viral disease, the Zang-system

[93]Korean Academy of Family Medicine, *Family Medicine*, Clinical Edition (Seoul: Gyechuk Munhwasa, 2003), pp. 1095-1096.

Inflammation Formula is more effective, as explained earlier. This is because it is a special virus with properties that differ from common viruses.

Ulcer Formula is commonly used for ulcerative diseases of the digestive tract, such as stomach ulcers, duodenal ulcers, and colon ulcers. Inflammatory diseases that affect only the superficial layer of the mucous membrane are treated with a Fu-system Inflammatory Formula (AsDt). However, when the superficial layer is destroyed and the underlying parenchymal cells die, leading to exposed blood vessels and bleeding, or when nerves are exposed causing severe pain, this Ulcer Formula (AsDtSr) should be used.

AsE'tSr 4:4:2, a Formula for gastric ptosis, is an extension of the 2-stage Formula, Vitality Formula, into a 3-stage Formula. In severe cases of gastric ptosis, the stomach may descend as far as the bladder. In such cases, the person needs to lie down on one's back in order for food to pass into the small intestine. When standing, food sags downward due to gravity, accumulating in the lower part of the stomach, causing a gurgling sound and preventing the food from moving into the small intestine. People with gastric ptosis need to be extremely cautious. In addition to treatment, performing handstands in the morning and evening can enhance the effectiveness of the treatment.

Gastric ptosis is a condition commonly seen in individuals with a Sueum Constitution, where the Stomach is the outer-most organ in Yin Field. For constitutions where E is the root, the 3-stage Formula EtA'tSr can be used in the ratio of 4:4:2 for treating gastric ptosis. Here, Et is the Basic Formula, A't is the Vitality Sub-formula, and Sr is the Mental Sub-formula.

Other 3-stage Formulae

Compound Formulae typically begin with a Basic Formula, though there are cases where they do not. One of the chronic stomach conditions is atrophic gastritis, a disease characterized by histological evidence of chronic atrophy of the stomach lining. For individuals with the Constitutions where "A" is the Disease-origin, the following Formula is used for treating atrophic gastritis: BsE'tSr 4:4:2. Here, "Bs" refers to Degeneration Sub-formula, "E't" refers to Vitality Sub-formula, and "Sr" refers to the Mental Sub-formula.

For degenerative joint diseases caused by the wear and tear of cartilage or bones, the appropriate Formula for degenerative joint disease should be applied. The "Degeneration Formula" does not begin with the Basic Formula but rather starts directly with the "Degeneration Sub-formula." For Constitutions where "A" is the Disease-origin, use the Formula B'sE'tS'r in the ratio of 5:5:1 or 4:4:2. The 5:5:1 ratio is used when pain is the primary symptom, while 4:4:2 is used when numbness is the main symptom. Here, B's is the Fu-system Degeneration Formula, E't is the Vitality Sub-formula, and S'r is the Fu-system Mental Sub-formula (Unit Formula to regulate the Triple Burner). Conversely, if E is the Disease-origin, the Formula is D'tA'sS'r in the ratio of 5:5:1 or 4:4:2.

This Formula is also used for conditions such as low blood pressure, anemia, poor blood circulation, dizziness, motion sickness, angina pectoris, and myocardial infarction. It is particularly effective in treating motion sickness and dizziness.

When Fu-system Basic Formula is used at the beginning of Compound Formula, there is a specific Formula for tide fever: A'sDtSr 5:5:1. A characteristic symptom of this fever is that it typically appears in the afternoon or at night and then subsides. In this case, you can use this fever Formula with the following ratios: 5 times Fu-system Basic Formula (A's), 5 times Fu-system Inflammation Sub-formula (Dt), and 1 time Mental Sub-formula (Sr).

There is a three-stage Formula used for high blood pressure or cerebral infarction, and this also begins with the Fu-system Basic Formula. For the Constitutions where A is the Disease-origin, the Formula is A'sD'tS'r 5:5:1. Here, A's is the Fu-system Basic Formula, D't is the Sterilization Sub-formula, and S'r is the Fu-system Mental Sub-formula.

Another example of using Fu-system Basic Formula is a Compound Formula for treating atopic dermatitis. It is commonly found in the Geumyang Constitution, so an example Formula for this Constitution is E'tBsS'r 4:4:2.

Here, E't is the Fu-system Basic Formula, Bs is the Fu-system Inflammation Sub-formula, and S'r is the Fu-system Mental Sub-formula. Atopic dermatitis is an allergic skin condition that occurs when individuals consume foods that do not suit their Constitutions, such as meat, wheat flour, dairy products, and spicy foods. Thus, it can only be cured if the treatment is combined with strict adherence to Constitutional Diet. Severe cases typically require continuous daily treatment for more than 6 months.

The 3-stage Formula used for conditions like gout or trigeminal neuralgia does not begin with the Basic Formula but rather with other Formula. For the Constitutions where "A" is the Disease-origin, the Formula is EtDtSr 5:5:1. Here, Et is for Zang-system Inflammation Sub-formula, Dt is for Fu-system Inflammation Sub-formula, and Sr is for Mental Sub-formula. Generally, Formulae start with Basic Formula, but for certain diseases, they often begin with a different Unit Formula instead of the Basic Formula. This tendency becomes more evident as the stage of the Formula increases. This can be interpreted as meaning that the more severe the disease, the more complex the pathology and the more abnormal the pathways involve.

Next, the Disc Formula can be further expanded and used as 4-stage Formula. This involves adding either Sterilization or Vitality Sub-formula to the Disc Formula. For example, it could be AsEtSrD't or AsEtSrE't in case of Disease-orgin A. The number of repetitions is 5:5:1:5 when the treatment target is focused on the Upper Burner of the body, and 5:5:5:1 when it is focused on the Lower Burner. When the target is the entire body or the middle of the body, the treatment with 5:5:5:5 can also be applied.

This is not a strict rule, but generally, when the Sterilization Sub-formula is added, it is used in acute cases with intense pain. In contrast, when the Vitality Sub-formula is added, it is used for chronic cases existing over a longer period of time. You can use this 4-stage Formula on one side and apply the Sterilization or Vitality Formula on the other side, similar to how it was used previously.

For example, it could be AsEtSrD't 5:5:1:5 / AsE't ana 4:2 for Upper Burner lesion, or AsEtSrE't 5:5:5:1 / AsE't cata 4:2 for Lower Burner lesion.

If you master how to use the Unit Formulae, you can create a wide variety of different Formulae.

Guidelines for the Number of Repetitions in Constitution-acupuncture

Constitution-acupuncture treatment involves a series of repeated procedures. The specific number of repetitions is based on Master Do-won Kuon's unique numerology, aimed at achieving the best possible outcome in a single treatment session. Performing fewer or more repetitions than his rule tends to reduce the effectiveness of the therapy. This approach is analogous to the optimal number five being significant in the theory of the Five Phases, which was discussed in Chapter 1. While theoretically different numbers could be chosen, the system theory suggests that the minimum balanced system, where Synchronizing and Antagonizing act symmetrically at the same time, is represented by the number five, making it optimal for system analysis. Likewise, in the context of Compound Formula in acupuncture, different numbers may be applied, but for most conditions, performing 4 or 5 repetitions is generally considered the minimum number needed to achieve the greatest therapeutic effect.

If the treatment begins with an odd number of repetitions, then odd numbers are applied consistently to all subsequent Unit Formulae. Conversely, if it starts with an even number, then even numbers are applied throughout the subsequent Unit Formulae. The standard treatment, known as "Basic Formula" to treat the Disease-origin, typically involves 4 or 5 repetitions. There is also a special Formula that repeats only the Basic Formula 6 times. This specific Formula is a hemostasis procedure, effective for treating all types of bleeding conditions.

As previously mentioned, the 2-stage of treatment employs the combination of Basic Formula and Sub-formula in the ratio of 4:2 or 5:1. For the Zang-system Inflammation Formula, the ratio is set at 5:1, while other 2-stage

Formulae typically follow the 4:2 ratio. However, it has been noted that there are exceptions where the ratio for the Zang-system Inflammation Formula is adjusted to 4:2, or other 2-stage Formula may use the 5:1 ratio instead.

For the 3-stage treatment, which includes the Mental Sub-formula in addition to the 2-stage treatment, the ratio of repetitions is typically set as follows: Basic Formula : Sub-formula : Mental Sub-formula = 4:4:2 or 5:5:1. Specifically, for painful conditions, the 5:5:1 ratio is used, and is primarily applied to the conditions involving symptom of excess (實證, Shizheng) or symptom associated with severe pain. The 4:4:2 ratio, on the other hand, is mainly applied to the conditions related to symptom of deficiency (虛證, Xuzheng) in the body or those accompanied by cold feeling or paralysis.

When determining the number of repetitions based on histological findings in Western medicine, the treatment protocol for cancer sets all the Unit Formulae at 5 repetitions for epithelial cell carcinoma (carcinoma) and 4 repetitions for sarcoma. This distinction is made based on the classification of the epithelial cells as belonging to the Yang (positive) and the connective or parenchymal tissues as belonging to the Yin (negative).

Cancer treatment typically involves stage 4 or stage 5 procedures. Therefore, the number of repetitions is set using the ratios like 4:4:4:4, 5:5:5:5 for 4-stage treatment, or 4:4:4:4:4, 5:5:5:5:5 for 5-stage treatment. If the tumor is located in a Zang-system organ, such as the liver or pancreas, use Zang-system Unit Formulae. For epithelial cell carcinoma, the procedure is repeated five times, whereas for sarcoma, it is repeated four times. In cases where the tumors are found in Fu-system, use the Fu-system Unit Formulae may be used. Here as well, the procedure is repeated 5 times for the epithelial cell carcinoma and 4 times for the sarcoma.

For very severe diseases, the entire Compound Formula may be repeated in its entirety. If an even number of repetitions has been used in the Compound Formula, it is repeated once more (double treatments). If an odd number of repetitions has been used in the Compound Formula, it is repeated twice more (triple treatments).

This is a commonly used procedure, but alternative methods of applying the Formulae are also possible. The Basic Formula does not necessarily have to be applied first; the sequence may vary depending on the specific condition being treated. All 64 cases of types ①, ②, ③, and ④, which were previously identified as the patterns of excessive imbalance, can be used for treating the specific diseases.

The number of repetitions specified above also is not an absolute rule; it simply represents a typical pattern of application. It is also possible to use the previous three-stage Compound Formulae in the ratio of 4:4:4 or 5:5:5. In some cases, ratios like 3:3:3, 2:2:2, or even 1:1:1 may also be used. The same principle can apply to 4-stage and 5-stage Compound Formulae. The main concern is determining which ratio is the most effective.

Tips for administering Compound Formulae

In the clinical application of Compound Formulae, when a patient presents with multiple overlapping conditions, different Compound Formulae can be administered simultaneously on each side of the patient. For example, as described above, Zang-system Inflammation Formula can be applied to the left side, while Sterilization Formula can be applied to the right side. This approach allows for efficient treatment of multiple conditions simultaneously.

One important point to note is that performing the procedure on both sides does not necessarily double the effect. Instead, it might dilute the therapeutic power of acupuncture targeted at a single disease.

In some cases, two or more Compound Formulae are applied consecutively on one side. At this level, the methods of application can be considered almost limitless. If two 5-stage Formulae are performed in succession, it results in 10-stage Formula (This is only used in special cases. Generally, the 5-stage Formula is the highest level of application). This approach is similar to a series connection in electrical circuits. Conversely, using Compound Formulae on both the left and right sides can be likened to a parallel connection.

If Constitution-acupuncture is performed incorrectly, it can be reversed. The incorrectly placed acupuncture point can be retreated, and the previous Following or Meeting Method can be undone. In other words, the Following

Method acupuncture is replaced with the Meeting Method acupuncture on the same acupoints, and vice versa. After that, the correct Formula can be applied again. In this respect, Constitutional Medicine is very logical, as everything aligns in a mathematical manner. Now, let's return to the principles of Compound Formulae.

Excessive imbalances of three Zang-Fu organs (4-Stage Compound Formulae)

Let's take the example of 'ABE', the second case in type ③ earlier, where the excessive imbalances occur in three Zang-Fu organs. This situation involves the excessive imbalances in Zang-Fu organs A, B, and E. In this case, you simply can apply the Unit Formulae to drain A and B, and then replenish E in sequence. When there are excessive imbalances involving three or more Zang-Fu organs, Mental Sub-formula should be used in the third step. Thus, after applying the Unit Formula for B, you should use the Mental Sub-formula, followed by the Unit Formula for E.

Let's take an example of Geumeum Constitution with the structure of "Lungs-Large Intestines Kidneys-Bladder Pancreas-Stomach Heart-Small Intestines Liver-Gallbladder," where, in the case of ABE, there are excessive imbalances involving the Lungs-Large intestines, Kidneys-Bladder, and Liver-Gallbladder. The treatment begins by addressing the Lungs-Large intestines, and Kidneys-Bladder, and the Mental Sub-formula, and then the Unit Formula for the Liver-Gallbladder.

In this case of excessive imbalances across all Zang-system organs in Geumeum Constitution, the Unit Formula of draining the Lungs, draining the Kidneys, regulating Pericardium, and replenishing the Liver can be applied. I have observed good results using this approach with the 5:5:5:5 ratio for treating palmar keratosis in a patient with Geumeum Constitution as follows[94]:

[94] My clinical case is as follows: Patient C, female, 35 years old at the time of visit. This patient complained that when exposed to cold wind, the skin on the inside of her fingers would keratinize, crack, bleed, and become painful. I initially tried a few 2-stage

KI10 (Yingu)c, LU5 (Chize)c, LR1 (Dadun)p, LU11 (Shaoshang)p — 5 repetitions

LU8 (Jingqu)c, KI7 (Fuliu)c, HT8 (Shaofu)p, KI2 (Rangu)p — 5 repetitions

PC3 (Quze)c, PC9 (Zhongchong)p — 5 repetitions

LU8 (Jingqu)c, LR4 (Zhongfeng)c, HT8 (Shaofu)p, LR2 (Xingjian)p — 5 repetitions

In case of all Fu-system organs' excessive imbalances for the Geumeum Constitution, the Unit Formula of draining the Large Intestines, draining the Bladder, regulating Triple Burner, and replenishing Gallbladder can be applied in sequence. Using the ratio of 4:4:4:4, the Compound Formula is as follows:

BL66 (Zutonggu)c, LI2 (Erjian)c, GB41 (Zulinqi)p, LI3 (Sanjian)p — 4 repetitions

LI1 (Shangyang)c, BL67 (Zhiyin)c, SI5 (Yanggu)p, BL60 (Kunlun)p — 4 repetitions

TB2 (Yemen)c, TB3 (Zhongzhu)p — 4 repetitions

LI1 (Shangyang)c, GB44 (Zuqiaoyin)c, SI5 (Yanggu)p, GB38 (Yangfu)p — 4 repetitions

Summing up, in the case of excessive imbalances involving the three Zang-Fu organs A, B, and E, the order of the Compound Formula is As → Bs → Sr → Et. Each Unit Formulae (As, Bs, Sr, and Et) has two variations, that is, Zang or Fu. Therefore, the total number of possible Compound Formulae is $2 \times 2 \times 2 \times 2 = 2^4 = 16$. The appropriate number of repetitions is typically set as 4:4:4:4 or 5:5:5:5. However, if the condition is predominantly affecting the Upper Burner or surface area, the ratio is adjusted to 4:4:2:4 or 5:5:1:5. Conversely, if the condition is

---

Compound Formulae and other high-stage Compound Formulae, but they did not seem to have much effect. Then, I applied the above-mentioned Compound Formula twice, and the condition improved immediately. The effect was quite rapid.

predominantly affecting the Lower Burner or deeper area, the ratio is adjusted to 4:4:4:2 or 5:5:5:1.

In general, the number of repetitions tends to be 5 (odd number) for Zang-system diseases and 4 (even number) for Fu-system diseases. However, it is difficult to apply this rule uniformly, as there are many exceptions. Each disease has an optimal number of treatments that yield better results, and this optimal number must be determined through careful reasoning and clinical experience.

Excessive imbalances in four Zang-Fu organs (5-Stage Compound Formulae)

Lastly, let's examine the case of excessive imbalances involving four Zang-Fu organs. In the example of 'ABDE', Zang-Fu A and B are excessively increased, while D and E are excessively decreased. Thus, the Compound Formula should be applied in the following sequence: As → Bs → Sr → Dt → Et.

For the Toeum Constitution ("Pancreas-Stomach Lungs-Large intestine Heart-Small intestine Liver-Gallbladder Kidneys-Bladder"), where all the Zang organs are imbalanced, applying each Unit Formula 5 times results in the following Compound Formula:

LU8 (Jingqu)c, SP5 (Shangqiu)c, KI10 (Yingu)p, SP9 (Yinlingquan)p — 5 repetitions

SP3 (Taibai)c, LU9 (Taiyuan)c, LR1 (Dadun)p, LU11 (Shaoshang)p — 5 repetitions

PC5 (Jianshi)c, PC3 (Quze)p — 5 repetitions

LU8 (Jingqu)c, LR4 (Zhongfeng)c, KI10 (Yingu)p, LR8 (Ququan)p — 5 repetitions

SP3 (Taibai)c, KI3 (Taixi)c, LR1 (Dadun)p, KI1 (Yongquan)p — 5 repetitions

As above, it is not just the Zang or only the Fu organs that cause excessive imbalance; there are also instances where both the Zang and Fu organs are mixed, leading to excessive imbalances. In such situations, a combination of Unit Formulae for the specific Zang and Fu organs involved can be used to correct the imbalances.

For example of Suyang Constitution ("Kidneys-Bladder Lungs-Large intestine Liver-Gallbladder Heart-Small intestine Pancreas-Stomach"), if there is a sequential imbalances affecting the Lungs, Stomach, Kidneys, and Small intestine, then the Unit Formulae for draining the Lungs, replenishing the Stomach, regulating the Triple Burner, draining the Kidneys, and replenishing the Small intestine can be used. If all four times are applied to the Unit Formulae, the Compound Formula can be as follows:

HT8 (Shaofu)p, LU10 (Yuji)p, KI10 (Yingu)c, LU5 (Chize)c — 4 repetitions

SI5 (Yanggu)p, ST41 (Jiexi)p, BL66 (Zutonggu)c, ST44 (Neiting)c — 4 repetitions

PC7 (Daling)p, PC5 (Jianshi)c — 4 repetitions

SP3 (Taibai)p, KI3 (Taixi)p, LU8 (Jingqu)c, KI7 (Fuliu)c — 4 repetitions

ST36 (Zusanli)p, SI8 (Xiaohai)p, LI1 (Shangyang)c, SI1 (Shaoze)c — 4 repetitions

If the Mental Sub-formula of Fu-system is applied, then use TB10 (Tianjing) p, TB1 (Guanchong) c — 4 repetitions.

General Compound Formulae

So far, we have explored the principles of Compound Formulae through specific examples. Upon closer examination of cases ①, ②, and ③ discussed above, it becomes evident that they are all encompassed within case ④. In fact, cases ①, ②, and ③ represent special cases of case ④. Specifically, if we take the first element of case ④, it corresponds to case ①; if we take the first two elements, it corresponds to case ②; and if we take the first three elements, it corresponds to case ③. Thus, case ④ serves as a generalization of all Compound Formulae. Please refer to the following table.

	Column 1	Column 2	Column 3	Column 4	Column 5	Column 6
Row A	AsBsSrDtEt	AsBsSrEtDt	AsDtSrBsEt	AsDtSrEtBs	AsEtSrBsDt	AsEtSrDtBs
Row B	BsAsSrDtEt	BsAsSrEtDt	BsDtSrAsEt	BsDtSrEtAs	BsEtSrAsDt	BsEtSrDtAs
Row D	DtAsSrBsEt	DtAsSrEtBs	DtBsSrAsEt	DtBsSrEtAs	DtEtSrAsBs	DtEtSrBsAs
Row E	EtAsSrBsDt	EtAsSrDtBs	EtBsSrAsDt	EtBsSrDtAs	EtDtSrAsBs	EtDtSrBsAs

Figure 3. General Compound Formulae

These 24 General Compound Formulae encompass all possible Compound Formulae. The symbols A, B, S, D, and E represent all types of Zang-Fu organs. When necessary, the Zang organ is denoted as A, B, S, D, and E, while the Fu organ is represented as A', B', S', D', and E'.

(Note: This table provides General Compound Formulae based on the assumption that a Zang-Fu of the same Qi is used only once. For instance, it is uncommon for a Compound Formula involving both A and A' to be used simultaneously in a single Compound Formula. If Zang and Fu organ of the same Qi are included in a single Compound Formula, the number of possible Compound Formulae can increase almost infinitely. Unexpectedly, such highly complex Formulae are often seen in clinical practice.)

In each cell of the table above, there is one General Compound Formula. Let's consider an example using the General Compound Formula in column 1 of row A. The General Compound Formula in this cell is AsBsSrDtEt. This formula addresses every case, ranging from an excessive imbalance in a single Zang-Fu organ to all possible excessive imbalances affecting up to four Zang-Fu organs.

If there is an excessive imbalance in one Zang organ, it can be treated with As alone. For imbalances involving two Zang organs, the treatment can be

AsBs, or AsBsSr if the Mental Sub-formula is included. For three organs, the Formula expands to AsBsSrDt. Finally, for imbalances across four organs, the Formula becomes AsBsSrDtEt. Thus, depending on the severity of the condition, any of the following Compound Formulae may be used: As (stage 1)→ AsBs (Stage 2)→ AsBsSr (Stage 3)→ AsBsSrDt (Stage 4)→ AsBsSrDtEt (Stage 5).

The General Compound Formula in each cell can replace specific Compound Formulae in all cases involving excessive imbalances across one Zang-Fu organ (A), two Zang-Fu organs (AB), three Zang-Fu organs (ABD), or four Zang-Fu organs (ABDE). Therefore, it can be concluded that a single General Compound Formula encompasses all Formulae across stages 1 to 5.

For example, a commonly used two-stage Formulae involves the first two Unit Formulae in column 3 of row A in the case of Mogyang, Geumeum, Suyang, and Toeum Constitutions where "A" out of the Zang-Fu Array "ABCDE" is the Disease-origin. Specifically, these are AsDt and AsD't, representing the Fu-system Inflammation Formula and Sterilization Formula, respectively. Similarly, in column 5 of row A, the first two Unit Formulae (AsEt and AsE't, representing the Zang-system Inflammation Formula and Vitality Formula, respectively) also form a two-stage Compound Foumulae.

For Constitutions like Geumyang, Mogeum, Toyang, and Sueum, where "E" is the Disease-origin, the first two Unit Formulae in column 3 of row E (EtBs and EtB's, representing the Fu-system Inflammation Formula and Sterilization, respectively), and the first two Unit Formulae in column 1 of row E (EtAs and EtA's, representing the Zang-system Inflammation Formula and Vitality Formula, respectively) form two-stage Compound Formulae.

Additionally, the Mental Formula is represented by AsSr for the Constitutions where A is the Disease-origin, and EtSr for the Constitutions where E is the Disease-origin (refer to the list of two-stage Compound Formulae in Figure 2).

Also, for the Disc Formula, which is representative of the 3-stage Formulae, in the case of the Constitutions where A is the Disease-origin, the first three Unit Formulae, AsEtSr in column 5 of row A becomes the Disc Formula. In the case of the Constitutions where E is the Disease-origin, the first three Unit Formulae in column 1 of row E, EtAsSr, form the Disc

Formula. In this way, all Compound Formulae that we can construct can be derived from this General Compound Formulae.

As shown in the table, there are only 24 General Compound Formulae. However, if you consider all the cases from stage 1 to 5, countless Compound Formulae can be derived. How many might there be?

Let's start by examining the case where all four Zang-Fu organs are excessively imbalanced (5-stage Compound Formulae). In the table above, each Formula is composed of five Unit Formulae, and each Unit Formula can be either Zang or Fu organ, giving us two possible scenarios for each. We can use this to calculate the total number of cases.

For example, in column 1 of row A, "A" can be either the Zang or Bu, "B" can also be the Zang or Bu, and the same applies to S, D, and E. Each of these has two possibilities. Thus, the number of possible combinations is $2 \times 2 \times 2 \times 2 \times 2 = 2^5 = 32$ (cases) for each General Compound Formula.

Therefore, since there are 32 cases for each of the 24 General Compound Formulae, we get a total of: $24 \times 2^5 = 768$ (cases). Thus, a total of 768 Compound Formulae (5-stage Compound Formulae) are theoretically possible when all four Zang-Fu organs are excessively imbalanced.

If three Zang-Fu organs are excessively imbalanced, we can use the first four Unit Formulae from each General Formula in the table above (4-stage Compound Formulae). For example, AsBsSrDt in row A of column 1, and DtEtSrAs in row D of column 5.

If two Zang-Fu organs are imbalanced, we can refer to the columns 1, 3, and 5 in the table (columns 2, 4, and 6 overlap with these columns). In this case, we use the first two Unit Formulae from the General Formulae (e.g., BsDt in row B of column 3, and EtDt in row E of column 5), which form 2-stage Compound Formula.

If we include the Mental Sub-formulae, we can take the first three Unit Formulae in sequence (3-stage Compound Formula). For example, BsDtSr in row B of column 3 and EtDtSr in row E of column 5 are possible cases.

If only one Zang-Fu organ is excessively imbalanced, we use the first Unit Formula from column 1 of the table (other columns overlap), resulting in a 1-stage Compound Formula (e.g., As, Bs, Dt, Et).

Moving to the next stage, let's consider the four-stage Compound Formulae. The four-stage Compound Formulae consist of 24 General Formulae. Each Unit Formula within a General Formula has two possibilities: Zang and Fu. Therefore, the total number of possible cases for the four-stage Compound Formulae (24 General Formulae of the four-stage) is: $2^4 \times 24 = 384$ cases.

Likewise, for the 3-stage Compound Formulae, the number of cases is $2^3 \times 12 = 96$ cases, and for the 2-stage Compound Formulae, the number of cases is $2^2 \times 12 = 48$ cases, and for the 1-stage Compound Formulae, the number of cases is $2 \times 4 = 8$ cases. From this, we can conclude that theoretically, up to 1,304 (= 8+ 48 + 96 + 384 + 768) Compound Formulae are possible when considering all stages combined.

This General Compound Formulae does not account for the cases where Zang and Fu with the same Qi are used simultaneously in a single Compound Formula. For instance, there is a Formula for the Suyang Constitution expressed as IsVIItIII'rVIIIt, which, when represented in the General Formula, corresponds to AsEtSrE't. So, this deviates from the General Formula table above. This is an example of the Unit Formulae that simultaneously addresses both the Lungs (E) and the Large intestine (E'), which belong to the same Qi, Metal, within a single Compound Formula, AsEtSrE't. It can be considered a combination of the Disc Formula and Vitality Sub-formula. The core Formula remains the Disc Formula, AsEtSr. This situation is a special case and is not very common. If we also include these exceptions, the total number of possible Formulae would far exceed the previously calculated 1,304 Compound Formulae.

Treating multiple diseases with one Compound Formula

Another important point is that a Compound Formula does not treat only a single disease. One Compound Formula functions like a category, encompassing all the diseases that fit within that category. In other words, regardless of the disease names, if they share the same pathology that aligns with a specific Compound Formula, then the entire group of diseases can be treated using that single Compound Formula. Consider the scope of the Disc Formula mentioned earlier. With just one Disc Formula, dozens of different diseases can be treated. Therefore, the number of diseases that can be addressed by the 1,304 Compound Formulae calculated earlier can be considered practically infinite.

Application example of the General Compound Formula

Let's look at an example of applying the General Formula using Toyang Constitution ("Pancreas-Stomach Heart-Small intestine Liver-Gallbladder Lungs-Large intestine Kidneys-Bladder"). In the General Formula above, let's arbitrarily select the case from row E of column 3, and apply it to the Toyang Constitution. The General Formula in row E of column 3 is EtBsSrAsDt.

For the 5-stage Formula, each Et, Bs, Sr, As, and Dt can have cases of excessive imbalances either of Zang or Fu. Thus, if we consider all possible cases, we get the following (a total of $2^5 = 32$ cases):

IXtIIIsIII'rVsVIIt	XtIIIsIII'rVsVIIt	IXtIVsIII'rVsVIIt	IXtIIIsIV'rVsVIIt
IXtIIIsIII'rVIsVIIt	IXtIIIsIII'rVsVIIIt	XtIVsIII'rVsVIIt	XtIIIsIV'rVsVIIt
XtIIIsIII'rVIsVIIt	XtIIIsIII'rVsVIIIt	IXtIVsIV'rVsVIIt	IXtIVsIII'rVIsVIIt
IXtIVsIII'rVsVIIIt	IXtIIIsIV'rVIsVIIt	IXtIIIsIV'rVsVIIIt	IXtIIIsIII'rVIsVIIIt
IXtIIIsIV'rVIsVIIIt	IXtIVsIII'rVIsVIIIt	IXtIVsIV'rVsVIIIt	IXtIVsIV'rVIsVIIt
XtIIIsIII'rVIsVIIIt	XtIIIsIV'rVsVIIIt	XtIIIsIV'rVIsVIIt	XtIVsIII'rVsVIIIt
XtIVsIII'rVIsVIIt	XtIVsIV'rVsVIIt	IXtIVsIV'rVIsVIIIt	XtIIIsIV'rVIsVIIIt
XtIVsIII'rVIsVIIIt	XtIVsIV'rVsVIIIt	XtIVsIV'rVIsVIIt	XtIVsIV'rVIsVIIIt

Figure 4. Example of applying the General Formula EtBsSrAsDt to Toyang Constitution

If you substitute the Unit Formulae of the Toyang Constitution here, all Compound Formulae in row E of column 3 can be easily derived. The Unit Formulae for the Toyang Constitution are as follows:

IX t = SP3(Taibai)c KI3(Taixi)c LU8(Jingqu)p KI7(Fuliu)p
III s = SP3(Taibai)c HT7(Shenmen)c LU8(Jingqu)p HT4(Lingdao)p
V s = HT8(Shaofu)c SP2(Dadu)c KI10(Yingu)p SP9(Yinlingquan)p
VII t = HT8(Shaofu)c LU10(Yuji)c KI10(Yingu)p LU5(Chize)p
X t = ST36(Zusanli)c BL40(Weizhong)c LI1(Shangyang)p BL67(Zhiyin)p
IV s = ST36(Zusanli)c SI8(Xiaohai)c LI1(Shangyang)p SI1(Shaoze)p
VI s = SI5(Yanggu)c ST41(Jiexi)c BL66(Zutonggu)p ST44(Neiting)p
VIII t = SI5(Yanggu)c LI5(Yangxi)c BL66(Zutonggu)p LI2(Erjian)p
III'r = PC8(Laogong)c PC3(Quze)p
IV'r = TB6(Zhigou)c TB2(Yemen)p

For example, if the Compound Formula (IXtIVsIV'rVsVIIIt) from row 5 of column 3 in Figure 4 is expressed as a specific Formula (with the number of repetitions set to 4), it is as follows:

SP3 (Taibai)c KI3 (Taixi)c LU8 (Jingqu)p KI7 (Fuliu)p
ST36 (Zusanli)c SI8 (Xiaohai)c LI1 (Shangyang)p SI1 (Shaoze)p
TB6 (Zhigou)c TB2 (Yemen)p
HT8 (Shaofu)c SP2 (Dadu)c KI10 (Yingu)p SP9 (Yinlingquan)p
SI5 (Yanggu)c LI5 (Yangxi)c BL66 (Zutonggu)p LI2 (Erjian)p

Among the 32 application examples of the Compound Formula, EtBsSrAsDt in Figure 4 above, IXtIIIsIII'rVsVIIt and XtIVsIV'rVIsVIIIt are the most frequently used Compound Formulae in 5-stage Formula for Toyang Constitution. The former is a 5-stage Formula consisting solely of Zang-system Unit Formulae, while the latter is a 5-stage Formula made up entirely of Fu-system Unit Formulae. These two Formulae are very important. With just these two Formulae, many severe diseases in the individuals with Toyang Constitution can be effectively treated. Based on this, the most typical treatment stages identified by me can be divided into Zang-system and Fu-system and can be expressed in General Formulae as follows.

Five-stage Formulae for Mogyang, Geumeum, Suyang, and Toeum Constitutions, where "A" is the Disease-origin:

Zang-system: AsDtSrEtBs
Fu-system: A'sD'tS'rE'tB's

Five-stage Formulae for Geumyang, Mogeum, Toyang, and Sueum Constitutions, where "E" is the Disease-origin:

Zang-system: EtBsSrAsDt
Fu-system: E'tB'sS'rA'sD't

I hope you can use these guidelines to create Formulae for various diseases. All possible Formulae are included in the General Compound Formulae shown in Figure 3. Initially, try treating by appropriately combining 2-stage or 3-stage Formulae. Once you get comfortable with this, you can create your own 4-stage or 5-stage Compound Formulae and attempt a treatment. The Formulae can be composed entirely of the Unit Formulae targeting the Zang-system, or it can consist solely of the Unit Formulae from the Fu-system. Alternatively, it can sometimes be created by appropriately mixing the Unit Formulae from both the Zang-system and the Fu-system. Depending on your understanding of physiology and pathology, you can develop an infinite variety of Formulae based on these principles.

In Eight-Constitution Medicine, if you know the Compound Formula for one Constitution, you can immediately obtain the desired treatment Formula for other Constitutions by converting the Zang-Fu using the above General Compound Formula. This is where the scientific nature of Eight-Constitution Medicine becomes evident. It exhibits the perfect regularity. The table for Zang-Fu conversion between the Constitutions is shown below. Zang and Fu in the same row can be converted interchangeably.

For example, the imbalances of the Liver and Pancreas in the Geumyang Constitution can be converted to the imbalances of the Liver and Pancreas in the Mogyang Constitution, the imbalances of the Lungs and Heart in the Geumeum and Mogeum Constitutions, the imbalances of the Kidneys and Heart in the Toyang and Suyang Constitutions, and the imbalances of the

Pancreas and Liver in the Toeum and Sueum Constitutions, respectively. Therefore, the same Formula can be applied to the diseases with the same pathology in other Constitutions if needed. The examples here all correspond to the Fu-system Inflammation Formula. Thus, if a specific disease is treated with a certain Formula for one Constitution, the same Formula can be applied to other Constitutions with the same disease, based on this conversion table.

Geumyang/ Mogyang	Geumeum/ Mogeum	Toyang/ Suyang	Toeum/ Sueum
Liver (I)	Lung (VII)	Kidney (IX)	Pancreas (V)
Pancreas (V)	Heart (III)	Heart (III)	Liver (I)
Pericardium (III')	Pericardium (III')	Pericardium (III')	Pericardium (III')
Lung (VII)	Liver (I)	Pancreas (V)	Kidney (IX)
Kidney (IX)	Kidney (IX)	Lung (VII)	Lung (VII)
Gallbladder (II)	L. intestine (VIII)	Bladder (X)	Stomach (VI)
Stomach (VI)	S. intestine (IV)	S. intestine (IV)	Gallbladder (II)
Triple Burner (IV')	Triple Burner (IV')	Triple Burner (IV')	Triple Burner (IV')
L. intestine (VIII)	Gallbladder (II)	Stomach (VI)	Bladder (X)
Bladder (X)	Bladder (X)	L. intestine (VIII)	L. intestine (VIII)

Figure 5. Eight-Constitution Zang-Fu conversion table

Compound Formulae: the world of freedom

I regard Compound Formulae as the world of freedom. From the definition of Constitution to the laws governing the exchange of Qis between Zang-Fu organs and the composition of Unit Formulae, this is a realm governed by strict mathematical principles, leaving no room for error. However, when it comes to the Compound Formulae, a vast open plain suddenly unfolds. While the derivation of the General Equation of the Compound Formulae is based on the clear principles, its specific application is highly flexible. It is a world where a wide range of methods are accepted, depending on the doctor's experience, intuition, sensitivity, solid theoretical foundation, and individual personality.

Thus, I compared the Unit Formulae to words, and the Compound Formulae to sentences made up of those words. Everyone knows the meaning of a word and has the option to use it, but the word alone cannot convey the sufficient meaning. This is because the quality of sentences formed from words with limited meanings is determined by the person's skill and writing ability, acquired through intensive training. In other words, while everyone knows the words that form the building blocks of language, the ability to combine them into elegant and precise sentences depends on the personal skill of the individual using those words.

Of course, the Unit Formula, which serves as a repository of precise words, is the most fundamental and essential premise. The Compound Formulae are a realm of freedom where you can fully express your individuality using these Unit Formulae! However, it is a freedom that exists within the strict order of the Zang-Fu Structure known as Constitution.

In Eight-Constitution Medicine, numerous Compound Formulae have been developed, ranging from minor ailments such as colds, digestive issues, headaches, and sprains to more severe conditions like herniated discs, hepatitis, cirrhosis, heart disease, stroke, immune system disorders, allergic diseases, and even malignant tumors. These Compound Formulae are widely used in the treatment of almost every disease that humans may suffer from. Most of them are included in the General Compound Formulae mentioned above.

However, the Compound Formulae currently in use represent only a small fraction of the General Compound Formulae. Eight-Constitution Medicine is truly a blue ocean with limitless possibilities. Countless Compound Formulae, whose effectiveness has yet to be explored, await the expertise of Eight-Constitution Medicine specialists.

CHAPTER 5

Constitution-acupuncture Formulary

CONSTITUTION-ACUPUNCTURE DOES NOT TARGET THE DISEASE. IT TARGETS YOURSELF.

CHAPTER 5

Constitution-acupuncture Formulary

The following data are Constitution-acupuncture Formulae frequently used in clinical practice. Some of these are what Master Doh-ol Young-oak Kim learned from Master Do-won Kuon, some are what I learned from fellow Korean Medicine doctors who study the Eight-Constitution Medicine, while others come from my firsthand experience treating many patients in my clinical practice. All the valuable data painstakingly collected have been compiled into an easy-to-read table.

Tracing back to the origins, most of this data was either directly published by Master Do-won Kuon, the founder of Eight-Constitution Medicine, through his clinical findings, or passed down by those close to him. This means that we owe a great debt to Master Do-won Kuon who dedicated his entire life to researching Eight-Constitution Medicine.

I hope that you will cherish this data and apply it well in your clinical practice. It will serve as valuable, gem-like information for Korean Medicine doctors specializing in Eight-Constitution Medicine, professors and students of Korean Medicine colleges, and researchers in the related fields.

Legend

The conventions used in the formulary introduced here are explained below. The Constitution Structure Formula is represented as "AA' BB' CC' DD' EE'," where A, B, C, D, and E refer to the Five Zang organs, and A', B', C', D', and E' refer to the Five Fu organs, which are in the complementary relationship with each other.

For the Geumeum, Toeum, Mogyang, and Suyang Constitutions, where A is the Disease-origin, the Unit Formula protocol is as follows.

As: Basic Formula
A's: Fu-system Basic Formula
Bs: Degeneration Sub-formula
B's: Fu-system Degeneration Sub-formula
Sr: Mental Sub-formula
S'r: Fu-system Mental Sub-formula
Dt: Fu-system Inflammation Sub-formula
D't: Sterilization Sub-formula
Et: Zang-system Inflammation Sub-formula
E't: Vitality Sub-formula

For the Geumyang, Toyang, Mogeum, and Sueum Constitutions, where E is the Disease-origin, the Unit Formula protocol is as follows.

Et: Basic Formula
E't: Fu-system Basic Formula
Dt: Degeneration Sub-formula
D't: Fu-system Degeneration Sub-formula
Sr: Mental Sub-formula
S'r: Fu-system Mental Sub-formula
Bs: Fu-system Inflammation Sub-formula
B's: Sterilization Sub-formula
As: Zang-system Inflammation Sub-formula
A's: Vitality Sub-formula

For convenience, in this formulary, the subscripts (s, r, t) of Unit Formulae are omitted and simply written as "A, A', B, B', S, S', D, D', E, E'." For example, in the formulary, BESD, which is a Formula for itching for those with Geumeum, Toeum, Mogyang, and Suyang Constitutions, involves the treatment in the following sequence with the Unit Formulae: Bs (Degeneration Sub-formula), Et (Zang-system Inflammation Sub-formula), Sr (Mental Sub-formula), and Dt (Fu-system Inflammation Sub-formula).

The number next to the Formula indicates the number of repetitions for each Unit Formula, based on my clinical experience and what is generally known or frequently applied. For example, it is written as 4424 for BESD, which means 4 times Bs, 4 times Et, 2 times Sr, and 4 times Dt.

In a two-stage Formula, the English lowercase letter "a" added to the end of the Formula stands for "ana," which indicates the Upper Burner treatment, while "c" stands for "cata," indicating the Lower Burner treatment.

In this formulary, the number of repetitions is indicated only for Constitutions where "A" is the Disease-origin (Geumyang, Toeum, Mogyang, Suyang). Likewise, the same number of repetitions applies for the Constitutions where "E" is the Disease-origin (Geumyang, Toeum, Mogeum, Suyang) as well.

In the actual clinical practice, Formulae (Compound Formulae) are written using Zang-Fu symbols for each Constitution as in the Figure 1 below. Here, it should be noted that the Zang-Fu organs (A, B, A', B') belonging to the Yang Field should be drained, while the Zang-Fu organs (D, E, D', E') belonging to the Yin Field should be replenished.

Zang-Fu	A	B	S	D	E	A'	B'	S'	D'	E'
Geumeum	VII	IX	III'	III	I	VIII	X	IV'	IV	II
Toeum	V	VII	III'	I	IX	VI	VIII	IV'	II	X
Mogyang	I	IX	III'	V	VII	II	X	IV'	VI	VIII
Suyang	IX	VII	III'	III	V	X	VIII	IV'	IV	VI
Geumyang	VII	V	III'	IX	I	VIII	VI	IV'	X	II
Toyang	V	III	III'	VII	IX	VI	IV	IV'	VIII	X
Mogeum	I	III	III'	IX	VII	II	IV	IV'	X	VIII
Sueum	IX	I	III'	VII	V	X	II	IV'	VIII	VI

Figure 1. Unit Formula Table Indicated with Zang-Fu Symbols for Each Constitution

For example, in the table above, the Zang "B" belongs to the Yang Field, so the Unit Formula is Bs. This corresponds to the Degeneration Sub-formula for Geumeum, Toeum, Mogyang, and Suyang Constitutions, and to the Fu-system Inflammation Sub-formula for Geumyang, Toyang, Mogeum, and Sueum Constitutions.

Additionally, since Fu "E'" belongs to the Yin Field, the Unit Formula is E't, which corresponds to the Vitality Sub-formula for Geumeum, Toeum, Mogyang, and Suyang Constitutions, and to the Fu-system Basic Formula for Geumyang, Toyang, Mogeum, and Sueum Constitutions.

Specific Unit Formulae can be easily obtained by replenishing or draining the relevant Zang or Fu (refer to the Unit Formulae table in Chapter 3).

If the Compound Formula BESD for pruritus, as mentioned above, is expressed using Zang-Fu symbols for the Mogyang Constitution, it would be "IX VII III' V" (refer to the Mogyang Constitution's row in the table shown above).

Draining Kidneys as Degeneration Sub-formula: SP3(Taibai)p KI3(Taixi) p LR1(Dadun)c KI (Yongquan)c

Replenishing Lungs as Zang-system Inflammation Sub-formula: SP3(Taibai)p LU9(Taiyuan)p LR1(Dadun)c LU11(Shaoshang)c

Regulating Pericardium as Mental Sub-formula: PC5(Jianshi)p PC3(Quze)c

Replenishing Pancreas as Fu-system Inflammation Sub-formula: LU8(Jingqu)p SP5(Shangqiu)p KI10(Yingu)c SP9(Yinlingquan)c

For other Constitutions, you can easily obtain the desired Compound Formulae using the same method in the table above.

The prescriptions disclosed here are primarily those discovered through Master Do-won Kuon's extensive clinical experience. While I was working at Doh-ol Clinic, I gathered materials related to Eight-Constitution Medicine from Master Doh-ol Young-oak Kim. I also collected the data from the seminars with Dr. Jae-jeong Park, the director of Dochoo Korean Medicine Clinic and fellow Korean Medicine doctors who attended the seminars, and from Mido Jhang's book, "*ECM Eleven Issues*," as well as from my own long-term clinical experience.

I believe that there should be countless Formulae in Dr. Do-won Kuon's archive, accumulated over his lifetime, that remain undisclosed to the world. I hope that these valuable resources should also be made public for the research of Eight-Constitution Medicine experts.

These Formulae in the following formulary table should be appropriately selected and applied by the specialists in Eight-Constitution Medicine, depending on the severity of the disease, the patient's condition, and individual characteristics.

Constitution-acupuncture Formulary

Constitutional Zang-Fu Structure Formula: [AA' BB' CC' DD' EE']

In this table, for the Geumeum, Toeum, Mogyang, and Suyang Constitutions with a Disease-origin of "A," it is advised to use the Formulae in the left column, while for the Geumyang, Toyang, Mogeum, and Sueum Constitutions with a Disease-origin of "E," it is advised to use the Formulae in the right column.

Disease & Symptom	Geumeum, Toeum, Mogyang, Suyang	Geumyang, Toyang, Mogeum, Sueum
abnormal viginal discharge	ADc 42	EBc
abnormal viginal discharge	AD'c 42	EB'c
acne	A'DS'/AD' 442/42	E'BS'/EB'
acne	ADS/AD'a 442/42	EBS/EB'a
acne	E'B'S'AD 44444	A'D'S'EB
allergic asthma	D'A'S'DE 55515	B'E'S'BA
allergic asthma	ADSE'B' 55515	EBSA'D'
allergic conjunctivitis	A'D'S'BE 55515	E'B'S'DA
allergic dermatitis	A'D'S'BD 44424	E'B'S'DB
allergic dermatitis	A'DS'D'E 44424	E'BS'B'A
allergic dermatitis	ADSE'B' 44424	EBSA'D'
allergic rhinitis	AE'SD 4424	EA'SB
allergic rhinitis	A'D'S'DE 44424	E'B'S'BA
allergic rhinitis	B'E'S'D' 4424	D'A'S'B'
allergic rhinitis	AE'S'D 4424	EA'S'B
allergy	D'A'S'DE 55555	B'E'S'BA
allergy	BESE'D' 55555	DASA'B'
amenorrhea	AD'S 442	EB'S
angina pectoris	BDSA/ADSD'E' 5515/55515	DBSE/EBSB'A'
angina pectoris	BE'S/ADa 551/42	DA'S/EBa
angina pectoris	BE'S/AEa 551/51	DA'S/EAa
angina pectoris	B'E'S'D' 5515	D'A'S'B'
ankylosing spondylitis	BESD'/AES 5555/551	DASB'/EAS
ankylosing spondylitis	ABSA'D' 55515	EDSE'B'
anxiety	A'D'S'B'E' 55555	E'B'S'D'A'
anxiety	AE/AS 51/51	EA/ES
arteriosclerosis	B'E'S'A 4444	D'A'S'E

arteriosclerosis	D'E'S' 442	B'A'S'
asthma	BESD'E' 55515	DASB'A'
asthma	D'E'S'EA 55515	B'A'S'AE
asthma	A'D'S'E'B' 55515	E'B'S'A'D'
asthma	BESD'A' 55515	DASB'E'
asthma	D'A'S'E'E 55515	B'E'S'A'A
asthma	EBSD'A' 55515	ADSB'E'
asthma (allergic)	A'D'S'DE 55515	E'B'S'BA
atopic dermatitis	A'D'S'B' 4424	E'B'S'D'
atopic dermatitis	BESD/A'D'S'B' 4424/4424	DASB/E'B'S'D'
atopic dermatitis	A'D'S'D 4424	E'B'S'B
atrophic gastritis	BE'S 442	DA'S
back pain	AESB 5555	EASD
back pain	AESE' 5555	EASA'
back pain	AESD' 5555	EASB'
back pain	AES/AE'c 551/42	EAS/EA'c
Behçet's Disease[95]	ADS/AD' 442/42	EBS/EB'
bile duct stones	AE' 42	EA'
bladder atony	AE'c 42	EA'c
blood circulation disorder	B'E'S'D' 4444	D'A'S'B
blood circulation disorder	AE'SD 4444	EA'SB
brain tumor	BE'SA 4424	DA'SE
bronchiectasis	DESB'A' 55515	BASD'E'
bronchiectasis	EBSD'A' 55515	ADSB'E'
bronchitis	D'A'S'DE 55515	B'E'S'BA

[95] Behçet's disease: A rare chronic inflammatory condition that causes inflammation in various organs of the body. The main symptoms include oral ulcers, genital ulcers, eye inflammation (uveitis), red nodules on the skin, joint pain, vasculitis, and central nervous system inflammation.

cartilage wear	ABS 551	EDS
cartilage wear	ABSB' 5555	EDSD'
cataract	D'A'S'B'E' 44424	B'E'S'D'A'
cataract	D'A'S'B'D' 44424	B'E'S'D'B'
cerebral hemorrhage	A'D'S'D 5515	E'B'S'B
cerebral hemorrhage	BDSD' 5515	DBSB'
cerebral hemorrhage	BDSE 5515	DBSA
cerebral infarction	E'BS'A 4424	A'DS'E
cerebral infarction (hypotension)[96]	BESA' 4424	DASE'
cerebral infarction (thrombus)[97]	AE'S 551	EA'S
chest congestion	B'E'S' 551	D'A'S'
cholecystitis, cholangitis, gallbladder cyst	AD/AD' 42/42	EB/EB'
chondromalacia[98]	AESB' 5555	EASD'
cirrhosis, hepatic cancer	BESDA' 55555	DASBE'
cirrhosis, hepatic cancer	BESDA 55555	DASBE
cirrhosis, hepatic cancer	AESDB 55555	EASBD
cold	AD'S/ADa 551/42	EB'S/EBa
cold hands and feet	AE'SD' 4424	EA'SB'
cold hands and feet	BE'SD 4424	DA'SB
cold lower abdomen	AE'SD 4442	EA'SB
cold with body aches	AD'S/AES 551/551	EB'S/EAS
constipation	ADSD'E' 44442	EBSB'A'
constipation	ADS/AD' 442/42	EBS/EB'
constipation	AD/AE' 42/42	EB/EA'

[96] Refers to cerebral infarction caused by low blood pressure.
[97] Refers to cerebral infarction caused by a blood clot.
[98] Chondromalacia: A condition that causes pain, a feeling of wear or tear, and swelling in the knee joint due to the softening and rupture of the cartilage under the patella.

constipation	AD/AD' 42/42	EB/EB'
cough	A'D'S'DE 55515	E'B'S'BA
cystitis, urethritis	ADc/AD'c 42/42	EBc/EB'c
degenerative arthritis	AE'S 551	EA'S
degenerative arthritis	BES 551	DAS
degenerative arthritis	E'B'S'A'D' 55555	A'D'S'E'B'
degenerative arthritis	ABSB'/AESD' 5555/5555	EDSD'/EASB'
degenerative arthritis	B'E'S' 551	D'A'S'
depression	B'E'S' 551	D'A'S'
depression	AE/ASa 51/51	EA/ESa
dermatitis	A'D'S'DE 44444	E'B'S'BA
diabetes	AE/ASa 51/51	EA/ESa
diabetes	A'D'S'E'B 55555	E'B'S'A'D
diarrhea	ADc/AD'c 42/42	EBc/EB'c
diplopia	ADS 442	EBS
dysautonomia	A'DS' 442	E'BS'
dysautonomia	B'E'S'D' 4444	D'A'S'B'
dysautonomia	A'D'S'B'E' 44444	E'B'S'D'A'
dysautonomia	D'E'S' 442	B'A'S'
dysmenorrhea	ADc 42	EBc
dysmenorrhea	AE'S/ADc 551/42	EA'S/EBc
dysmenorrhea	AES/ADS 551/442	EAS/EBS
edema	ADSD'E' 55555	EBSB'A'
edema (diabetic)	A'D'S'E'B 55555	E'B'S'A'D
endometritis	BESD' 4442	DASB'
endometritis	BESD 4442	DASB
epilepsy	ADS 551	EBS
esophagitis, plum pit Qi	ADa/ASa 51/51	EBa/ESa

esophagitis, plum pit Qi	ADS/AD'a 442/42	EBS/EB'a
esophagitis, plum pit Qi	ADS/AE'a 442/42	EBS/EA'a
esophagitis, plum pit Qi	AE'a 42	EA'a
esophagitis, plum pit Qi	A'D'S'B'/ADS 4424/442	E'B'S'D'/EBS
facial cramps[99]	AES 551	EAS
facial palsy	AESE' 5515	EASA'
facial palsy	A'DS'E 5515	E'BS'A
facial pain	AES/AD'a 551/42	EAS/EB'a
facial pain	EDSD'A' 55515	ABSB'E'
facial pain	AES/AD'S 551/442	EAS/EB'S
facial pain	AES 551	EAS
foamy urine	AEc/ASc 51/51	EAc/ESc
frequent urination	B'A'SEE' 55555	D'E'SAA'
frostbite	ADS/AD' 442	EBS/EB'
frozen shoulder	AESD'/AE'a 5515/42	EASB'/EA'a
frozen shoulder	BDSE' 5515	DBSA'
frozen shoulder	AES 551	EAS
frozen shoulder	E'ASD'/AES 5515/551	A'ESB'/EAS
Fu-system Inflammation	AD 42	EB
gastric cancer	A'D'S'E'B' 55555	E'B'S'A'D'
gastric cancer	A'D'S'E' 5555	E'B'S'A'
gastric ulcer	ADS/AD' 442/42	EBS/EB'
gastritis	AD/AD' 42/42	EB/EB'
gastritis (helicobacter pylori)	ADS/AD' 442/42	EBS/EB'
gingivitis, periodontitis	ADa/AD'a 42/42	EBa/EB'a
gingivitis, periodontitis	AES/AD'a 551/42	EAS/EB'a
glaucoma	A'D'S'E 4424	E'B'S'A
glomerulonephritis	A'D'S'DB 55555	E'B'S'BD

[99] Symptoms of muscle spasms in the eyelids, lips, etc.

glomerulonephritis	ADc/ASc 51/51	EBc/ESc
goiter	ADa/AD'a 42/42	EBa/EB'a
gout	ADSEB' 55555	EBSAD'
gout	BESD' 5555	DASB'
gout	ADSE'B' 55555	EBSA'D'
gout	EDSA'B' 55555	ABSE'D'
hand tremors	ABSE' 5515	EDSA'
hand tremors	BE'SD' 4424	DA'SB'
hand tremors	AES 551	EAS
headache	AES 551	EAS
headache (low-energetic)	BE'SD' 5555	DA'S'B'
headache (neurogenic)	A'D'S'B'E' 55555	E'B'S'D'A'
heart disease	B'E'S'D' 5515	D'A'S'B'
hematuria (renal)	AEc 51	EAc
hemorrhage	A 6	E
hemorrhoids, fistula	ADc/AE'c 42/42	EBc/EB'c
hemorrhoids, fistula	ADS 442	EBS
hepatitis	AE/ASa 51/51	EA/ESa
hernia	AE'S 442	EA'S
herniated disc	AESE'/AE' 5555/42	EASA'/EA'
herniated disc	AES/AD 551/42	EAS/EA'
herniated disc	AESD'/AE' 5555/42	EASB'/EA'
herniated disc	AES 551	EAS
herniated disc	AESD' 5555	EASB'
herniated disc	AES/AE' 551/42	EAS/EA'
hordeolum (stye)	ADa/AD'a 42/42	EBa/EB'a
hoarse voice	BESD/ADa 4424/42	DASB/EBa

hoarse voice[100]	ADa/AE'a 42/42	EBa/EA'a
hyperhidrosis (palmar and plantar)	AE/ASa 51/51	EA/ESa
hypertension	A'D'S'B'E' 55555	E'B'S'D'A'
hypertension	BDSE 5555	DBSA
hypertension	A'D'S'D 5555	E'B'S'B
hyperthyroidism	BDSE 4424	DBSA
hyperthyroidism	ADa/AD'a 42/42	EBa/EB'a
hypotension	DES 551	BAS
hypotension	BES 442	DAS
hypotension	B'E'S' 442	D'A'S'
hypotension	BESA' 4424	DASE'
hypotension	BE'SD' 4424	DA'SB'
hypothyroidism	ADa/AE'a 42/42	EBa/EA'a
impotence	AES/AE' 551/42	EAS/EA'
infertility	BE'SD' 4442	DA'SB'
infertility	ADc 42	EBc
influenza	AD'S/A'D'S'E'B' 551/55555	EB'S/E'B'S'A'D'
influenza	AD'S/AES 551/551	EB'S/EAS
influenza	A'D'S'E'B' 55555	E'B'S'A'D'
insomnia	A'D'S'B'E' 55555	E'B'S'D'A'
irritable colitis	ADS/AD'c 442/42	EBS/EB'c
joint edema	ADSD'E'/AES 55555/551	EBSB'A'/EAS
kinetosis (motion sickness)	B'E'S' 442	D'A'S'
lateral epicondylitis	AES/AE'a 551/42	EAS/EA'a
lateral epicondylitis	AES/AD'a 551/42	EAS/EB'a

[100] Symptoms of hoarseness or difficulty making sounds.

loss of energy	AE'S 442	EA'S
loss of energy	BE'S 442	DA'S
Lou Gehrig's Disease[101]	BESAE' 55555	DASEA'
lupus (SLE)[102]	DASBE 55555	BESDA
menopausal syndrome	A'DS' 551	E'BS'
mental Formula	AS 51	ES
mucosal ulcer	A'D'S'B' 4444	E'B'S'D'
myalgia	AES 551	EAS
myasthenia gravis	ABSE' 5515	EDSA'
myeloma	DASB 5555	BESD
myomas	ADc/AD'c 42/42	EBc/EB'c
Ménière's Syndrome[103]	AESDA' 55555	EASBE'
obesity	ADSD'E' 55555	EBSB'A'
ocular pain, pink eye	AE/ASa 51/51	EA/ESa
osteomyelitis	AESD' 5555	EASB'
otitis media	BE'SD' 4424	DB'SB'
otitis media	B'DS'D' 4424	D'BS'B'
otitis media	BESD' 4424	DASB'
otitis media	BDSD' 4424	DBSB'
otitis media	BESA' 4424	DASE'

[101] Lou Gehrig's Disease: A condition that refers to amyotrophic lateral sclerosis (ALS). Named after Lou Gehrig, a famous American Major League Baseball player who was diagnosed with this disease in 1939, it causes muscle weakness, atrophy, and loss of motor function. Symptoms include speech difficulties, swallowing difficulties, breathing difficulties, and progressive paralysis.

[102] Systemic lupus erythematosus: A chronic inflammatory autoimmune disease that affects various organs of the body, including connective tissue, skin, joints, blood, and kidneys. Symptoms include general weakness, fatigue, rash, mouth ulcers, joint pain, fever, weight changes, headache, hair loss, chest pain when breathing, swelling of the lower extremities, and Raynaud's phenomenon.

[103] Ménière's syndrome: A chronic disease of the inner ear that causes symptoms such as vertigo, tinnitus, hearing loss, and a feeling of stuffiness in the ears.

otitis media	BDSE' 4424	DBSA'
otitis media	AD'S/AD' 442/42	EB'S/EB'
otitis media	ADS/AD' 442/42	EBS/EB'
otitis media	ADa/AD'a 42/42	EBa/EB'a
otitis media	BD'SD 4424	DB'SB
ovarian cyst	ADc/AD'c 42/42	EBc/EB'c
ovarian cyst	AES/ADc 551/42	EAS/EBc
ovulation disorder	BE'SD' 4442	DA'SB'
palmar keratosis[104]	ABSE 5555	EDSA
pancreatic cancer	ADSEB 55555	EBSAD
pancreatitis	AE/ASa 51/51	EA/ESa
panic disorder	A'D'S'B'E' 55555	E'B'S'D'A'
paresthesia (pins and needles)	AES 551	EAS
paresthesia (pins and needles)	A'D'S'B'E' 55555	E'B'S'D'A'
paresthesia[105]	AE'SD 5555	EA'SB
Parkinson's disease	BDSD'A 55515	DBSB'E
Parkinson's disease	AA'SE' 5515	EE'SA'
pelvic inflammatory disease	AESD' 5551	EASB'
pelvic peritonitis	BESD 5551	DASB
pharyngitis	ADa/AD'a 42/42	EBa/EB'a
pins and needles	A'DS' 442	E'BS'
pins and needles	A'D'S'B'E' 44444	E'B'S'D'A'
pins and needles	AES 551	EAS
pins and needles	AE'S 442	EA'S
pituitary tumor	BE'SA 4424	DA'SE

[104] When the cold autumn wind blows, the skin on the palms and fingers becomes keratinized, and in severe cases, it cracks and bleeds.

[105] Symptoms of paresthesia and decreased sensation (desensitization) in the body.

postpartum wind	BE'SD' 4424	DA'SB'
postpartum wind	AES 551	EAS
prostatic hypertrophy	BESA 4444	DASE
prostatic hypertrophy	ADSE' 4444	EBSA'
prostatic hypertrophy	B'A'SEE' 55555	D'E'SAA'
prostatitis	ADc/AD'c 42/42	EBc/EB'c
prostatitis	AD'S 442	EB'S
prostatitis	ADSE' 4444	EBSA'
prostatitis	BESD 4444	DASB
prostatitis	BESD' 4444	DASB'
pruritus	BESD 4424	DASB
psoriasis	ADSE'B' 44444	EBSA'D'
psoriasis	E'B'S'A' 4444	A'D'S'E'
ptosis (stomach-colon), hernia	AE'S 442	EA'S
pulmonary asthenia	AE'a/AEa 42/42	EA'a/EAa
pulmonary fibrosis[106]	BESD'A' 55515	DASB'E'
pulmonary tuberculosis	AD'a 51	EB'a
purpura	A'D'S'DB 44444	E'B'S'BD
purpura	BESE'A' 44444	DASA'E'
pyelonephritis (edema)[107]	AEc/ASc 51/51	EAc/ESc
Ramsay-Hunt Syndrome[108]	AES/AD'S 551/551	EAS/EB'S
Raynaud's Syndrome[109]	AES/AE' 551/42	EAS/EA'

[106] Pulmonary fibrosis: A disease that causes fibrosis of the lung tissue. Symptoms include shortness of breath, chronic dry cough, fatigue, weight loss, and muscle pain.

[107] The Formula is used when pyelonephritis or resulting edema is severe.

[108] Ramsay-Hunt syndrome: A condition in which shingles and facial paralysis occur simultaneously.

[109] Raynaud's syndrome: A condition that occurs when blood vessels in the fingertips, toes, nose, and earlobes constrict excessively and abnormally when exposed to cold, vibration, or stress (psychological changes). The extremities, such as the fingertips and toes, become pale, and sensory abnormalities like numbness or pain may occur.

renal failure	A'D'S'B 5551	E'B'S'D
renal failure	A'D'S'B' 5551	E'B'S'D'
renal failure	DESB 5551	BASD
renal failure (edema)[110]	ADSD'E'/A'D'S'B' 55551/5551	EBSB'A'/E'B'S'D'
retinitis	ADS 442	EBS
rheumatoid arthritis (RA)	ADSB/BE'S 5555/551	EBSD/DA'S
rheumatoid arthritis (RA)	ADSD'E' 55555	EBSB'A'
rheumatoid arthritis (RA)	ADSE'B' 55555	EBSA'D'
rheumatoid arthritis (RA)	E'B'S'A'D' 55555	A'D'S'E'B'
rhinitis	ADa/ADa' 42/42	EBa/EB'a
rhinitis	BESD/AD 4424/42	DASB/EB
rhinitis (allergic)	D'A'S'DE 55515	B'E'S'BA
salpingitis	BESD 4442	DASB
shoulder pain	BDSE' 5515	DBSA'
sinusitis	D'A'S'DE 44424	B'E'S'BA
sinusitis	AD'S/AD' 442/42	EB'S/EB'
sinusitis	BESD' 4424	DASB'
sinusitis	BDSE' 4424	DBSA'
sinusitis	BESDA' 44424	DASBE'
sinusitis	BESD/ADa 4424/42	DASB/EBa
sinusitis	B'DS'D' 4424	D'BS'B'
sinusitis	BE'SD' 4424	DB'SB'
sinusitis	BD'SD 4424	DB'SB
sinusitis	BESA' 4424	DASE'
sinusitis	ADa/AD'a 42/42	EBa/EB'a
sinusitis	ADS/AD' 442/42	EBS/EB'
sinusitis	BDSD' 4424	DBSB'

[110] The Formula is used when kidney failure or resulting edema is severe.

sinusitis	AE'SD 4424	EA'SB
skin cracks	ABSE 5555	EDSA
spinal compression fracture	ABSB'/AES 5555/551	EDSD'/EAS
spinal instability	BESD' 5555	DASB'
spinal instability[111]	BESD 5555	DASB
spinal stenosis	BESE'A 55555	DASA'E
spinal stenosis	BESDA 55555	DASBE
spinal stenosis	BESDA' 55555	DASBE'
splenomegaly	AE/ASa 51/51	EA/ESa
sputum	BESD 5515	DASB
Sterilization Formula	AD' 42	EB'
stomatitis	ADa/AD'a 42/42	EBa/EB'a
stroke (cerebral hemorrhage)	BDSE/AES 4424/551	DBSA/EAS
stroke (cerebral hemorrhage)	BDSE/A 4424/6	DBSA/E
stroke (cerebral infaction)	BDSE/D'E'S'A' 4424/4424	DBSA/B'A'S'E'
stroke (cerebral infaction)	BDSE/DESA' 4424/4424	DBSA/BASE'
stroke (cerebral infaction)	AE'SD 4424	EA'SB
stroke (cerebral infaction)	AE'S'D 4424	EA'S'B
stroke (cerebral infaction)	BDSE/BESA' 4424/4424	DBSA/DASE'
TMJ disorder[112]	AES/AD'a 551/42	EAS/EB'a
TMJ disorder	AES/AE'a 551/42	EAS/EA'a

111 A condition in which the stability of the spine is reduced due to the weakening of the muscles and ligaments that support the spine.

112 A disease that occurs in the temporomandibular joints (TMJ), commonly referred to as temporomandibular joint disease.

TMJ disorder	AES 551	EAS
tenosynovitis[113]	BDS 551	DBS
thrombus	BE'SA 4444	DA'SE
thrombus	AE'S 442	EA'S
thyroid disease	A'D'S'E'B 44424	E'B'S'A'D
tidal fever	A'D'S'D 4444	E'B'S'B
tidal fever[114]	A'DS' 442	E'BS'
tinnitus, hearing loss	AD'S 551	EB'S
tinnitus, hearing loss	AESDA' 55515	EASBE'
tinnitus, hearing loss	AD'S 551	EB'S
tinnitus, hearing loss	AESDA' 55515	EASBE'
tinnitus, hearing loss	BESD' 5515	DASB'
tinnitus, hearing loss	DESA' 5515	BASE'
tonsillitis (severe)	A'D'S'E'B' 44424	E'B'S'A'D'
trigeminal neuralgia	AES 551	EAS
trigeminal neuralgia	EDSD'A' 55515	ABSB'E'
ulcer (stomach, mucosa)	ADS/A'D'S'B' 442/4444	EBS/E'B'S'D'
ulcer (stomach-colon)	ADS 442	EBS
uresis, polyuria, incontinence	AE'c/ADc 42/42	EA'c/EBc
uresis, polyuria, incontinence	ADS/AE'S 442/442	EBS/EA'S
uresis, polyuria, incontinence	AES/AE'c 551/42	EAS/EA'c
uresis, polyuria, incontinence	B'A'SEE' 44442	D'E'SAA'
uresis, polyuria, incontinence	ADc 42	EBc
uresis, polyuria, incontinence	AEc 51	EAc

[113] Tenosynovitis: Inflammation of the synovial membrane surrounding tendons, causing movement disorders such as pain, swelling, and muscle weakness. It often occurs in the shoulder joint.

[114] A symptom in which hot flashes come and go periodically. It mainly occurs in menopausal syndrome, but can also occur in other diseases.

urethritis	ADc/AD'c 42/42	EBc/EB'c
urinary stones	AE'c/ADc 42/42	EA'c/EBc
urticaria (allergic)	D'A'S'DE 44444	B'E'S'BA
urticaria (food poisoning)	AD/AD' 42/42	EB/EB'
urticaria (food poisoning)	AE/AD' 51/42	EA/EB'
uterine ptosis	ADc/AE'c 42/42	EBc/EB'c
vertebral (spinal) disease	AES 551	EAS
vertigo	B'E'S' 442	D'A'S'
viral disease	AD'S 551	EB'S
Vitality Formula	AE' 42	EA'
vitiligo	ADS/AD' 442/42	EBS/EB'
Zang-system Inflammation	AE 51	EA

Simple Constitution-acupuncture Formulary

For convenience, let me introduce a very simple Constitution-acupuncture formulary for quick use. The abbreviation rules are as follows:

K: Basic Formula, Q: Fu-system Basic Formula, G: Degeneration Sub-formula, R: Fu-system Degeneration Sub-formula, P: Mental Sub-formula, T: Fu-system Mental Sub-formula, F: Fu-system Inflammation Sub-formula, Z: Zang-system Inflammation Sub-formula, S: Sterilization Sub-formula, V: Vitality Sub-formula

Disease & Symptom	Formula
abnormal vaginal discharge	KFc 42
abnormal vaginal discharge	KSc 42
acne	QFT/KS 442/42
acne	KFP/KSa 442/42
acne	VRTKF 44444
allergic asthma	SQTFZ 55515
allergic asthma	KFPVR 55515
allergic conjunctivitis	QSTGZ 55515
allergic dermatitis	QSTGF 44424
allergic dermatitis	QFTSZ 44424
allergic dermatitis	KFPVR 44424
allergic rhinitis	KVPF 4424
allergic rhinitis	QSTFZ 44424
allergic rhinitis	RVTS 4424
allergic rhinitis	KVTF 4424
allergy	SQTFZ 55555
allergy	GZPVS 55555
amenorrhea	KSP 442
angina pectoris	GFPK/KFPSV 5515/55515

angina pectoris	GVP/KFa 551/42
angina pectoris	GVP/KZa 551/51
angina pectoris	RVTS 5515
ankylosing spondylitis	GZPS/KZP 5555/551
ankylosing spondylitis	KGPQS 55515
anxiety	QSTRV 55555
anxiety	KZ/KP 51/51
arteriosclerosis	RVTK 4444
arteriosclerosis	SVT 442
asthma	GZPSV 55515
asthma	SVTZK 55515
asthma	QSTVR 55515
asthma	GZPSQ 55515
asthma	SQTVZ 55515
asthma	ZGPSQ 55515
asthma (allergic)	QSTFZ 55515
atopic dermatitis	QSTR 4424
atopic dermatitis	GZPF/QSTR 4424/4424
atopic dermatitis	QSTF 4424
atrophic gastritis	GVP 442
back pain	KZPG 5555
back pain	KZPV 5555
back pain	KZPS 5555
back pain	KZP/KVc 551/42
Behçet's Disease	KFP/KS 442/42
bile duct stones	KV 42
bladder atony	KVc 42
blood circulation disorder	RVTS 4444
blood circulation disorder	KVPF 4444

brain tumor	GVPK 4424
bronchiectasis	FZPRQ 55515
bronchiectasis	ZGPSQ 55515
bronchitis	SQTFZ 55515
cartilage wear	KGP 551
cartilage wear	KGPR 5555
cataract	SQTRV 44424
cataract	SQTRS 44424
cerebral hemorrhage	QSTF 5515
cerebral hemorrhage	GFPS 5515
cerebral hemorrhage	GFPZ 5515
cerebral infarction	VGTK 4424
cerebral infarction (hypotension)	GZPQ 4424
cerebral infarction (thrombus)	KVP 551
chest congestion	RVT 551
cholecystitis, cholangitis, gallbladder cyst	KF/KS 42/42
chondromalacia	KZPR 5555
cirrhosis, hepatic cancer	GZPFQ 55555
cirrhosis, hepatic cancer	GZPFK 55555
cirrhosis, hepatic cancer	KZPFG 55555
cold	KSP/KFa 551/42
cold hands and feet	KVPS 4424
cold hands and feet	GVPF 4424
cold lower abdomen	KVPF 4442
cold with body aches	KSP/KZP 551/551
constipation	KFPSV 44442
constipation	KFP/KS 442/42
constipation	KF/KV 42/42
constipation	KF/KS 42/42

cough	QSTFZ 55515
cystitis, urethritis	KFc/KSc 42/42
degenerative arthritis	KVP 551
degenerative arthritis	GZP 551
degenerative arthritis	VRTQS 55555
degenerative arthritis	KGPR/KZPS 5555/5555
degenerative arthritis	RVT 551
depression	RVT 551
depression	KZ/KPa 51/51
dermatitis	QSTFZ 44444
diabetes	KZ/KPa 51/51
diabetes	QSTVG 55555
diarrhea	KFc/KSc 42/42
diplopia	KFP 442
dysautonomia	QFT 442
dysautonomia	RVTS 4444
dysautonomia	QSTRV 44444
dysautonomia	SVT 442
dysmenorrhea	KFc 42
dysmenorrhea	KVP/KFc 551/42
dysmenorrhea	KZP/KFP 551/442
edema	KFPSV 55555
edema (diabetic)	QSTVG 55555
endometritis	GZPS 4442
endometritis	GZPF 4442
epilepsy	KFP 551
esophagitis, plum pit Qi	KFa/KPa 51/51
esophagitis, plum pit Qi	KFP/KSa 442/42
esophagitis, plum pit Qi	KFP/KVa 442/42

esophagitis, plum pit Qi	KVa 42
esophagitis, plum pit Qi	QSTR/KFP 4424/442
facial cramps	KZP 551
facial palsy	KZPV 5515
facial palsy	QFTZ 5515
facial pain	KZP/KSa 551/42
facial pain	ZFPSQ 55515
facial pain	KZP/KSP 551/442
facial pain	KZP 551
foamy urine	KZc/KPc 51/51
frequent urination	RQPZV 55555
frostbite	KFP/KS 442
frozen shoulder	KZPS/KVa 5515/42
frozen shoulder	GFPV 5515
frozen shoulder	KZP 551
frozen shoulder	VKPS/KZP 5515/551
Fu-system Inflammation	KF 42
gastric cancer	QSTVR 55555
gastric cancer	QSTV 5555
gastric ulcer	KFP/KS 442/42
gastritis	KF/KS 42/42
gastritis (helicobacter pylori)	KFP/KS 442/42
gingivitis, periodontitis	KFa/KSa 42/42
gingivitis, periodontitis	KZP/KSa 551/42
glaucoma	QSTZ 4424
glomerulonephritis	QSTFG 55555
glomerulonephritis	KFc/KPc 51/51
goiter	KFa/KSa 42/42
gout	KFPZR 55555

gout	GZPS 5555
gout	KFPVR 55555
gout	ZFPQR 55555
hand tremors	KGPV 5515
hand tremors	GVPS 4424
hand tremors	KZP 551
headache	KZP 551
headache (low energetic)	GVPS 5555
headache (neurogenic)	QSTRV 55555
heart disease	RVTS 5515
hematuria (renal)	KZc 51
hemorrhage	K 6
hemorrhoids, fistula	KFc/KVc 42/42
hemorrhoids, fistula	KFP 442
hepatitis	KZ/KPa 51/51
hernia	KVP 442
herniated disc	KZPV/KV 5555/42
herniated disc	KZP/KF 551/42
herniated disc	KZPS/KV 5555/42
herniated disc	KZP 551
herniated disc	KZPS 5555
herniated disc	KZP/KV 551/42
hordeolum (stye)	KFa/KSa 42/42
hoarse voice	GZPF/KFa 4424/42
hoarse voice	KFa/KVa 42/42
hyperhidrosis (palmar and plantar)	KZ/KPa 51/51
hypertension	QSTRV 55555
hypertension	GFPZ 5555

hypertension	QSTF 5555
hyperthyroidism	GFPZ 4424
hyperthyroidism	KFa/KSa 42/42
hypotension	FZP 551
hypotension	GZP 442
hypotension	RVT 442
hypotension	GZPQ 4424
hypotension	GVPS 4424
hypothyroidism	KFa/KVa 42/42
impotence	KZP/KV 551/42
infertility	GVPS 4442
infertility	KFc 42
influenza	KSP/QSTVR 551/55555
influenza	KSP/KZP 551/551
influenza	QSTVR 55555
insomnia	QSTRV 55555
irritable colitis	KFP/KSc 442/42
joint edema	KFPSV/KZP 55555/551
kinetosis (motion sickness)	RVT 442
lateral epicondylitis	KZP/KVa 551/42
lateral epicondylitis	KZP/KSa 551/42
loss of energy	KVP 442
loss of energy	GVP 442
Lou Gehrig's Disease	GZPKV 55555
lupus (SLE)	FKPGZ 55555
menopausal syndrome	QFT 551
mental Formula	KP 51
mucosal ulcer	QSTR 4444
myalgia	KZP 551

myasthenia gravis	KGPV 5515
myeloma	FKPG 5555
myomas	KFc/KSc 42/42
Ménière's Syndrome	KZPFQ 55555
obesity	KFPSV 55555
ocular pain, pink eye	KZ/KPa 51/51
osteomyelitis	KZPS 5555
otitis media	GVPS 4424
otitis media	RFTS 4424
otitis media	GZPS 4424
otitis media	GFPS 4424
otitis media	GZPQ 4424
otitis media	GFPV 4424
otitis media	KSP/KS 442/42
otitis media	KFP/KS 442/42
otitis media	KFa/KSa 42/42
otitis media	GSPF 4424
ovarian cyst	KFc/KSc 42/42
ovarian cyst	KZP/KFc 551/42
ovulation disorder	GVPS 4442
palmar keratosis	KGPZ 5555
pancreatic cancer	KFPZG 55555
pancreatitis	KZ/KPa 51/51
panic disorder	QSTRV 55555
paresthesia (pins and needles)	KZP 551
paresthesia (pins and needles)	QSTRV 55555
paresthesia	KVPF 5555
Parkinson's disease	GFPSK 55515
Parkinson's disease	KQPV 5515

pelvic inflammatory disease	KZPS 5551
pelvic peritonitis	GZPF 5551
pharyngitis	KFa/KSa 42/42
pins and needles	QFT 442
pins and needles	QSTRV 44444
pins and needles	KZP 551
pins and needles	KVP 442
pituitary tumor	GVPK 4424
postpartum wind	GVPS 4424
postpartum wind	KZP 551
prostatic hypertrophy	GZPK 4444
prostatic hypertrophy	KFPV 4444
prostatic hypertrophy	RQPZV 55555
prostatitis	KFc/KSc 42/42
prostatitis	KSP 442
prostatitis	KFPV 4444
prostatitis	GZPF 4444
prostatitis	GZPS 4444
pruritus	GZPF 4424
psoriasis	KFPVR 44444
psoriasis	VRTQ 4444
ptosis (stomach-colon), hernia	KVP 442
pulmonary asthenia	KVa/KZa 42/42
pulmonary fibrosis	GZPSQ 55515
pulmonary tuberculosis	KSa 51
purpura	QSTFG 44444
purpura	GZPVQ 44444
pyelonephritis (edema)	KZc/KPc 51/51
Ramsay-Hunt Syndrome	KZP/KSP 551/551

Raynaud's Syndrome	KZP/KV 551/42
renal failure	QSTG 5551
renal failure	QSTR 5551
renal failure	FZPG 5551
renal failure (edema)	KFPSV/QSTR 55551/5551
retinitis	KFP 442
rheumatoid arthritis (RA)	KFPG/GVP 5555/551
rheumatoid arthritis (RA)	KFPSV 55555
rheumatoid arthritis (RA)	KFPVR 55555
rheumatoid arthritis (RA)	VRTQS 55555
rhinitis	KFa/KFQ 42/42
rhinitis	GZPF/KF 4424/42
rhinitis (allergic)	SQTFZ 55515
salpingitis	GZPF 4442
shoulder pain	GFPV 5515
sinusitis	SQTFZ 44424
sinusitis	KSP/KS 442/42
sinusitis	GZPS 4424
sinusitis	GFPV 4424
sinusitis	GZPFQ 44424
sinusitis	GZPF/KFa 4424/42
sinusitis	RFTS 4424
sinusitis	GVPS 4424
sinusitis	GSPF 4424
sinusitis	GZPQ 4424
sinusitis	KFa/KSa 42/42
sinusitis	KFP/KS 442/42
sinusitis	GFPS 4424
sinusitis	KVPF 4424

skin cracks	KGPZ 5555
spinal compression fracture	KGPR/KZP 5555/551
spinal instability	GZPS 5555
spinal instability	GZPF 5555
spinal stenosis	GZPVK 55555
spinal stenosis	GZPFK 55555
spinal stenosis	GZPFQ 55555
splenomegaly	KZ/KPa 51/51
sputum	GZPF 5515
Sterilization Formula	KS 42
stomatitis	KFa/KSa 42/42
stroke (cerebral hemorrhage)	GFPZ/KZP 4424/551
stroke (cerebral hemorrhage)	GFPZ/K 4424/6
stroke (cerebral infaction)	GFPZ/SVTQ 4424/4424
stroke (cerebral infaction)	GFPZ/FZPQ 4424/4424
stroke (cerebral infaction)	KVPF 4424
stroke (cerebral infaction)	KVTF 4424
stroke (cerebral infaction)	GFPZ/GZPQ 4424/4424
TMJ disorder	KZP/KSa 551/42
TMJ disorder	KZP/KVa 551/42
TMJ disorder	KZP 551
tenosynovitis	GFP 551
thrombus	GVPK 4444
thrombus	KVP 442
thyroid disease	QSTVG 44424
tidal fever	QSTF 4444
tidal fever	QFT 442
tinnitus, hearing loss	KSP 551
tinnitus, hearing loss	KZPFQ 55515

tinnitus, hearing loss	KSP 551
tinnitus, hearing loss	KZPFQ 55515
tinnitus, hearing loss	GZPS 5515
tinnitus, hearing loss	FZPQ 5515
tonsillitis (severe)	QSTVR 44424
trigeminal neuralgia	KZP 551
trigeminal neuralgia	ZFPSQ 55515
ulcer (stomach, mucosa)	KFP/QSTR 442/4444
ulcer (stomach-colon)	KFP 442
uresis, polyuria, incontinence	KVc/KFc 42/42
uresis, polyuria, incontinence	KFP/KVP 442/442
uresis, polyuria, incontinence	KZP/KVc 551/42
uresis, polyuria, incontinence	RQPZV 44442
uresis, polyuria, incontinence	KFc 42
uresis, polyuria, incontinence	KZc 51
urethritis	KFc/KSc 42/42
urinary stones	KVc/KFc 42/42
urticaria (allergic)	SQTFZ 44444
urticaria (food poisoning)	KF/KS 42/42
urticaria (food poisoning)	KZ/KS 51/42
uterine ptosis	KFc/KVc 42/42
vertebral (spinal) disease	KZP 551
vertigo	RVT 442
viral disease	KSP 551
Vitality Formula	KV 42
vitiligo	KFP/KS 442/42
Zang-system Inflammation	KZ 51

CHAPTER 6

Diagnosis of Constitution

DIAGNOSIS OF CONSTITUTION IS A PROCESS OF DISCOVERING YOURSELF.

CHAPTER 6

Diagnosis of Constitution

Diagnosis of Eight-Constitution Medicine starts with Diagnosis of Constitution. Diagnosing Constitution helps determine one's condition based on the Constitution. By identifying the Constitution, you can devise an optimal treatment strategy to find the cause of the person's disease, understand one's pathology, and determine how to address the disease effectively.

There are several techniques for diagnosing Constitution. In addition to the "four diagnostic methods (四診)" of looking, listening, asking, and touching (望聞問切), there is a questionnaire method, which tests various questions about Constitution, a method of using a standardized morphological typology, and a method using electrical or electronic devices, or even using a computer.

However, the most important diagnostic method in Eight-Constitution Medicine is the Constitutional pulse diagnosis. It was first introduced in the thesis written by Do-won Kuon in 1965. It is quite different from the traditional pulse diagnosis. To summarize, it is as follows:

Constitutional pulse-feeling process

1. Grab the pulse of the patient's left hand with the doctor's right fingers and the pulse of the patient's right hand with the doctor's left fingers.
2. Place the doctor's index finger on the radial artery, next to the highest bone part on the palm side of the patient's radial styloid process.

3. The doctor's index finger should be placed like a bridge between the upward slope of the area grasped in step 2 and the line of the flexor carpi radialis muscle. The tip of the finger should almost touch the palmaris longus muscle.
4. After adjusting the feeling of the index finger so that the radial artery can be observed, the doctor places the second and third fingers in the same order and aligns them.
5. In this way, the doctor holds the patient's pulse and muscles together with three fingers applying equal pressure.
6. If the patient's muscles have good elasticity, press the patient's pulse and muscles vertically as strongly as possible. If the patient's muscles lack elasticity, pull and press toward the patient's radius, and find to determine which finger has the pulse remaining until the end.
7. If the same reaction continues to appear even after repeating the pulse examination of the left and right hands two or three times, the doctor diagnoses the Constitution according to the pulse diagram.

It is quite difficult to understand the pulse-feeling procedure just from the explanation in this paper. This is because it can be interpreted differently depending on the viewing angle. The more practical pulse-feeling method, along with specific diagram of the pulse and detailed explanations, is shown later.

8 Constitutions Pulse Diagram

The paper presents a pulsation diagram along with this pulse-feeling method. This pulse diagram was later revised into a new version that reflects more three-dimensional and dynamic aspects. The revised pulse diagram is as follows:

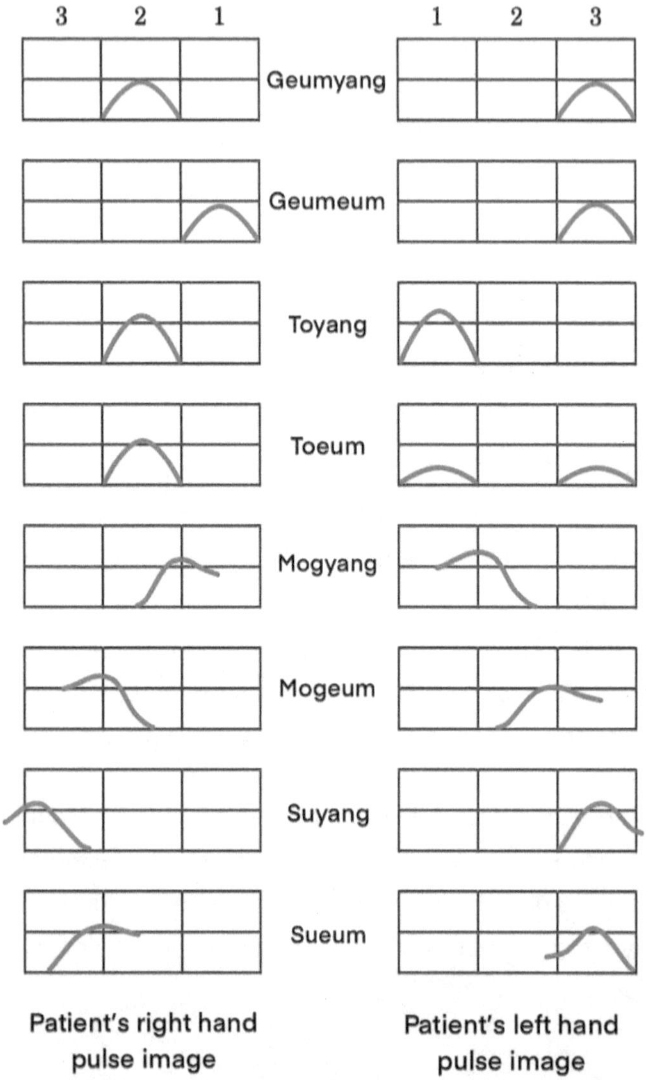

Figure 1. Pulse Diagram of the Eight Constitutions

Zone 1 is where the doctor's index finger is located, zone 2 the middle finger, and zone 3 the ring finger. The right hand pulse refers to the pulse in the patient's right arm, and the left pulse the patient's left arm.

Practical method of Constitutional pulse-feeling

This pulse-feeling method is quite difficult and requires a lot of perseverance. The tips for actual clinical practice are as follows:

Place in order the index finger (zone 1), the middle finger (zone 2), and the ring finger (zone 3) on the radius about 2 cm apart from the wrist (see Figure 1 above and Figure 2 below). Press down with all three fingers until the three pulses stop beating, then relax and decrease the pressure little by little and observe which pulse beats first. When pressing on the pulse, the flexor carpi radialis tendon is pulled toward the radius and attached to the radius. It is important to keep the radial artery positioned between the radius and this muscle tendon to prevent it from slipping.

When performing the pulse-feeling, the patient should be lying in the supine position, facing upward. If the pulse is taken in any other position, the results may not be accurate. Constitutional pulse diagnosis is a highly delicate process that can be influenced by even minor changes in posture. Therefore, it is best conducted when the patient is as still as possible.

1. The key to Constitutional pulse diagnosis lies in the patient's left hand. First check if a pulse is present in zone 3 of the left wrist. If a pulse is detected in this area, it suggests one of the following Constitutions: Geumyang, Geumeum, Suyang, or Sueum. If there is no pulse in zone 3, then the patient likely belongs to one of the following Constitutions: Toyang, Toeum, Mogyang, or Mogeum. If the pulse is felt in zone 3, then examine the patient's right hand to further differentiate among the Geumyang, Geumeum, Suyang, and Sueum Constitution.
2. If a pulse is also detected in zone 3 of the right hand, the patient likely has Suyang or Sueum Constitution. If the pulse is felt beating in Zone 3 and extends beyond its outer boundary, it suggests a Suyang Constitution. If it feels beating in zone 3 and moving over to zone 2, it indicates Sueum Constitution. A pulse that moves fluidly like this is called "flowing pulse."

3. If the pulse remains stationary in zone 2 of the right hand, it indicates a Geumyang Constitution. If it stays in zone 1, it suggests Geumeum Constitution. A pulse that beats while staying in place is called "fixed pulse." The Constitutions of Geumyang, Geumeum, Toyang, and Toeum are associated with the fixed pulse, whereas the Constitutions of Mogyang, Mogeum, Suyang, and Sueum are associated with the flowing pulse. Thus, the pulse for Mogyang, Mogeum, Suyang, and Sueum extends across two zones.
4. If the initial pulse felt in the patient's left hand is in zone 1 rather than zone 3, it usually indicates Toyang or Toeum Constitution. However, a caution is needed, as the Toeum Constitution may also show a slight beating in zone 3. Statistically, the Toyang Constitution is more common than the Toeum Constitution, so diagnosis often leans toward the Toyang Constitution. In the right hand, the Toyang or Toeum Constitution typically presents as the fixed pulse in zone 2, with the Toyang pulse being slightly stronger.
5. If the pulse is detected in zone 2 of the left hand, the patient likely has Mogyang or Mogeum Constitution. The Mogyang pulse moves from zone 2 to zone 1, while Mogeum pulse moves from zone 2 to zone 3. Both are classified as the flowing pulses, so careful observation is needed.

The above is one of the practical methods used to measure the Constitutional pulse in actual clinical practice. However, it is important to develop the method that is most optimal for the practitioners themselves. This is presented only as a reference example.

These pulses of Eight-Constitutions are literally the image of pulsation. The pulses are not in the one-to-one relation to the separate Zang-Fu organs, but rather the overall image of the characteristic pulsation of each Constitution. That is, there are just the overall eight types of pulsation, which emerges as the images fused and merged from Zang-Fu Structures of each Constitution in the beating of the radial artery. Therefore, do not try to understand it as the direct relationship with the Six Zangs and Six Fus. The truth is always distorted by over-interpreting things that deviate from the original meaning.

Practice of Eight-Constitution pulse diagnosis

The following picture is an example of the Eight-Constitution pulse diagnosis. Examine it carefully and practice repeatedly to learn the correct Constitutional Pulses.

[Preparation]

Hold the patient's left hand with both of the doctor's hands and align it so that the radial artery is well exposed. At this time, the patient's elbow should be naturally slightly bent, and the wrist should be held slightly tilted back. Then, position the patient's arm at a slight incline with the bed (preparation step 1).

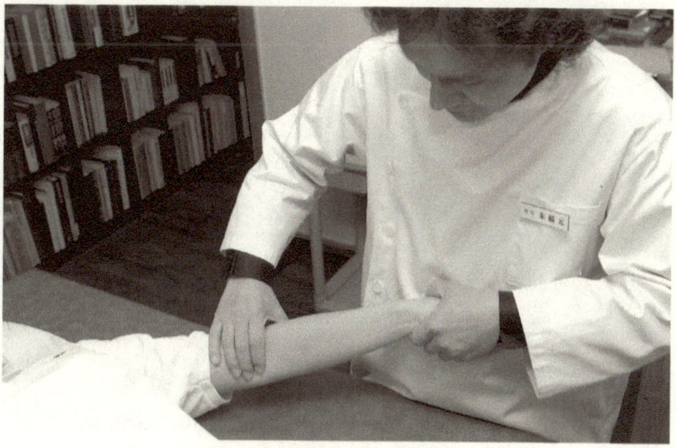

Figure 2. Eight-Constitution pulse diagnosis (preparation step 1)

Place your index, middle, and ring fingers in order on the slope of the radius. At this time, it is important to keep the three fingers neatly aligned. Instead of holding the pulse at the tip of the fingers, it is better to hold it between the first joint of the finger and the area where the fingerprint is formed (preparation step 2).

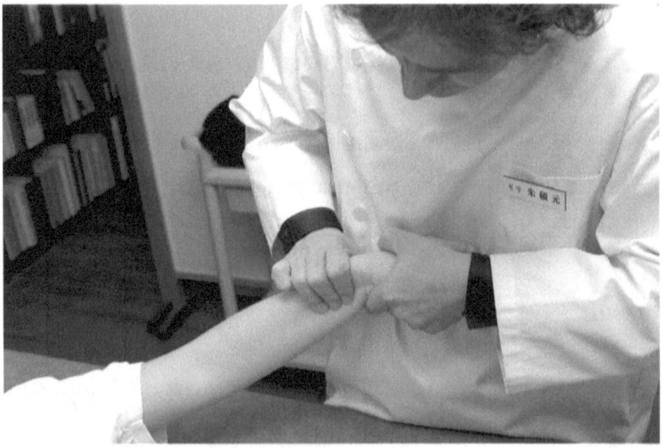

Figure 3. Eight-Constitution pulse diagnosis (preparation step 2)

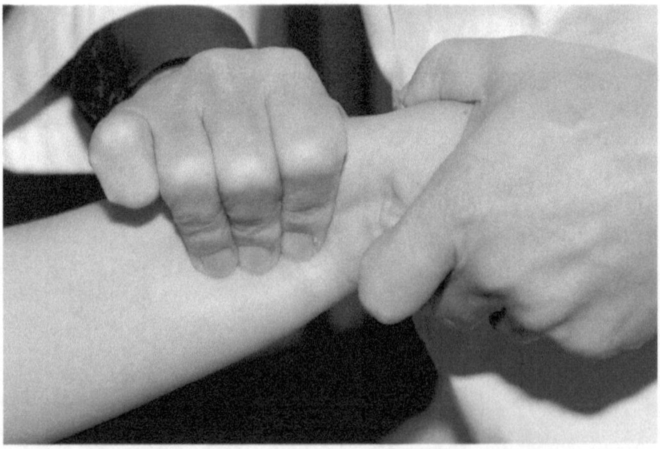

Figure 4. Eight-Constitution pulse diagnosis
(the moment of actual pulse-feeling)

Press all three fingers equally and firmly on the patient's left hand at the same time. The most important factor is to apply even pressure. If the pressure is not equal, regardless of how many other requirements are met, the result will be ineffective. When pressing, it is important to apply the pressure while pulling the flexor carpi radialis tendon toward the radius. Pay close attention to the first joint of the finger, as it is tilted back quite a bit. The pulse is not held at the tips of the fingers, but between the first joint of the distal phalanges and the fingerprint area. Press hard enough to make the pulse disappear due to the pressure, then hold for about 3 to 5 seconds. Afterward, slightly decrease and relax the pressure and closely observe which finger the pulse beats first. The pulse of the finger that beats first is the Constitutional pulse. The same method is used to feel the pulse in the patient's right hand.

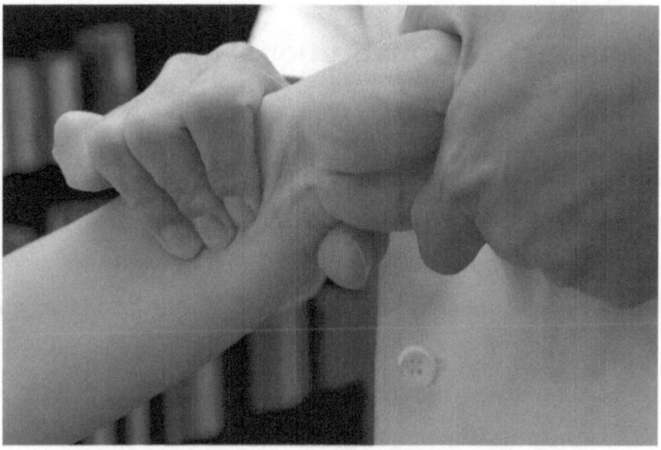

Figure 5. Eight-Constitution pulse diagnosis (view from below)

Grab the patient's wrist tightly with your thumb to support the pressure of your fingers evenly. The picture shows the wrist slightly raised for the photo, but in reality, you should lower it.

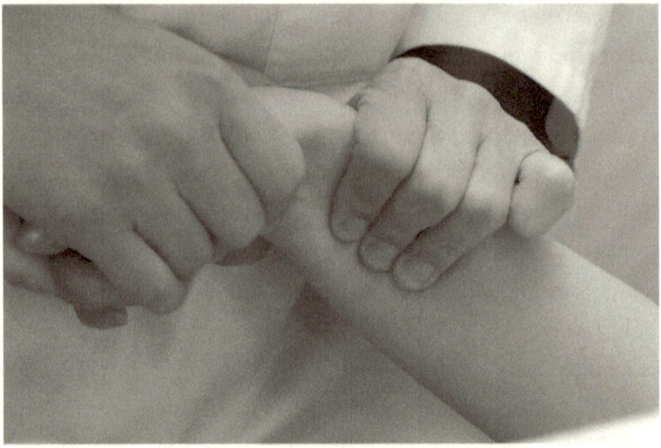

Figure 6. Eight-Constitution pulse diagnosis of the right hand
(The pulse-feeling method is the same as the left hand.)

The Importance of Constitutional diagnosis

The diagnosis of the Eight Constitutions is very important. This is because all treatments in Constitutional Medicine begin with the diagnosis of the Constitution. All of the above Unit and Compound Formulae are meaningful only when an accurate diagnosis of the Constitution is made. No matter how well you understand the theory of Constitution or how many Formulae you know, it is meaningless if you cannot diagnose a person's Constitution. Therefore, you should always prioritize and not neglect the practice of Constitutional pulse diagnosis.

Diagnosis of the Eight Constitutions includes other common diagnostic methods, such as visual examination (diagnosis by sight), palpation (diagnosis by touch), auscultation (diagnosis by hearing), and the most basic diagnostic method, interview. It is a good idea to conduct the diagnosis by these methods simultaneously. This is because, in many cases, it can be easily diagnosed using the simple methods such as looking, touching, hearing, or asking. And you will need to constantly develop your own unwavering techniques and know-how to accurately diagnose the Constitution.

CHAPTER 7

Constitution-acupuncture Treatment

ALL PROFESSIONAL ACTIVITIES REQUIRE PHYSICAL DISCIPLINE, AND CONSTITUTION-ACUPUNCTURE TREATMENT IS NO EXCEPTION.

CHAPTER 7

Constitution-acupuncture Treatment

The treatment method of Constitution-acupuncture is very unique compared to other acupuncture techniques. Unlike general acupuncture techniques, in which needles are inserted into the skin or muscles and left there for a certain period of time, no needle remains in the flesh. Instead, it is a unique technique where a combination of Unit Formulae (Compound Formula) is instantly applied (the needle is sticked in and pulled out instantly) in the serial order to address the Zang-Fu organs causing excessive imbalance in the corresponding Constitution. This acupuncture method is specific to Eight-Constitution Medicine and does not exist anywhere else in the world. It is a procedure based on sophisticated calculations, similar to mathematics, considering the dynamics of Synchronizing and Antagonizing of the Five Phases derived from the Zang-Fu Structure of the Constitution. The goal is to decrease what is excessive and increase what is lacking.

Let's learn about Constitution-acupuncture tools

For Constitution-acupuncture treatment, a special needle tube designed for instantaneous needling is used. The function of this needle tube has been constantly improved through design changes. The needle that goes into the needle tube is recommended to have a diameter of 0.25 mm and a length of 30 mm. Depending on the practitioner's preference, thinner or thicker needles may be used, but in my case, 0.25 mm thickness delivers the best needle feel. The length must be 30 mm because the needle tube is manufactured to fit the needle of this length. The shape of the acupuncture tube and needles are shown in the following picture.

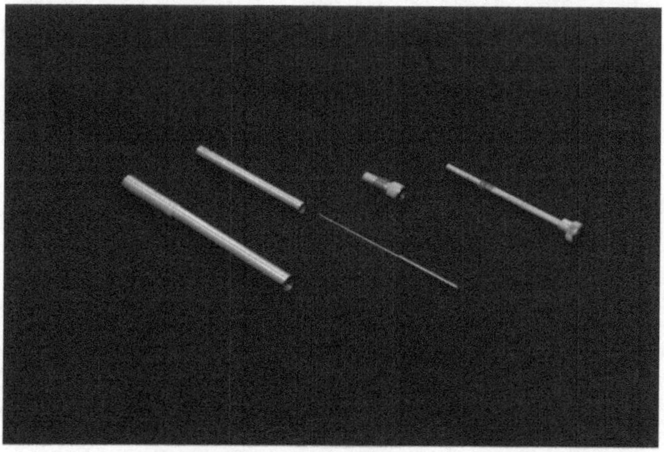

Figure 1. Component parts of the needle tube and needle

The picture above shows the parts that make up the needle tube and the needle. The leftmost part is the outer tube, which forms the outermost part of the needle tube. Next is the needle mount, where the needle is inserted. Then, there is the needle that goes into the needle mount, followed by the tightening screw that connects to the outer tube, and finally a pestle (head-like handle shape) tube, which is used when applying acupuncture on the needle with the index finger of your right hand. This explanation is based on the assumption of the right-handed person. When these components are assembled, they look like the following picture.

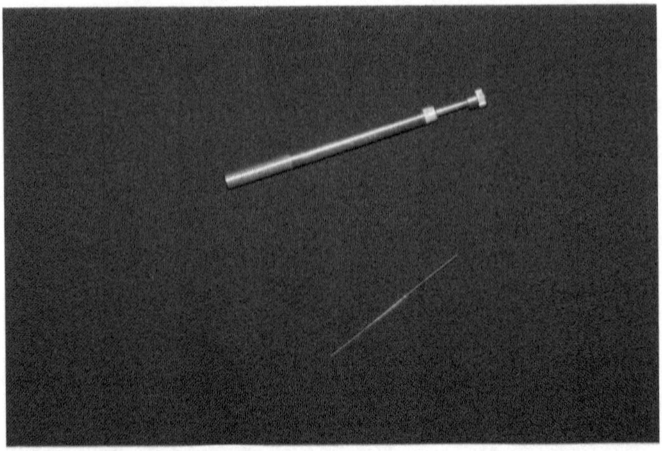

Figure 2. Assembled acupuncture tube and needle

The parts of the needle tube are assembled with screws, so they must be tightened properly. Otherwise, they may come loose during the

Constitution-acupuncture treatment process. The needle tube should always be thoroughly disinfected to maintain a clean and sterile condition.

Preparation for Constitution-acupuncture practice

The acupuncture tube has a knurled section about 2 cm long at the end. This part is held with the thumb and forefinger of the left hand, and the pestle of the acupuncture tube is pulled upward with the thumb and forefinger of the right hand. The middle and ring fingers of the right hand support the body of the acupuncture tube. The following picture shows the needle tube being held correctly and placed on the treatment area. The pictures below show treatment procedures using the Constitution-acupuncture tool, demonstrated by me.

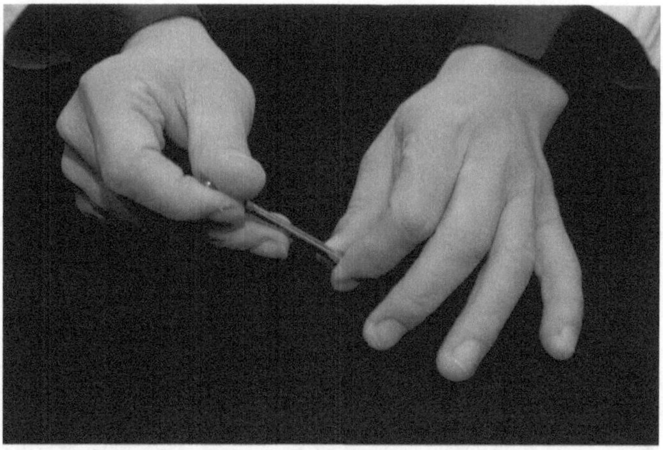

Figure 3. Constitution-acupuncture treatment (preparatory stage)

Pull the needle back and hold it with your right thumb and forefinger. Also, use both hands to support the needle tube so that it does not shake.

3 Steps of Constitution-acupuncture treatment

As shown in Figure 3, hold the needle tube and place it at a 45-degree angle to the treatment area in preparation for inserting the needle. The tips for applying the acupuncture needle are as follows:

① Tilt the index finger of your right hand back.
② Lightly and momentarily tap the pestle of the needle tube using the snap of your index finger and wrist.
③ At the same time as snapping the pestle, grab its head with the thumb and forefinger of your right hand and pull it back. At this time, the needle tube is slightly lifted backward due to inertia. When applying and removing the needle, support the needle tube well so that it does not shake left or right.

For the good Constitution-acupuncture treatment, it must be performed so that these three movements are carried out almost simultaneously and in a flexible, continuous motion, like lightning. This is easier said than done, but quite difficult at first. You can't master it right away. First, place something like a rubber plate with a texture similar to the muscles of the human body and start practicing with separate movements. Look at the following picture.

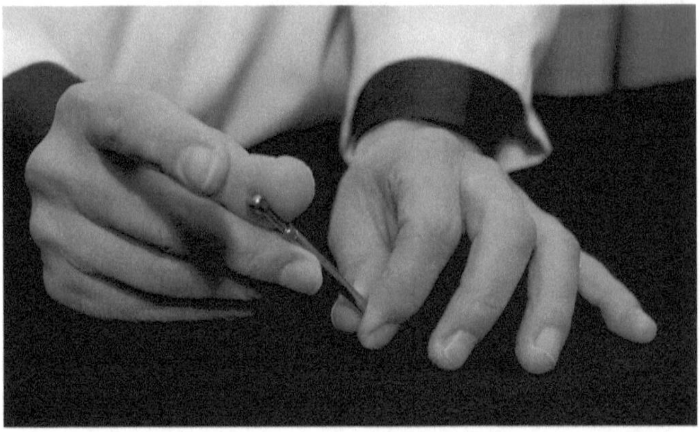

Step 1: Tilt the index finger of your right hand back. The right thumb continues to support the pestle. The left hand should also support the end of the needle tube to prevent it from shaking when applying the needle.

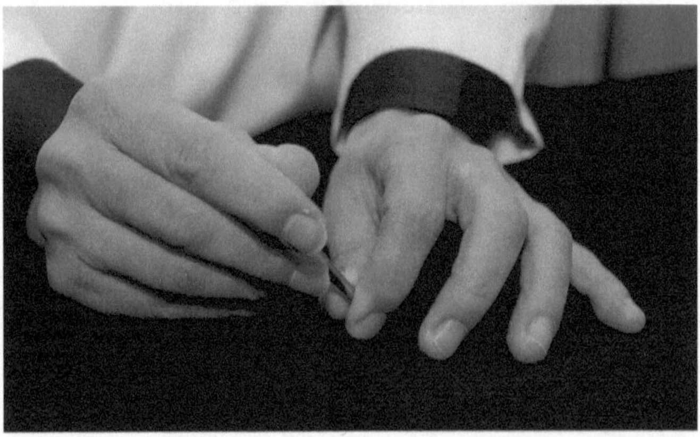

Step 2: Instantly hit the pestle of the needle tube. When striking, you must use a quick wrist snap to strike swiftly. Do not push. When the needle tube shakes while pushing, the tip of the

needle may bend. In fact, this often happens in the early stages of Constitution-acupuncture treatment when treating a patient.

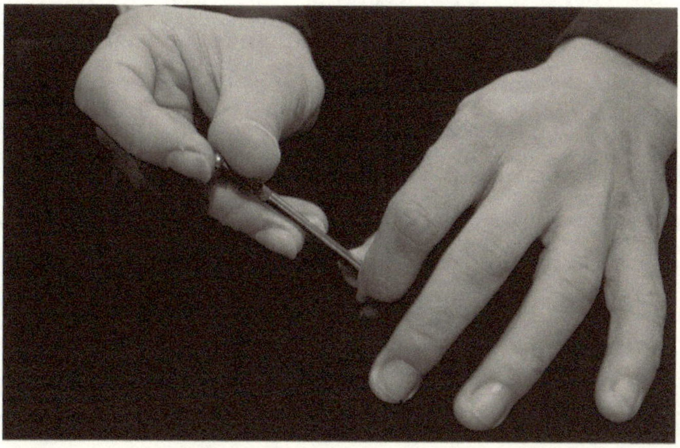

Step 3: Grab the pestle head of the acupuncture tube and pull it back. At this time, due to inertia, the needle tube and the hand holding it are naturally lifted backward. Here, for convenience, the three steps ①, ②, and ③ are explained separately, but in the actual practice, these three steps occur instantaneously, so they should be considered as almost simultaneous actions.

Figure 4. Three steps of Constitution-acupuncture treatment

Constitution-acupuncture treatment is one of the acupuncture methods that is performed extremely superficially, as it aims to move in and out of the Zang-Fu acupoints on the skin at a depth of approximately 1 to 2 mm from the surface. Therefore, it is performed for completely different purpose from those ordinary acupuncture techniques, which physically stimulate the skin, subcutaneous muscles, or nerves usually deep much more than Constitution-acupuncture treatment.

Constitution-acupuncture method is never an acupuncture technique that physically stimulates the skin, muscles, or nervous tissue. Although it may appear that way externally, its purpose is to transmit the signals of the Five Phases—Wood, Fire, Earth, Metal, and Water—that regulate the Five Zangs and Five Fus, essentially conveying vital information. Therefore, no matter how shallow the Constitution-acupuncture treatment is, if it is above the threshold that our body can accept as a signal, it is recognized as meaningful information. That is, though you apply more pressure, the effect would not be proportionally stronger, and though you apply less pressure, the effect would not be proportionally weaker. What is important is how rhythmically and accurately the needle is inserted to the appropriate depth. The signal consists of only two types: one is plus, and the other is minus. A plus sign refers to the Following Method, where the needle is applied in the same direction as the meridian's travel direction, while a minus sign refers to the Meeting Method, where the needle is placed in the opposite direction of the meridian's travel.

Practice!

Although the Constitution-acupuncture is performed in this shallow depth, it can be quite painful to patients for beginners to apply Constitution-acupuncture treatment. This is because they lack the skills to handle the needle tube and often end up inserting it deeper than necessary. Of course, the effect remains the same, but it is better to practice acupuncture frequently to become more skilled and to make the patient feel a slight tingling sensation. When performing the procedure on young children, they are particularly sensitive to pain, so advanced techniques are required to ensure that the procedure is performed as gently as possible, minimizing the pain.

Also, the areas where Constitution-acupuncture needles are applied are often difficult spots to insert acupuncture needles, such as the fingertips, toes, crooks, and elbows, etc. Additionally, the skin in these areas is either thick or sensitive, so the pain is stronger. That is why skilled acupuncture technique is required. How do you reach that level? There is only one answer: practice, practice, practice. If you practice like that, at some point, you will suddenly have an "Aha!" moment when you can get the hang of it. When you reach a level of mastery, you can delicately control the depth at which the needle enters the skin. Of course, don't forget—it's all about practice!

At first, practice the acupuncture technique using a latex-like rubber plate, imagining the acupuncture points in your mind and reiterating the number of repetitions. It would be even better if you have a human body model or a doll made of rubber-like material. Make it a habit to repeat accurately, paying attention to the things such as how to hold the needle tube, the angle between the needle tube and the treatment area, and the appropriate timing of hand movements.

Example of Constitution-acupuncture treatment

Now, let's look at an example of applying Constitution-acupuncture through the Geumeum Constitution, one of the Eight Constitutions, in more detail. Let's take as an example the Basic Formula for Geumeum Constitution. The Basic Formula for Geumeum Constitution is a Unit Formula that targets the Lungs and consists of KI10 (Yingu), LU5 (Chize), LR1 (Dadun), and LU11 (Shaoshang). The acupuncture is performed in the following order.

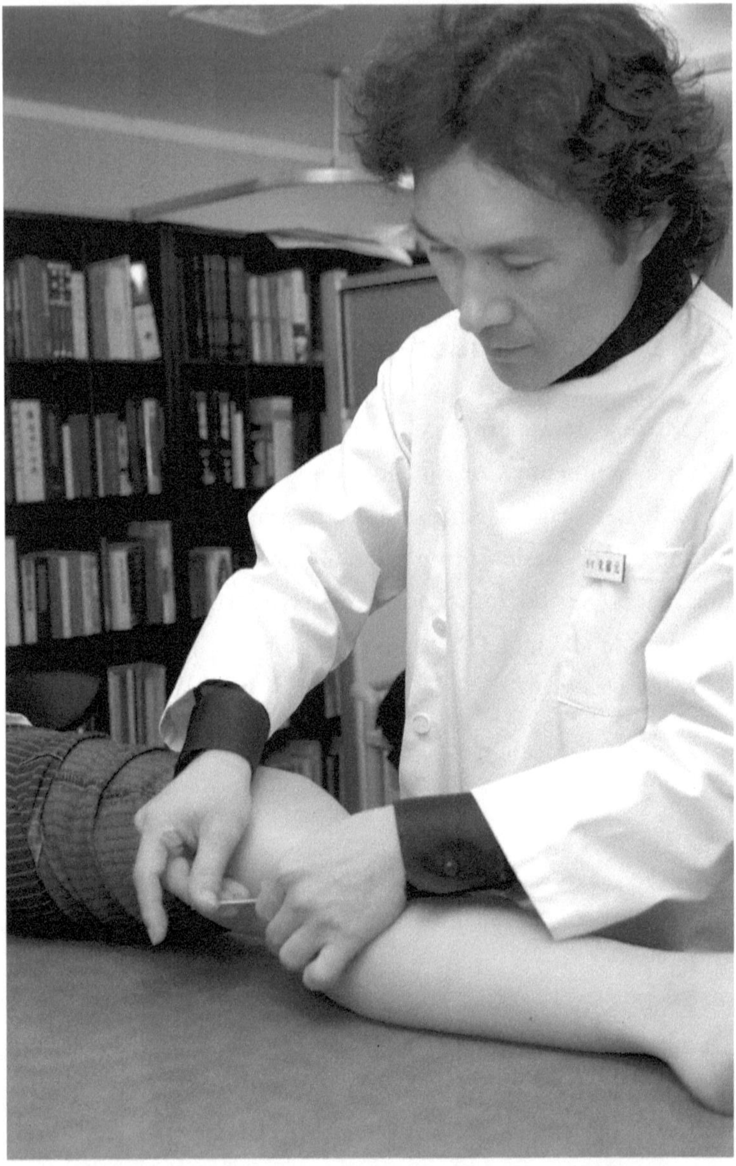

① Apply the Meeting Method on KI10 (Yingu) point, which serves as Water point for the Liver meridian, in the direction to the foot, which is opposite to the direction of movement of the Liver meridian. At this time, point the tip of the needle tube toward the toe and maintain an angle of 45 degrees to the treatment surface.

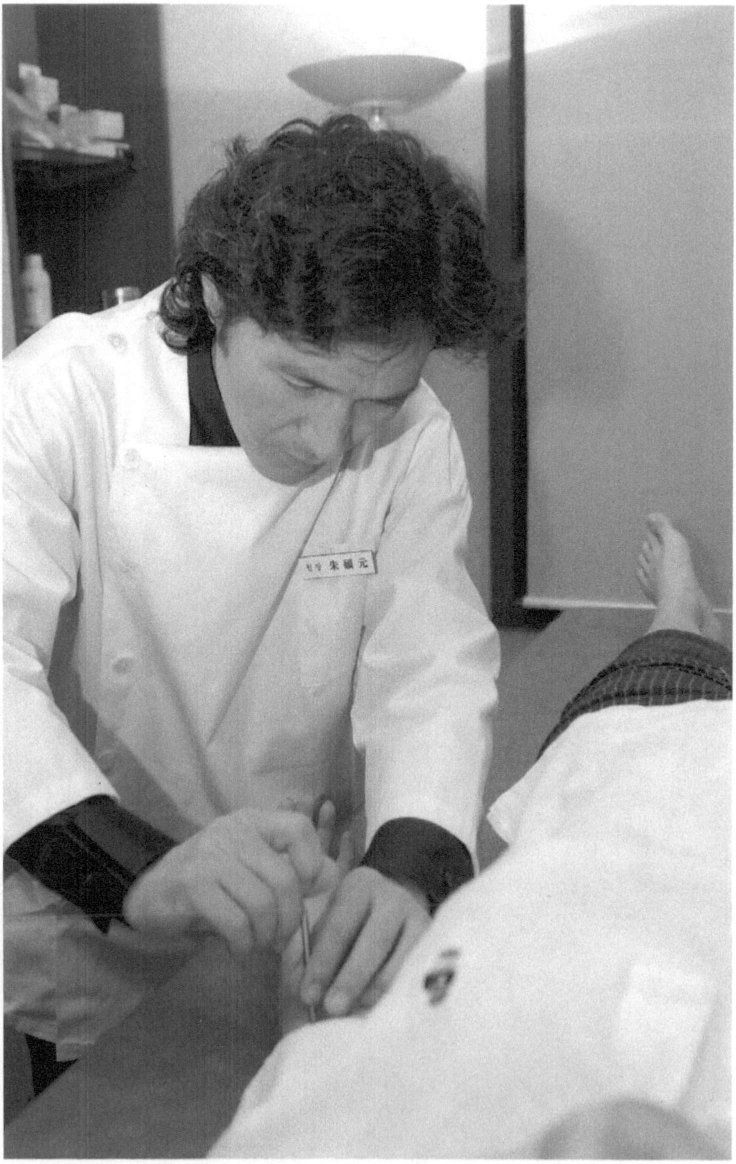

② Apply the Meeting Method on LU5 (Chize) point, which serves as Water point for the Lung meridian, in the direction to the body (torso), which is opposite to the direction of movement of the Lung meridian.

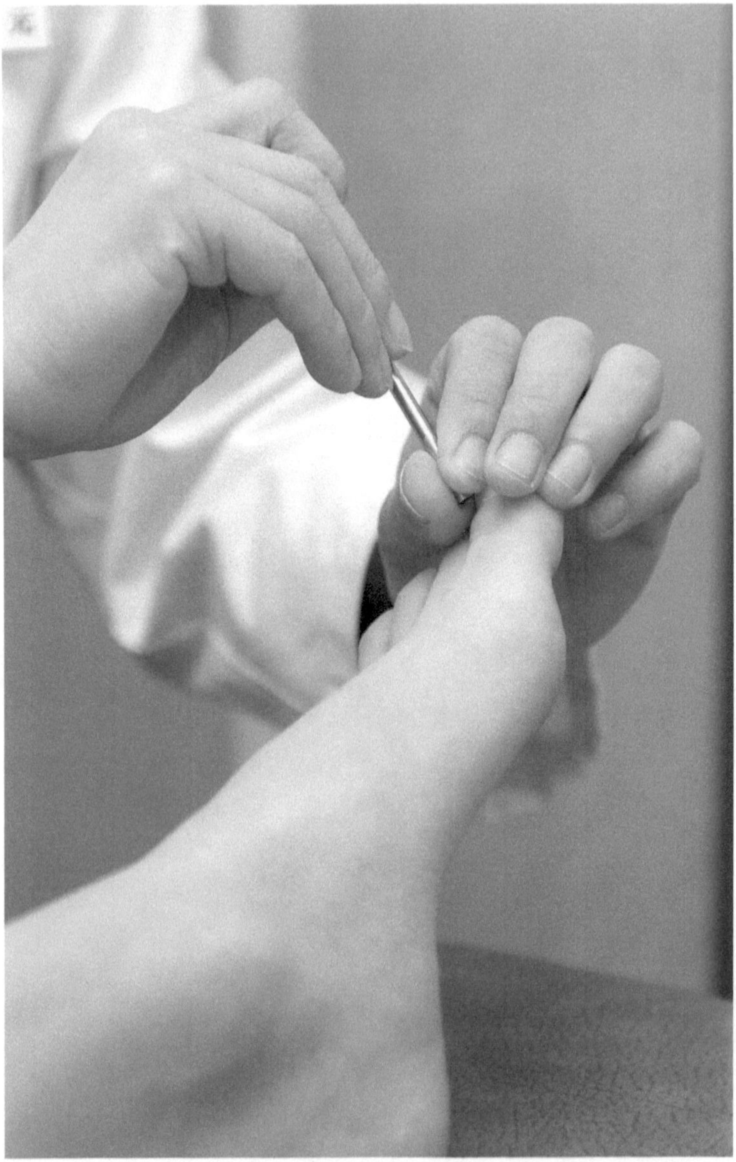

③ Apply the Following Method on LR1 (Dadun) point, Wood point of the Liver meridian, facing toward the body in the same direction as the movement of the Liver meridian.

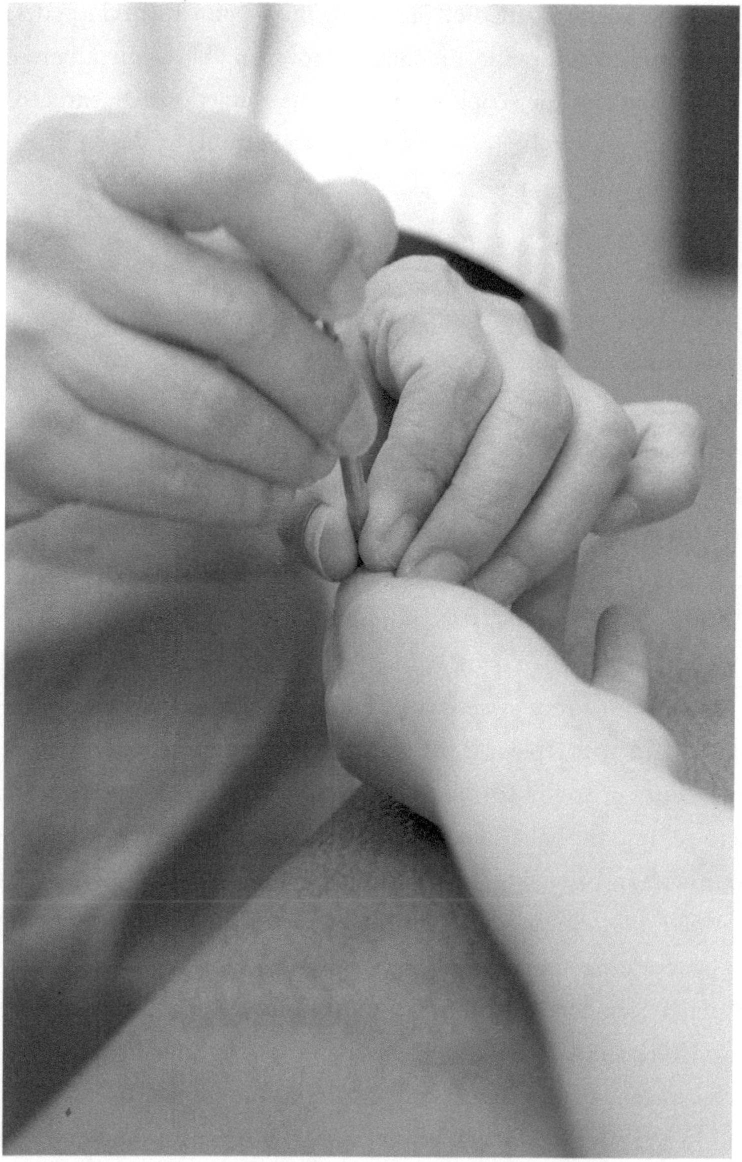

④ Apply the Following Method on LU11 (Shaoshang) point, a Wood point of the Lung meridian, in the same direction as the movement of the Lung meridian, toward the fingertip.

Figure 5. Basic Formula acupuncture treatment for Geumeum Constitution

You must follow the method of holding the acupuncture tube as described above, carefully consider the direction of movement of the meridians, ensure the correct angle of the acupuncture tube, and practice frequently to apply it calmly and quickly. If you repeat the Basic Formula as shown in Figure 5 above 5 times, you can repeat ①, ②, ③, and ④ five times in that order. That is, ①, ②, ③, ④ (1st time), ①, ②, ③, ④ (2nd time), ①, ②, ③, ④ (3rd time), ①, ②, ③, ④ (4th time), and ①, ②, ③, ④ (5th time).

Next, let's look at an example of actually performing the Compound Formula based on the example above. Let's treat inflammatory disease of the stomach, which is a condition that many people suffer from. This prescription can be treated with the Fu-system Inflammation Formula, which is a two-stage Formula. The Formula consists of 4 times Basic Formula and 2 times Fu-system Inflammation Sub-formula. You can apply the Fu-system Inflammation Formula with 4 times Unit Formula (VIIs) to drain the Lungs and 2 times Unit Formula (IIIt) to replenish the Heart.

First, repeat KI10 (Yingu) c, LU5 (Chize) c, LR1 (Dadun) p, and LU11 (Shaoshang) p 4 times as shown in Figure 5 above. Next, repeat the Unit Formula (IIIt) that replenish the Heart, KI10 (Yingu) c, HT3 (Shaohai) c, LR1 (Dadun) p, and HT9 (Shaochong) p, repeating the process twice. You need to get into the habit of counting the number of repetitions in this order in your head and applying them accurately.

Constitution-acupuncture treatment uses a method of amplifying the effect by repeating Unit Formula, so when performing high-level Compound Formula, a considerable number of repetitions are made. For example, if a 5-stage Compound Formula is repeated 5 times, the number of needlings for Unit Formulae of two Zang-Fu organs in the Yang Field, and two Zang-Fu organs in the Yin Field (a total of four Zang-Fu organs) would be 4 x 5 x 4 = 80 (times), and the number of needlings for Unit Formulae of Pericardium or Triple Burner would be 2 x 5 = 10 (times), resulting in a total of 90 needlings. If the 5-stage Formula is performed on both the left and right sides, the number of needlings could reach as many as 180 times. Imagine performing 180 needlings in one procedure! It can be expected that this will result in a very strong amplification effect. Therefore, the higher the level of the Formula, the more serious disease it is used to treat. However, high-stage Formulae are not necessarily the solution. As Je-ma Lee said, a serious illness should be treated with a heavy treatment, and a mild illness should be treated with a mild treatment.

Any procedure always requires skill, and since it involves our body, it is crucial to stick to the basics when first learning Constitution-acupuncture so that it becomes ingrained in your body without even realizing it. I hope that through sincere training, while remaining faithful to the basics, you become a master of Constitution-Acupuncture.

CHAPTER 8

Clinical Cases of 8 Constitutions (Medical Essay)

EVEN IF IT IS THE SAME DISEASE, ITS SYMPTOMS CAN VARY FROM PATIENT TO PATIENT, MUCH LIKE A RAINBOW. DIFFERENCES IN ILLNESS EXIST BOTH BETWEEN INDIVIDUALS AND WITHIN THE SAME INDIVIDUAL. THE DISTINCTION BETWEEN DISEASES RESIDES IN REPETITION.

CHAPTER 8

Clinical Cases of 8 Constitutions (Medical Essay)

The following is clinical cases of the Eight Constitutions. Among the numerous clinical cases, memorable and special cases have been selected. In general, there are not many patients with such special cases compared to other patients. However, no matter how ordinary the disease, there are not many cases where treatment is so easy. In some cases, the process of treating a disease resolves dramatically, in other cases, it resolves with much difficulty, and in some cases, it ends in a less-than-satisfactory manner.

Most of the diseases we suffer from are not actually caused by external factors. They are "self-inflicted." Even though we clearly know that certain foods are not good for us, we eat them under various excuses. We fail to properly control our emotions, allowing ourselves to constantly wander in a swamp of stress. We neglect to train our bodies and become lazy. These are what ultimately leads us to illness. Disease is what "manifests itself" as a revolt caused by our body when its exit is blocked. Therefore, "I" am the cause of the disease. Illness is the sad cry of my body, a cry that I have brought upon myself. Danjae Chae-ho Shin (1880-1936, a historian and an independence movement activist against Japanese rule over Korea in the early 20th century), in his book *Joseon Sanggosa* (*Ancient History of Korea*), stated that history is "the struggle between self and non-self," but this is not true when it comes to diseases. Illness is the struggle between "self and self." The enemy is always within myself. In the clinical cases of the Eight

Constitutions that I am introducing here, you will witness this reality countless times.

Treating an illness is actually not as easy as you might think. It is often said that "politics is a living thing." This means that politics is not a fixed entity but rather a dynamic, ever-changing process, much like a living organism. Similarly, the human disease and the human body that copes with it are living things. They are like an unpredictable, nonlinear function that moves constantly, engaging in an endless and fierce battle. Through the specific cases presented here, readers will be able to vividly experience how the diseases of the Eight Constitutions occur, what symptoms they show, and how they are treated, as if they were witnessing these events right before their eyes.

My treatment method disclosed in these clinical cases is generally consistent with the treatment method introduced in the Principle of Compound Formulae in Chapter 4. However, as a result of my own approach, there are often cases that deviate from the standard treatment (this is generally true regarding the number of repetitions for the Formulae or the treatment location on the left or right). This is because, as long clinical trials accumulate, ad hoc and transformative treatments emerge unexpectedly or naturally. Therefore, please keep in mind that there may be some different treatment processes from what I discussed in the Principle of Compound Formulae. Beginners are advised to establish a standard treatment framework, first.

The principles of Eight-Constitution Medicine are very strict and detailed, but creative deviations are allowed in the treatment process, as long as they operate within those principles. Constitution-acupuncture is literally a world of freedom with no limits. As long as it does not deviate from the premise of the Constitutional Zang-Fu Structure, it offers an infinite space that can accommodate all possible treatments without limitation. I hope practitioners can freely explore and expand the possibilities of treatment within the framework of this Constitutional Zang-Fu Structure.

When we get sick, our body temporarily loses its order of life. If you become seriously ill or have a chronic illness, it becomes complete chaos. It is just the battlefield as in *Sun Tzu's Art of War* where advanced tactics and stratagems are more evident. It is a fierce battleground where the disease threatening health and the power of life seeking to restore it face off dramatically. The series of "Challenge and Response" mentioned by Arnold J. Toynbee (1889–1972) is clearly unfolding. The variations of disease and treatment are manifesting as a panorama of dialectics—thesis, antithesis, and synthesis—proposed by Georg Wilhelm Friedrich Hegel (1770–1831). The process of our body restoring its own order through the treatment of the Eight Constitutions in that extreme battle is sometimes mysterious, sometimes beautiful, and sometimes majestic. By participating in the thrilling combat within our bodies, readers will be able to understand Eight-Constitution Medicine in more depth. So, let's dive into the time-space of living life right now!

Geumyang Constitution's Clinical Cases

[Geumyang Case 1] Eight-Constitution Medicine Is The Sacred Site for Vocalists

* Patient: Mr. G, 43 years old at the time of visit
* Chief complaints: Recurrent stomatitis and stinging sensation of the tongue

The patient was a vocalist in the classical music field, such as opera, who was prone to stomatitis and frequently suffered from it. For professional singers, these symptoms can be quite annoying.

I diagnosed him with Geumyang Constitution. Since the oral cavity, the treatment area, belongs to the Fu-system and the Upper Burner, treatment was performed using the Fu-system Inflammation Formula in a 4:2 ratio (the numbers in parentheses indicate the ratio) with ana-puncture on the right and the Sterilization Formula in a 4:2 ratio with ana-puncture on the left. The specific acupoint names and methods are as follows.

Constitution-acupuncture: R. I V (ana 42) / L. I VI (ana 42)

The specific acupoint names are as follows:

[Right] Fu-system Inflammation Formula for Upper Burner
* LU8 (Jingqu) c, LR4 (Zhongfeng) c, KI10 (Yingu) p, PC3 (Quze) p - repeat 4 times.
* LU8 (Jingqu) c, LU8 (Jingqu) c, SP5 (Shangqiu) c, SP5 (Shangqiu) c, KI10 (Yingu) p, SP9 (Yinlingquan) p - repeat 2 times.

[Left] Sterilization Formula for Upper Burner
* LU8 (Jingqu) c, LR4 (Zhongfeng) c, KI10 (Yingu) p, PC3 (Quze) p - repeat 4 times.
* LI1 (Shangyang) c, LI1 (Shangyang) c, ST45 (Lidui) c, ST45 (Lidui) c, BL66 (Zutonggu) p, ST44 (Neiting) p - repeat 2 times.

The patient was completely cured with this prescription in just one session! In fact, this result is remarkable, especially when you often witness many people around you who suffer from chronic stomatitis.

He returned to my clinic one month later, this time for swollen, sore throat. Since the throat also belongs to the Fu-system and is located in the Upper Burner, it was treated with the same prescription as the first session. Again, it was completely cured in just one session.

The fact that the different diseases are cured with the same treatment is like the "principle of identity" in philosophy. This is because it focuses on the common properties hidden behind different phenomena. However, the trend of modern philosophy actually emphasizes "difference" rather than identity. In some ways, Constitutional Formulae seem to go against this trend and pursue uniformity. However, if we consider that the same disease is treated differently depending on the Constitution, the perspective changes completely. This is because it focuses on difference rather than sameness. In this way, sameness and difference coexist.

The patient in this case responded well to Constitution-acupuncture treatment. Stomatitis and sore throat, which had been chronic conditions for this patient that are typically not easy to treat, were easily cured with one treatment session each using the same two-stage Formula.

The Geumyang Constitution has the Zang-Fu Structure consisting of "Lungs-Large intestine Pancreas-Stomach Heart-Small intestine Kidneys-Bladder Liver-Gallbladder." Since the Lungs are the outermost organ in the Yang Field, a healthy person with Geumyang Constitution leads to good lung capacity and abundant vocal volume, making it the optimal Constitution for vocal music. However, if a singer frequently consumes a diet that is not suitable for the Constitution, excessive imbalance may occur, leading to inflammation of the vocal cords and, in severe cases, vocal nodules which can be detrimental to the singer. Individuals with vocations such as vocalists or singers often face the issue with their vocal cords, making it difficult to sing. Constitutional therapy is highly effective in addressing and resolving these problems.

Singer Baek-ho Choi (1950~) once shared that his health significantly improved after being diagnosed with the Geumyang Constitution and receiving Constitutional treatment. He proudly states that not only is his health better, but his vocal cords—vital to a singer—are in much better condition than they were in his prime, allowing him to sing even better now. As a result, he refers to himself as an "8-Constitution evangelist," enthusiastically sharing his genuine advocacy for Eight-Constitution Medicine with everyone he meets. As I have always admired him as a singer, I looked into his live performances and carefully compared his past to present performances. His vocal control, including pitch, volume, and high notes, was more stable than before. The song such as his early classic, "My Heart Has No Place to Go," was performed even at a higher pitch than when he was younger. Considering that he is well over 70 years old now in 2024, this is quite incredible.

Musical actress Joo-hyun Ok (1980~) is also an advocate of the Eight-Constitution Medicine. After being diagnosed with Mogyang Constitution, she mentioned that by thoroughly following the Mogyang Constitution's regimen, she got healthy and improved her vocalizations, and has maintained a consistently good voice. Many patients who visit my clinic often come after hearing about the Eight Constitutions from her.

In fact, individuals with the Mogyang Constitution, like Joo-hyun Ok, may face many challenges as singers when viewed from the perspective of the Zang-Fu Structure. This is because, in the Mogyang Constitution's Zang-Fu Structure of "Liver-Gallbladder Kidneys-Bladder Heart-Small Intestine Pancreas-Stomach Lungs-Large Intestine," the Lungs are the outermost Zang in the Yin Field and have the lowest potential within the Structure. However, this can be overcome by following a thorough Constitutional regimen. This is because the regimen can significantly elevate the potential of the Lungs to their optimal state. And just like the vocalist mentioned in this clinical case 1, the problems that cannot be resolved on their own can be easily addressed through the professional treatment based on the Eight Constitutions. Constitutional Medicine is a balancing approach that brings our body to its optimal state. I believe singer Joo-hyun Ok has successfully overcome her vocalization issues, a weakness of her Mogyang Constitution, through Constitutional Medicine.

In my clinical practice, I have quite extensive experiences treating vocal cord issues in vocalists and singers using Eight-Constitution Medicine.

One notable case involved Kim, who was once Korea's leading female trot singer. She urgently called me on a holiday, distressed because her voice had stopped functioning after her first performance of the day. She was performing at the Jangchung Gymnasium, and with one more performance to go, she desperately requested my help, saying it was an emergency.

I quickly grabbed my acupuncture kit and rushed to the venue. Kim had a Geumyang Constitution, so I applied Constitution-acupuncture tailored to Geumyang. Her voice recovered, and she was able to complete her second performance successfully.

I also recall treating fellow performers at that time, including some of the leading singers of the same genre—Mr. Hyun, Mr. Nam, and musical actress Park—providing them with Constitutional diagnoses and Constitution-acupuncture treatments.

Notably, singer Hyun had recently suffered a serious accident during another performance. While navigating on the dark stage, he misstepped and fell off, resulting in his ribs fracture. His torso was wrapped in bandages, and each time he sang, the contraction and relaxation of the intercostal muscles, which are essential for breathing, caused excruciating pain in the thoracic area. Through my Eight-Constitution acupuncture treatment, his pain was significantly alleviated, enabling him to complete his performance successfully, too.

That day stands out as a pivotal moment in my Eight-Constitution clinical journey, as I had the opportunity to treat the four singers who were iconic figures in Korea's music scene—all in a single day.

[Geumyang Case 2] Restoring Radiant Skin

* Patient: Ms. G, 9 Years old at the time of visit
* Chief complaints: Severe inflammation and dead skin buildup on the face and body caused by atopic dermatitis

An elementary school girl came to my clinic with atopic dermatitis all over her face. The lesion was severe not only on the face, but also on the entire body, including the limbs and torso. Her mother said that after frequently visiting the swimming pool that winter, her atopic dermatitis worsened. Before that, it, being not severe, would come on and go away, but this time it doesn't get better and keeps getting worse. When she laid down on the treatment bed to get a diagnosis, dead skin cells fell from her entire body like snow and piled up on the bed surface. It seemed like the treatment would take quite a long time.

Atopic dermatitis often develops when you frequently consume foods that are not suited to your Constitution, particularly meat, flour-based foods, spicy foods, and dairy products. It seems that the girl's predisposition to atopic dermatitis had accumulated due to her diet pattern that was not aligned with her Constitution, and the increased exposure to the disinfectant used in the pool water, resulting from her frequent swimming, likely acted as a trigger, causing the atopic dermatitis to flare up in earnest. The treatment process was as follows.

Feb 28, 20XX. Entered treatment. The Formula for atopic dermatitis was prescribed differently for the right and left sides.

Geumyang Constitution-acupuncture: R. II VI IV' X (4444) / L. II VI IV' V (4444)

To describe it in detail, on the right side, the Fu-system Basic Formula, Sterilization Sub-formula, Fu-system Mental Sub-formula, and Fu-system Degeneration Sub-formula were treated four times each. On the left side, the Fu-system Basic Formula, Sterilization Sub-formula, Fu-system Mental

Sub-formula, and Fu-system Inflammation Sub-formula were treated four times each.

After the treatment for a while, I explained the characteristics of Geumyang Constitution to the girl and her mother and provided them with the detailed instructions on diet, including the Constitutional Diet. Severe skin diseases, such as atopic dermatitis, require a strict Constitutional Diet; otherwise, treatment can be quite difficult. Even if the treatment progresses well, it often worsens quickly if the patient consumes even a small amount of food that is not suitable for Constitution. The child and her mother listened attentively to my advice and left.

March 2, 20XX. The patient visited my clinic two days later, reporting that the condition had slightly worsened. She mentioned that the condition seemed to have deteriorated due to discontinuing Western medicine. It is common to experience withdrawal symptoms when stopping Western medicine abruptly, which often leads to a temporary worsening of the condition. Therefore, it is important to inform patients that atopic dermatitis may worsen during the early stages of treatment, so both the patient and the doctor can continue the treatment without hesitation. I treated her with the same Constitution-acupuncture treatment and advised them to adhere strictly to the Constitutional Diet.

March 4, 20XX. The patient came back to my clinic two days later and reported having a difficult time with itching at night. Overcoming this hurdle is essential for the fundamental treatment of atopic dermatitis. The Constitutional regimen was emphasized once again, and the same treatment continued.

March 5, 20XX. The patient visited my clinic the following day and mentioned that she slept well because the itching had decreased. I felt that improvement was happening faster than expected. There was hope. The same Constitution-acupuncture Formula was applied.

March 6, 20XX. The patient reported scratching a little the previous day. The same prescription procedure was followed.

March 7, 20XX. The patient visited the next day and mentioned that she had scratched slightly. She also noted that the scabs were starting to form on the skin. This is a positive sign, as it indicates that the process of oozing and overlapping inflammation is decreasing. The same prescription procedure continued.

March 9, 20XX. The patient visited two days later, reporting gradual improvement. Many scabs had fallen off and disappeared, and the itching was almost gone! This is a significant change. Atopic dermatitis is challenging to treat because it often recurs due to constant itching and scratching. When the itching stops, the scratching ceases, and the additional inflammation no longer occurs, allowing the patient to progress toward healing. The same prescription procedure was followed.

March 12, 20XX. Three days later, the patient reported that fewer dead skin cells were falling off, and the skin was regenerating where the dead skin cells had fallen. She still felt some itching at night. The same prescription procedure was followed.

March 14, 20XX. Two days later, the patient reported improvement. The same prescription procedure was followed.

March 18, 20XX. Four days later, the patient reported further improvement. The same prescription procedure continued.

March 20, 20XX. Two days later, less dead skin was falling off. The same prescription procedure was followed.

March 25, 20XX. Five days later, the patient mentioned that upon waking up in the mornings, she used to experience dead skin cells falling off and skin oozing, but this was now happening less frequently. The same prescription procedure was followed.

March 26, 20XX. The next day, the patient reported that she was now able to sleep without scratching much. The same prescription procedure continued.

April 4, 20XX. The patient had been visiting every 2-3 days, but today she visited my clinic 9 days after the last treatment. Although some dead skin cells remained on the face, the itching had decreased significantly, and the skin had improved greatly. Therefore, the frequency of visits became less. The same prescription procedure was followed.

April 18, 20XX. This time, the patient visited my clinic after 14 days. She reported that the atopic dermatitis had decreased significantly in most areas of the body, including the face and legs. The same prescription procedure was followed.

July 6, 20XX. After almost two and a half months, the patient's mother visited my clinic alone. She thanked me for the treatment and reported that her daughter had improved significantly. End.

This patient was completely cured with a total of 15 Constitution-acupuncture treatments, from the first visit to the final treatment. Contrary to my initial expectations, it was a successful case that was treated relatively quickly.

Atopic dermatitis is not an easy disease to treat. In particular, patients who visit my clinic often come after long-term use of harsh drugs like steroids in Western dermatology clinics, making it more difficult to treat them.

Therefore, it is best to prevent atopic dermatitis by consistently following a regimen that suits one's Constitution. The most important preventive measure is adhering to a healthy diet, that is, Constitutional Diet.

However, in addition to food, there are other factors that can worsen atopic dermatitis. Stress is a major factor, aside from food. This is easily confirmed by observing that students' atopic dermatitis worsens significantly during exam periods. Other factors, such as fine dust and climate, can also have a significant impact on the disease.

Meals from outside, rather than home-cooked meals—such as eating out—are also a major culprit that worsens atopic dermatitis. Even if you order food that suits your Constitution, eating out often exacerbates atopic dermatitis. The most likely reason is the use of MSG (monosodium glutamate) or various other chemical seasonings. Many patients unanimously report that their atopic dermatitis worsens quickly after eating something from outside. If possible, it is recommended to maintain a clean diet at home.

Construction materials are unexpectedly one of the factors that can cause atopic dermatitis. A few years ago, a male student visited my clinic with severe atopic dermatitis. Initially, the cause was unclear, but when his father thought about it, he realized that his son had developed the disease after moving into a new apartment. Specifically, the harmful chemicals released from various building materials used in the new apartment were responsible for triggering his son's condition.

This patient had already tried various treatments, including hospital care, herbal medicine, supplements, etc. However, none of the prescribed medications and supplements worked, and some even worsened his condition. Then, after hearing about my reputation, the family visited my clinic.

I diagnosed the patient with Geumyang Constitution and began treating his atopic dermatitis using Geumyang Constitution-acupuncture Formula and Constitutional decoction. While some improvement was seen with this treatment, the progress was quite slow.

The issue was the chemicals in the new apartment, which continued to affect the patient. Despite cleaning all the spaces in the apartment thoroughly and trying various remedies like cypress tree phytoncide (well-known for removing harmful substances), nothing worked. However, his father, firmly determined to resolve the issue, researched various solutions to eliminate the harmful chemicals in the new apartment. To support his desperate efforts to cure his son, I, with a glimmer of hope, recommended using pine wood to address his son's atopic dermatitis, as pine trees are beneficial for the Geumyang Constitution. Eventually, the father decided to take a drastic step to purchase high-quality pine wood.

With a heavy heart, the father went to a woodworking shop and bought numerous pine boards. He then covered the entire inside of his son's room with the pine wood boards, replacing the wallpaper. The transformation of the room was astounding, turning it into a log cabin, even though the apartment itself was a concrete building.

Surprisingly, this method worked wonders. The change was remarkable. In fact, I had suggested this pine wood solution with some doubts, so I had never imagined it would be so effective. The harmful chemicals in the apartment were blocked by the pine wood barrier, preventing the atopic dermatitis-causing agents from entering the boy's skin or respiratory system. With this added protection, the Constitution-acupuncture treatment began to work more effectively.

I concluded that the situation dramatically improved by supplementing the Wood Qi of the pine trees, which helped balance the lack of Wood Qi in the Geumyang Constitution.

The Geumyang Constitution, along with the Geumeum Constitution, is particularly vulnerable to chemical toxic substances. As demonstrated by this patient, harmful substances not only from building materials but also from sources such as factory or automobile exhaust, fine dust, pesticides, chemical components in dyes, the smell of cosmetics or perfumes, chemical seasonings in food, and even synthetic fibers used in everyday fabrics can significantly affect people with this Constitution.

In more severe cases, electromagnetic waves also play a role. Electromagnetic waves emitted from devices such as computers, mobile phones, and even ATM machines can cause significant issues. One patient with the Geumyang Constitution experienced headaches merely from turning on the microwave. Even after retreating to the master bedroom, which was the farthest from the kitchen where the microwave was located, the headache persisted.

The most extreme case I encountered in my clinical practice involved a patient who could not tolerate electromagnetic waves from fluorescent lights. This individual eventually moved to a remote area in a deep mountain valley in Gangwon-do Province, far from the distractions of civilization. There, he lived in isolation, using an oil lamp and cultivating vegetable gardens on his own. In severe cases, the Geumyang Constitution may require a lifestyle completely disconnected from modern civilization.

[Geumyang Case 3] Leave Liver Disease to Eight-Constitution Medicine

* Patient: Mr. G, office worker, 57 years old at the time of visit
* Chief complaints: Hepatic cancer, allergic rhinitis

The patient visited my clinic during his treatment for liver cancer at a local hospital. The previous year, he was diagnosed with the disease, received chemotherapy, and underwent embolization[115] once. He had been suffering from chronic hepatitis B for a long time. One day, feeling unwell, he underwent a liver ultrasound at a primary medical institution. After discovering abnormal findings, he was transferred to K University Hospital, where he was diagnosed with the liver cancer. This is a typical case that chronic hepatitis B progressed over time and eventually developed into liver cancer. He had a history of frequent drinking alcohol in his younger years but quit it immediately after being diagnosed with the disease, as he was so scared of its fatal consequences. He had also quit smoking about 17 years ago. In addition to the liver cancer, he had been suffering from allergic rhinitis at that time.

Oct 13, 20XX. 13. The first treatment began with the following basic two-stage Formulae:

R. I VII (51) / L. I V (42)

A Zang-system Inflammation Formula (5:1) was applied to the right, and a Fu-system Inflammation Formula (4:2) was applied to the left. Combining these two Formulae in this way is a prescription method that I devised a long time ago. Explaining the significance of the Formula, treatment for the Liver, which belongs to the Zang system, and treatment for the Stomach, which is part of the digestive system, were performed simultaneously. Although liver cancer is a serious disease, I began treatment at a basic stage of the Formulae—so to speak, using a "starting-engine-like" approach.

The Zang-system Inflammation Formula on the right aims to correct excessive imbalances of the Liver and Lungs. The Fu-system Inflammation Formula on the left addresses the imbalances of the Liver and Pancreas. This Fu-system Inflammation Formula can be seen as a prescription for treating "Liver and Pancreas Disharmony (肝脾不和)," a common pathology in Oriental medicine that affects the digestive system.

---

[115] A medical procedure that blocks blood flow to a specific area. In this context, it refers to a treatment that targets and kills cancer cells by blocking the blood vessels supplying the liver cancer lesion.

After performing Constitution-acupuncture in this manner, I prescribed an additional Constitutional decoction to replenish the Liver and provided detailed explanations of important dietary tips for the Geumyang Constitution, including the Constitutional Diet. A disease like liver cancer affects the central detoxification organs, making the Constitutional Diet crucial. This is because by minimizing the energy spent on detoxifying harmful foods, the liver can focus more on healing itself. The patient was strongly advised to adhere to the Constitutional Diet.

October 15, 20XX. Two days later, the patient returned to my clinic with a bright expression on his face and reported that he felt much more at ease. This is a very positive sign, as it clearly indicates that even low-level treatment has been effective. In fact, as soon as the patient walked through the door of the treatment room, I could read his facial expression and confidently predict a favorable prognosis.

With this progress, I decided to shift the treatment into a higher gear. For the prescription, I developed a unique combination:

R. I VII (51) / L. V III' VII IX I (55555)

On the right side, I continued with the Zang-system Inflammation Formula as before. On the left side, I applied a series of Formulae in the following order, repeating each Unit Formula five times: Fu-system Inflammation Sub-formula, Mental Sub-formula, Zang-system Inflammation Sub-formula, Degeneration Sub-formula, and Basic Formula. The final Basic Formula serves as a Unit Formula that replenishes the Liver, structuring the prescription to target the liver specifically.

Typically, the five-stage cancer Formula is written in the following sequence: Basic Formula → Fu-system Inflammation Sub-formula → Mental Sub-formula → Zang-system Inflammation Sub-formula → Degeneration Sub-formula. However, in my prescription, I followed the same cyclical order but placed the Basic Formula to replenish the Liver in the last. This adjustment was made intentionally to get the desired treatment effect. I also advised him with particular emphasis on compliance with the Constitutional Diet.

October 19, 20XX. The patient returned and reported that his breathing had become much easier following the last treatment. In most cases of liver disease, including liver cancer, the Liver Qi fails to communicate properly, leading to stagnation (Liver Qi stagnation) and symptoms such as thoracic and flank congestion, which makes breathing difficult. With the stagnation removed, his breathing had eased. This is a significant indicator that acupuncture treatment is so effective for his liver-related conditions.

The patient also mentioned that his voice had improved. This suggests that the excessive imbalance of the Lungs in the Yang Field has decreased, indicating a transition to a more physiological imbalance or a more appropriate state of imbalance.

October 22, 20XX. He reported a significant decrease in fatigue and felt less tired upon waking in the morning, indicating that the liver treatment continued to be effective. However, he mentioned experiencing frequent urination, which he said had worsened after receiving anticancer drug injections, specifically chemotherapy. The same Constitution-acupuncture treatment was continued.

October 25, 20XX. The patient stated that his body felt very light. He also shared that he no longer felt short of breath and could take deeper breaths. Based on his feedback, it was clear that the treatment was progressing rapidly. The same Constitution-acupuncture treatment was performed.

October 27, 20XX. The patient reported feeling good overall. The same Constitution-acupuncture treatment procedure was maintained.

October 29, 20XX. The patient shared that his physical condition was stable. He reflected on his prior experience with treatment at Western hospitals, stating that it caused him significant pain without improving his condition. He reminisced that this led him to search for health-related books at a bookstore, where he discovered my book and decided to visit my clinic to seek treatment from me. After undergoing Constitutional treatment, he expressed feeling as though he was truly living again. He mentioned that he was sleeping well and no longer felt tired. The patient's decision to pursue this treatment could be described as an "excellent choice." The same Constitution-acupuncture prescription was continued.

November 1, 20XX – December 11, 20XX. The patient continued visiting my clinic every two or three days, reporting consistent improvement in his health. The same Constitution-acupuncture prescription was maintained, and a second Constitutional decoction was provided on November 1st.

Following this period, the patient did not visit my clinic but managed his health independently through adherence to Constitutional regimen.

August 3, the following year. Nearly nine months later, the patient returned to my clinic, reporting that his body felt completely normal. He added that the symptoms he described as "earthworms in the body" had disappeared. Patients sometimes use an unusual expressions to describe their symptoms. In Oriental medicine, this sensation is referred to as "uijugam" (蟻走感), which translates literally to "a feeling of ants crawling." In Western medicine, this phenomenon is termed formication, which also originates from the sensation of ants crawling. It is fascinating that both Eastern and Western medicine describe this sensation with reference to ants.

Western medicine usually associates symptoms like these with dopaminergic factors such as Parkinson's disease or restless leg syndrome; neuropathies such as diabetic neuropathy, shingles, or fibromyalgia; or hormonal changes such as those seen in menopausal syndrome.

In Oriental medicine, such symptoms are typically attributed to conditions like Qi deficiency, Blood deficiency, Phlegm, or preliminary Wind-struck symptom (preliminary stroke symptoms). In this patient's case, the symptoms seemed to stem from Wind-struck symptom caused by Blood deficiency. According to Chinese medical classic, the Liver's function is described as "Gan-cang-xue" (肝藏血), which means storing blood and regulating its flow. Similarly, Western medicine identifies nutrient synthesis as one of the liver's primary functions, aligning with the Oriental medicine perspective of the Liver's role in managing blood function. In severe conditions such as liver cancer, the Liver's blood-storing function is significantly impaired, often resulting in blood deficiency throughout the body.

The disappearance of the patient's "earthworm crawling" sensation can be interpreted as a sign that the Liver's blood-storing function has been restored, coinciding with the resolution of the liver cancer.

The patient firmly stated that, during the time he did not visit my clinic, he adhered strictly to the Constitutional Diet, following it 100%. He even took packed meals to work to ensure compliance. This demonstrates the determined effort to overcome his liver cancer, a life-threatening illness, by fully committing to the prescribed regimen. The same Constitution-acupuncture prescription was maintained for the treatment.

August 27, 20XX. The patient visited my clinic after almost a month and reported that his body was still in good condition. The same Constitution-acupuncture prescription was used for the treatment.

September 17, 20XX. The patient returned to my clinic after three weeks, reporting that his rhinitis had worsened due to the seasonal changes in weather. Nevertheless, my prescription remained unchanged. This decision was based on the fact that his liver cancer is a much more critical condition than his rhinitis.

The patient had not visited my clinic since the beginning of the year but resumed visits in August. Rather than attending regularly, he now only visits when specific symptoms or conditions arise. This demonstrates that he has made significant progress in recovering from the liver cancer.

September 24, 20XX. One week after his previous visit, the patient reported that his rhinitis had improved and that the symptoms of eye pain had disappeared. In the classic of Oriental medicine, there is a saying, "Gan-zhu-mu" (肝主目), which means "The liver governs the eyes." In Oriental medicine, the condition of the eyes is often seen as a reflection of Liver health. This improvement can be interpreted as part of the healing response, the recovery from the liver cancer. The same Constitution-acupuncture prescription was again performed.

October 15, 20XX. The patient visited my clinic and shared the results of the recent CT scan, which showed that his liver was clear. His blood test results were also normal! This incredible news came exactly one year after he first visited my clinic on October 13 of the previous year and began the treatment for liver cancer.

This year, his visits were intermittent rather than frequent, meaning his actual treatment period was approximately two months long, from October

13 to December 11 of last year. During this time, a total of 16 Constitution-acupuncture treatments were performed, and two Constitutional decoctions were prescribed. This outcome is nothing short of extraordinary.

Diseases affecting the liver often respond less effectively to Western medicine than anticipated. The liver, as the central organ responsible for detoxification, struggles to process Western medications effectively when its detoxification function is impaired due to the disease. This often leads to unexpected side effects. However, Eight-Constitution Medicine employs acupuncture points and Constitutional decoctions tailored specifically to an individual's Constitution, enabling highly effective treatment of the liver disease without these unforeseen side effects. The remarkable efficacy of Constitutional Medicine for liver-related conditions was clearly demonstrated in this patient's case.

Geumeum Constitution's Clinical Cases

[Geumeum Case 1] Testimony

* Patient: Ms G, 53 years old at the time of visit
* Chief complaints: Megacolon with gas accumulation in the abdomen causing significant bloating.

The patient constantly experienced bloating in her abdomen and described feeling as though she was on the brink of death. She was a relatively petite woman, standing 144 cm tall and weighing 38 kg, yet her abdomen swelled dramatically, resembling that of a full-term pregnant woman—protruding enormously like a mountain. She endured this excruciating condition by relying on hospital-prescribed medications such as Agiocur Pregranules[116] and Polybutine tablets,[117] which provided only temporary relief from her agonizing symptoms. These treatments did not address the root issue but merely served as a stopgap measure to manage symptoms spiraling out of control.

In addition to megacolon, she suffered from multiple issues with her colon, including numerous diverticula and adenomas that required surgical removal. Her family history was also concerning, as her mother had passed away from colon cancer, suggesting a hereditary predisposition to such diseases. Despite her struggles, she shouldered the considerable burden of serving as a district manager at her local cathedral, which imposed significant physical strain on her fragile health.

---

[116] It is a granule made from psyllium and psyllium husk, used as a herbal medicine to treat constipation, abdominal distension, abnormal intestinal fermentation, and hemorrhoids. Psyllium (車前子) refers to the seeds of the plantain plant (psyllium), which was commonly found in the past along unpaved roads frequented by carts and carriages. This is how it earned its name, meaning "seeds before a carriage."

According to Je-ma Lee's *Donguisusebowon*, psyllium is classified as a Soyangin (Toyang or Toeum Constitutions) herbal medicine and is primarily used to stimulate Kidney function and promote diuresis. However, in this context, its high fiber content is utilized to address constipation and reduced intestinal motility.

[117] A medication used to alleviate digestive dysfunction and irritable bowel syndrome, as well as to treat habitual vomiting, constipation, and diarrhea in children.

While her colon condition was her most critical issue, she also battled several other ailments, including allergic rhinitis, insomnia, and reflux esophagitis—any of which would be serious conditions on their own for most individuals.

Her Constitution was diagnosed with Geumeum. The Zang-Fu Structure of the Geumeum Constitution consists of the following Zang-Fu organs: "Lungs-Large intestine Kidneys-Bladder Pancreas-Stomach Heart-Small intestine Liver-Gallbladder."

In Constitutional Medicine, it is noted that in Yin Constitutions, the Fu-system organs often exert more dominant influence on physiology or pathology than the Zang-system organs. For Geumeum Constitution, the Large intestine is the outermost organ in the Yang Field. Master Do-won Kuon described the Geumeum Constitution as "the Constitution with the longest Large intestine." Geumeum patients often report that during colonoscopies, doctors remark on their unusually long colons. This sometimes annoys the doctors doing the endoscopy, as navigating through the rectum, descending colon, transverse colon, ascending colon with a tiny camera becomes time-consuming and physically taxing, especially if the large intestine is long and convoluted, as is typical for people with the Geumeum Constitution.

This patient seemed to have lived without understanding her Constitution and had unknowingly consumed foods unsuitable for it. Furthermore, the excessive stress from burdensome responsibilities—particularly from her volunteer work—combined with the emotional ups and downs of her life had likely contributed significantly to the development of her megacolon.

According to Do-won Kuon, individuals with the Geumeum Constitution should especially avoid anger. Intense anger in such individuals can lead to serious conditions like Parkinson's disease or myasthenia gravis, both of which affect the neuro-muscular system. Je-ma Lee also described a condition similar to myasthenia gravis in his discussion of "Jie-yu-zheng" (解㑊症) in *Donguisusebowon*. He emphasized that such diseases could be cured by avoiding deep sorrow and severe anger. While myasthenia gravis or dyskinesia causes weakness in skeletal muscles, it seemed that the stress in this patient had caused functional weakness in her large intestine.

I provided the patient with a detailed explanation of the Constitutional regimen, including the structure and characteristics of the Geumeum Constitution and dietary recommendations tailored to it. Treatment was then initiated based on these principles.

January 22, 20XX. The first day I began treating her with a simple Fu-system Inflammation Formula. Constitutional decoction was also prescribed to aid bowel movements.

R. VII III (42)

On the right side, the Basic Formula and Fu-system Inflammation Sub-formulae were administered in a 4:2 ratio. Although the Large Intestine belongs to the Fu-system, the treatment was not directed to the Lower Burner since she was under stressful circumstances, which could affect the Heart located in the Upper Burner. A thorough adherence to the Constitutional Diet was strongly recommended, and the treatment for the first day was concluded.

January 24, 20XX. Two days later, she returned to my clinic. She mentioned feeling somewhat more comfortable after the treatment and expressed how much better she felt after the acupuncture. Her response to the 2-stage Formula was quite promising. Confident in the treatment, I upgraded the prescription to a 5-stage Compound Formula (repeated 3 times per Unit Formula for each side) as follows:

R. VIII IV IV' II X (33333) / L. VII III III' I IX (33333)

On the right side, a Fu-system 5-stage Formula was applied, while on the left, a Zang-system 5-stage Formula was used. The prescription was designed to regulate all Five Zangs and Five Fus.

Jan 26, 20XX. She diligently visited my clinic every two days, as instructed. She reported feeling better and noted that despite being tired from moving around a lot on Friday, she felt it manageable. The same Constitution-acupuncture prescription as the previous session was administered.

Jan 28, 20XX. She reported feeling very comfortable, which indicates that the symptom of the intestinal distention was alleviating. Constitution-acupuncture was again performed using the same prescription.

Jan 29, 20XX. She began visiting my clinic daily, seemingly recognizing the efficacy of the treatment. On this day, she reported feeling hunger for the first time after having no appetite for a long time. This is definitive evidence that the treatment is effective, as appetite represents the most fundamental instinct for survival. The same Constitution-acupuncture prescription was applied.

Jan 30, 20XX. She returned to my clinic a day later and reported gaining a taste for food and improvement in her intestinal condition. She also noted a reduction in dizziness, a sign that digestive function, nutrient absorption, and blood circulation were improving. The same prescription was used.

Feb 1, 20XX. She said her intestines felt even more comfortable, and it seemed her overall condition was improving, giving the impression that the treatment was gaining momentum. The same prescription was applied.

Feb 2, 20XX. She woke up coughing due to cold symptom. She mentioned wanting to exercise because her abdomen felt stronger but decided to stay inside due to the cold. Treatment was continued with the same prescription.

Feb 8, 20XX. She visited my clinic for the first time in six days. As soon as she entered the treatment room, she recounted a strange experience she had a few days ago. She had diarrhea after lunch on Saturday, and afterward, her bowels churned throughout the night, keeping her awake. At the same time, she passed an enormous amount of gas through her anus. She described it as if her intestines, which had been bloated like a giant balloon, had burst, releasing a massive amount of gas in an exodus. Afterward, her stomach pain disappeared! Feeling relieved, she resumed her vigorous activities. (Her extraordinary experience sounded like a religious testimony of faith.) She interpreted this process as the expulsion of poison.

Megacolon, in essence, is a condition where the large intestine becomes completely paralyzed due to certain factors, stops moving, and swells up like a huge balloon. Her mystical experience symbolized a significant breakthrough in her treatment. The same Formula as before was continued.

Feb 11, 20XX. She reported feeling very healthy. The same treatment was maintained.

Feb 16, 20XX. She mentioned that she had been very busy for the past four days. Although she felt exhausted from overexertion, she noted that her intestines did not exhibit any pain. This indicated that her bowel movements were functioning normally. The same Constitution-acupuncture prescription was applied, and an additional Constitutional decoction was prescribed.

She visited my clinic once more but did not return after that. Once the root cause of her visit to Joowonjang Clinic—the megacolon—was resolved, she discontinued the treatment on her own.

[Geumeum Case 2] Between Geumeum and Geumyang

* Patient: Ms. Y, 50 years old at the time of visit
* Chief Complaints: Unable to sleep due to insomnia and experiencing ringing in the ears (tinnitus).

The patient traveled from a distant local city, approximately two hours by car, to visit Joowonjang Clinic. Patients who pay a call on my clinic from afar tend to present with complex or difficult-to-treat conditions. At the time of visit, she was being treated for lupus (systemic lupus erythematosus or SLE) at a local Western hospital, taking steroids and anti-malarial drugs. Concurrently, she was receiving Constitution-acupuncture treatment at another Eight-Constitution Clinic in her area.

The issue was that she had been diagnosed with Geumyang Constitution at the clinic. Geumyang Constitution! It may seem inconsequential since both Geumyang and Geumeum Constitutions belong to the broader "Geum (Metal) Constitution" category (Taeyangin). Indeed, since more than 90% of their fundamental Constitutional traits are identical, there may not be significant issues when applying proper Constitutional dietary guidelines or eligible Sasang decoction treatments. If the prescribed Sasang medication suits the patient's condition, improvement is possible even with such a different diagnosis.

However, the problem arises in Constitution-acupuncture treatment. This is because the Zang-Fu structures of the Geumyang and Geumeum Constitutions differ, resulting in different acupuncture points for achieving the targeted Zang-Fu balance. The structural differences between these two Constitutions are as follows:

* Geumyang: Lungs-Large Intestine Pancreas-Stomach Heart-Small Intestine Kidneys-Bladder Liver-Gallbladder
* Geumeum: Lungs-Large Intestine Kidneys-Bladder Pancreas-Stomach Heart-Small Intestine Liver-Gallbladder

Both Constitutions share the outermost Zang-Fu organs in the Yang and Yin Field (Lungs and Liver), reflecting the similar Constitutional traits of the Geum Constitution category. However, the arrangements of the other three pairs of Zang-Fu organs differ, altering the overall topography of the Zang-Fu structure and, consequently, altering the Unit Formula needed to balance this structure as well. The impact of this difference on this patient will be discussed during the treatment process.

This patient also had cataracts caused by steroid treatment (methylprednisolone), leading to astigmatism—a typical example of the vulnerability of the Geumeum Constitution to drugs. Such cases are common in clinics specializing in Eight-Constitution Medicine, highlighting the limitations of pharmaceutical interventions, which, I regret to say, may do more harm than good.

She also complained of persistent skin itchiness. For this, she had been receiving treatment at the local Eight-Constitution Clinic. However, her astigmatism worsened, prompting her to discontinue treatment in December of the previous year. The astigmatism appeared to be a side effect of Geumyang Constitution-acupuncture treatment.

Despite thoroughly undergoing Geumyang regimen and receiving Constitution-acupuncture again at the local clinic in September of the same year, her symptoms began to worsen. By October, her menstruation became irregular, and she started experiencing early morning tremors after the acupuncture sessions there. The side effects from Geumyang acupuncture were evident. However, it was perplexing that the practitioner continued to treat her as a Geumyang patient, and the patient also adhered to this misdiagnosis. Despite her complaints to the doctor, she continued receiving treatment under the same Constitution, Geumyang, due to the practitioner's unwavering confidence in his Constitutional diagnosis. This underscores the significant influence of a doctor's authority on patients. I believe that doctors should be clearly aware of this dynamic and interact with patients accordingly.

The patient had a history of myasthenia gravis, which developed suddenly in her early 20s. She underwent a thymectomy, after which the condition was cured. In cases of myasthenia gravis, tumors or thickening in the thymus can be present, and removing the tumor reportedly leads to improvement in 50-85% of cases. This medical history also supports the conclusion that she belongs to the Geumeum Constitution.

Nov 28, 20XX. I diagnosed her with the Geumeum Constitution and treated her with the following Constitution-acupuncture prescription:

R. VII I (51) / L. VIII IV IV' X II (55555)

The Zang-system Inflammation Formula was applied to the right side, and the Formula for autonomic dysfunction was applied to the left side. Detailed dietary instructions for Geumeum Constitution were explained, and Constitutional decoction was prescribed.

Nov 29, 20XX. The patient reported sleeping well but was unsure about any significant improvement. The same Constitution-acupuncture prescription was continued.

Dec 2, 20XX. The patient reported that the tinnitus stopped on the day she received the acupuncture. She was especially pleased to have her first clear and complete bowel movements, producing golden-colored stool, which I was sure was a crucial positive outcome. However, the patient admitted to drinking a can of beer around midnight on Saturday before going to bed. The following morning, she experienced severe itching in her legs, leading to excessive scratching, and felt intense nausea, almost vomiting.

It is often observed that humans are prone to neglect their regimen even when they feel slightly better. Patients faithfully adhere to the instructions when ill, but as soon as they feel some improvement, they think, "I should be fine now," and break their dietary or lifestyle regimen. Such lapses inevitably lead to side effects, hardships, and regret. The importance of strictly following the Constitutional Diet was strongly re-emphasized to her. Treatment continued with the same prescription.

Dec 4, 20XX. The patient reported occasional episodes of fecal incontinence and mentioned waking up at 2 am the previous day. Individuals with the Geumeum Constitution are prone to experiencing issues with the large intestine. Irritable bowel syndrome (IBS) is also a common complaint in this Constitutional type.

As a marker of wellness in the Geumeum Constitution, I take note of the phrase "Daebyeonwangda" (大便旺多), meaning "abundant and healthy bowel movements." When health improves, the stool becomes plentiful and passes comfortably. Patients with Geumeum Constitution often express concern, saying, "I'm passing so much stool! Is my body failing to absorb what I eat?" No, that is not the case. Having large, quick, and effortless bowel movements is a sign of perfect health in individuals with the Geumeum Constitution. The same Constitution-acupuncture prescription was administered.

Dec 11, 20XX. After a week, the patient complained that the tinnitus had returned. Since my clinic is far away, the patient once again received Geumyang Constitution-Acupuncture at the nearby Eight-Constitution Medicine clinic in her hometown, and this was the result. I was speechless. While being treated for the Geumeum Constitution here, the patient visited another clinic and received treatment for the Geumyang Constitution again! I asked the patient for the full story.

Although the patient said she had improved after being diagnosed with the Geumeum Constitution and receiving treatment at Joowonjang Clinic, the doctor at the other clinic insisted that the patient was definitely of the Geumyang Constitution. The patient felt compelled to receive Geumyang Constitution-acupuncture treatment again (For a patient, a doctor's words can feel absolute like this).

Isn't the most reliable evidence the improvement in the patient's condition? Is there any clearer proof than this? I respect the doctor's sincere judgment, but doctors are human too, right? I also make mistakes sometimes. When that happens, I just correct them quickly. A best doctor, I believe, is not someone who can cure every disease but someone who quickly identifies and addresses mistakes to provide effective treatment. Confucius once said: "Do not hesitate to correct your mistakes!"

Constitutional diagnosis is not the goal; it is merely a step in treating the disease. If errors arise in the process, they must be corrected immediately. Dogma is a dangerous thing. Medieval dogmatism led to many people being burned at the stake. The dogmatism of Eight-Constitution Medicine can also harm the patients. In fact, all medical dogmas can harm the patients. We must awake from the slumber of dogmatism and listen to the patient's earnest appeals. The same prescription was used for treatment.

Dec 12, 20XX. The patient reported that she slept very well! There was no itching, and she slept without scratching even once. However, she said the tinnitus was still loud in the morning. Even so, I was thrilled simply because she could sleep well!

The patient also shared that while most people feel better after visiting hot springs, she felt worse, as though she might die. Hot springs are not suitable for people with Geumeum Constitution (saunas are also harmful). Surprisingly, however, she said she felt great after visiting an outdoor hot spring in Japan. She remembered that taking a hot spring bath in the open air while it was snowing was indescribably pleasant. It seems that the cold air of the snowy mountains subdued the hyperactivity of her lungs and helped balance her Zang-Fu organs. For people with Geumeum Constitution, outdoor hot springs in the cold environments can be recommended.

The patient also mentioned that whenever she returned from hiking, her face would turn red, and her condition would worsen. Besides the Geumyang Constitution, the Geumeum Constitution is also not well-suited for mountain climbing. This is because the high oxygen saturation in mountainous environments overstimulates the lungs of people with highly active lungs.[118] For those with this Constitution, walking on flat ground is better than hiking.

Dec 13, 20XX. The patient reported sleeping very well again. She also said the itching had disappeared, and there was no longer any lingering discomfort. Unfortunately, the tinnitus persisted. This was deeply regrettable, as it could have been treated effectively. However, I expect improvement if the patient continues with Geumeum Constitution treatment. The same Constitution-acupuncture prescription was followed.

Afterward, this patient occasionally visited Joowonjang Clinic when traveling to Seoul, but did not attend it regularly. I heard that her primary symptoms have been alleviated to much extent, and the patient maintains good health through her Constitutional regimen in her local area. However, I think it is unfortunate that the tinnitus had recurred. I sincerely hope the patient does not undergo Geumyang Constitution-acupuncture treatment again.

---

[118] Captain Seong-taek Hong, a world-renowned climber and explorer who became the first person in the world to conquer all five poles (Everest, North Pole, South Pole, Bering Strait, and Greenland), once shared an anecdote about his experiences. This is a story about a Sherpa who often assisted him during his climbs in the Himalayas. To express his gratitude, Captain Hong invited the Sherpa to Korea. He showed him Korea's scenic spots and treated him to delicious Korean cuisine. While in Korea, he suggested he visit Seoraksan Mountain together, one of Korea's most famous mountains.

They climbed Mt. Seoraksan together, but something strange happened. While Everest (8,848m) — over 8,000 meters above sea level — had been a breeze, climbing Mt. Seorak (1,708m), which is less than 2,000 meters above sea level, turned out to be quite a struggle for the Sherpa. After some time, the Sherpa gave up, saying it was too difficult to climb it.

What kind of mystery is this? This phenomenon can only be explained through Constitutional Medicine. The Sherpa may have had Geumyang or Geumeum Constitution. These "Metal" Constitutions are characterized by the highest Lung Potentials. On a mountain like Mt. Seoraksan, which has high oxygen saturation due to its dense forestation, Lung function can become overstimulated, causing breathing difficulties. The Sherpa's Constitution was likely optimized for the Himalayas, where oxygen is scarce.

In my clinic, I have seen many cases of individuals with Geumyang or Geumeum Constitutions who enjoyed hiking but developed health issues or struggled with mountain climbing. Therefore, it is recommended that people with Geum Constitution avoid hiking in such environments and instead walk on flat terrain.

[Geumeum Case 3] Eliminating Allergies

* Patient: Ms. O, kindergarten student, 6 years old at the time of visit.
* Chief Complaints: Allergic dermatitis, itchy skin, and rashes.

This child, living in a distant city in Gyeonggi Province, presented with skin rashes and severe itching after consuming flour-based foods and snacks. Such reactions seemed to occur frequently. She had suffered from allergic dermatitis from a very young age. The first allergic outbreak occurred after consuming powdered milk. Subsequently, she developed allergies to various foods, including beef, milk, and eggs, and once required a visit to the emergency room after consuming walnuts. As a result of these issues, she was exclusively breastfed as an infant.

Once allergies develop, they tend to recur. Among immune cells, there are specialized lymphocytes called memory cells that carry antibodies to neutralize or destroy previously encountered antigens (substances—such as microorganisms, environmental pollutants, and others—causing disease). These memory cells, including memory B cells and memory T cells, retain this information. They vigilantly protect our bodies and enable a swift immune response when the same harmful microorganisms or substances invade again. This is the basis of the immune mechanism. Vaccines, for example, work by introducing antigens in advance, essentially "sparring" with the immune system to form memory cells and create immunity.

Ironically, allergies are a side effect of this immune mechanism. When allergens enter the body, the immune system should ideally neutralize and eliminate them, restoring the body to its normal state after the threat is managed. However, for some reason, the immune system fails to return to its baseline and instead remains in a heightened "Class A emergency alert state," as if it's preparing for a massive invasion. This overreaction resembles mobilizing an entire army to capture a single spy in the demilitarized zone. Instead of handling the situation with a small company or battalion, the immune system escalates to deploying divisions or even an entire corps. While the "spy" (allergen) may be neutralized, collateral damage occurs, harming "allied forces" (the body's own tissues). In severe cases, the immune system mistakenly identifies allies as enemies, leading to tragic situations where it attacks its own body.

In essence, allergies are an excessive immune response. The immune system becomes overly sensitive and reactive. This heightened sensitivity doesn't just affect the immune system; it also impacts the person emotionally. People with severe allergies often become anxious about their environment, as eating even slightly unsuitable food, inhaling a small amount of fine dust, or experiencing a minor change in temperature can trigger allergic reactions. Such constant vigilance can alter a person's personality. This is particularly distressing when allergies develop in young children, as it affects their ability to enjoy childhood fully. A child who should be carefree and joyful may instead live in constant worry, like this young girl.

Most allergies in children are caused by food. Unfortunately, many of the foods this child enjoyed were constitutionally unsuitable for her, such as candy, biscuits, bread, milk, cake, noodles, and ramen—all of which were allergens to her. One might wonder how a child can enjoy a happy childhood under such restrictions. Unfortunately, she must constantly monitor what she eats; however, this vigilance is necessary for the sake of her health.

I explained the characteristics of the Geumeum Constitution to the family and provided dietary guidelines and precautions suited to this Constitution. The following outlines the treatment process.

April 18, 20XX. Since the patient was a child, two stages of basic treatment were initially performed. The prescription was as follows:

R. VII I (51) / L. VII III (42)

The treatment targeted Zang-system Inflammation Formula on the right side and Fu-system Inflammation Formula on the left side.

April 29, 20XX. The patient was advised to visit my clinic every two days, however, due to unforeseen circumstances, the visit was delayed by 11 days. Her mother reported that the child's skin was worsening and that when fine dust levels were high, the child experienced excessive phlegm production, nearly to the point of vomiting. The same prescription was used for treatment.

May 21, 20XX. The next visit occurred nearly a month later. However, there was a positive response to Constitution-acupuncture. Her mother shared that the skin allergy on the child's thighs had completely disappeared following the previous Constitution-acupuncture treatment.

June 23, 20XX. After exposure to excessive air conditioning, the child developed a cough and a clear runny nose, indicating a cold. The same prescription was used for treatment.

June 25, 20XX. Her mother reported that the cough subsided immediately after the previous acupuncture treatment. However, phlegm was still present. The same Constitution-acupuncture prescription was administered.

July 12, 20XX. After playing in water, the child developed a cough and nasal congestion. The same prescription was applied.

Nov 14, 20XX. After eating a vegetable cake, the child's skin developed a chicken-skin-like texture (goose bumps), prompting a return visit to my clinic. Constitution-acupuncture was administered using the same prescription.

Dec 12, 20XX. Her mother reported intermittent skin itching, causing the child to scratch. The same Constitution-acupuncture prescription was used.

Dec 19, 20XX. The child was stricken with a flu, experiencing a cough and severe phlegm. Constitution-acupuncture was performed using the same prescription.

Feb 24, 20XX (next year). While in Phuket, Thailand, the child vomited after eating buttered potatoes and developed dermatitis on the legs and arms. The same Constitution-acupuncture treatment was administered.

Mar 28, 20XX. Her mother reported that the child's skin became clear after the previous acupuncture session.

This child responded remarkably well to my treatment, with symptoms typically resolving after just one session each time. However, symptoms reappeared immediately when the child consumed foods unsuitable for her Constitution. I often find myself wishing that the child's memory cells could experience "amnesia" to forget their allergic triggers!

Whenever the child experienced allergy or cold symptoms, she returned to Joowonjang Clinic for treatment. Life is a process, and health is ultimately part of that ongoing journey. In this sense, there is no such thing as "completion" of health.

Toyang Constitution's Clinical Cases

[Toyang Case 1] Who Said Toyang Constitution's Stomach Is the Strongest?

* Patient: Ms. B, 47 years old at the time of visit
* Chief Complaints: Persistent indigestion and a sour taste in the mouth.

This patient came from a distant southern region of Korea. I presume that her visit to my clinic was driven by sheer desperation. Her initial complaint was a complete inability to digest, even to the point where water could not be tolerated. Her condition was so severe that she reported hearing a constant sloshing sound in her stomach. Despite this, she had much gluttony and continued to eat excessively. The problem was that after eating, she was unable to digest food properly, which caused intense stomach pain and left her immobile. While her appetite was strong, her stomach simply could not handle it.

Recently, she developed a persistent sour taste in her mouth, as if she had eaten an excessive number of tangerines, even though she hadn't touched any. This, too, caused considerable discomfort.

In individuals with Toyang Constitution, the structure of the Zang-Fu organs is: "Pancreas-Stomach Heart-Small intestine Liver-Gallbladder Lungs-Large intestine Kidneys-Bladder." Since the Pancreas-Stomach is positioned as the outermost Zang-Fu of the Yang Field, the Pancreas and Stomach, the pivotal organs of the digestive system, possess the highest potential. Naturally, one might expect such individuals to have exceptional digestive abilities. However, having the "highest potential" of Zang-Fu does not always equate to the optimal function. If the Pancreas-Stomach becomes overly dominant, digestion can paradoxically become impaired. This is consistent with the patient's recent experience of being unable to digest even water properly.

Thus, common assumptions that people with Toyang Constitution have robust digestive systems and can eat anything need to be reconsidered. These traits hold true only when the Constitutional Zang-Fu organs are well-balanced. Otherwise, digestion can be severely impaired, as seen in this case. When the Zang-Fu organs are well-balanced, digestion is manageable for any Constitutions. Even individuals with the lowest Pancreas-Stomach potential, such as those with Suyang or Sueum Constitutions, can digest well if the Zang-Fu organs are physiologically balanced. The key lies in whether the Zang-Fu balance is in the state of equilibrium.

When I informed the patient that she had a Toyang Constitution, she was taken aback. This individual had deeply ingrained misconceptions about her constitutional type and had outright rejected the possibility of being classified as Toyang Constitution. Her lifestyle reflected this belief. Misdiagnoses at the Eight-Constitutions clinics she had previously visited only reinforced this misunderstanding. In one clinic, she was diagnosed with Mogyang Constitution, and in another, with Sueum Constitution.

In Constitutional Medicine, a misdiagnosis renders treatment completely ineffective. When the diagnosis is incorrect, all treatments—including medications, acupuncture, and dietary adjustments—are futile and may even result in adverse effects. In Eight-Constitution Medicine, the Constitutional treatment is considered a kind of "all-or-nothing" approach. If the diagnosis is accurate, the results can be transformative; if not, everything fails.

I took considerable time explaining and persuading the patient to accept her Toyang Constitution. I advised her to adopt the Toyang Constitution-specific diet, avoiding hot (in temperature) foods and consuming cold (in temperature) foods. Due to common belief, she had been rigorously avoiding cold foods out of fear that her body could not handle them. Mysteriously, when she ate cold foods, she used to experience indigestion, feverish symptoms, and an overall physical decline.

The patient repeatedly asked if eating cold foods was genuinely safe. I reassured her that it was not only safe but also necessary for her recovery, provided she followed the Toyang Contitution-based diet meticulously. Thus began the treatment journey for this challenging Toyang Constitution patient.

Jan 15, 20XX. Acupuncture treatment was administered as follows:

R. IX V (51) / L. X VI (42)

On the right side, Zang-system Inflammation Formula was used, and on the left side, a Formula specifically designed by me was applied. The treatment targeted the Pancreas (right side) and Stomach (left side). In addition to the acupuncture treatment, Constitutional decoction was prescribed to treat Pancreas-Stomach, that is, the digestive system.

Jan 17, 20XX. She made a long-distance call instead of visiting my clinic. I strained my ears, anxiously hearing her voice on the other end of the phone.

"The bloating has eased, and the sour taste in my mouth is gone!" said she enthusiastically. Then she added "Even when I eat cold foods, I no longer feel feverish!"

I was overjoyed—perhaps even more than she was—because her own words validated the accuracy of my diagnosis. Moments like this bring profound happiness and make all the stress melt away like snow under the sun. It's these moments that make being a doctor incredibly rewarding.

Jan 23, 20XX. She returned to my clinic a week after the phone call. I found her face lit up with a smile. She shared her experiences enthusiastically, as if she were chatting with a friend.

"What's really surprising is that my makeup doesn't float!"

She conveyed that her daughter even remarked on how her makeup remained perfect, even after three hours. Honestly, I don't fully understand what it means for makeup not to float. Perhaps it means that her skin is in better condition and retains makeup well. Regardless, what matters is that the patient is happy and feeling better. As a man, I may never fully grasp the significance of this, but it's enough to know that she is pleased.

She also shared that the sour taste in her mouth disappeared immediately after obeying Constitutional Diet. Such rapid improvement reflects the marvelous power of the Constitutional Diet. She repeatedly mentioned how much better she was feeling. Hearing such positivity doesn't tire me at all; in fact, it's a welcome relief compared to patients who constantly talk about pain, suffering, and discomfort. Her words were like sweet whispers—like a chocolate for my ears.

Jan 27, 20XX. On this day, she didn't visit my clinic but called instead.

Unfortunately, this time the news wasn't positive. She reported excessive sweating in her hands and blurred vision. She assured me that she was sticking to the foods beneficial for the Toyang Constitution, such as red bean water, barley tea, cucumbers, carrots, cabbage kimchi, and oat flour. I encouraged her to continue and emphasized the importance of taking her Constitutional decoction and adhering more thoroughly to the Constitutional Diet.

Feb 4, 20XX. She called again to share an update. The sensation of something being stuck in her eye had completely disappeared, and she proudly reported feeling significantly healthier. She assessed that her recent discomfort was likely "Myeonghyeon" (瞑眩), a healing reaction. Interestingly, she had already reached this conclusion on her own and shared her medical interpretation with me, which felt somewhat awkward for a medical doctor like me. While it felt a bit strange to be relieved of the doctor's obligation to explain the reaction, I was happy nonetheless. As the saying goes, when the patient is happy, everything is okay, no matter what.

After this phone call, I heard nothing more from her. This was unexpected, as patients like her would often call at any time to ask questions or provide updates on their condition. On the contrary, she abruptly stopped reaching out. That's okay—I take it as a sign that she's doing well.

Looking back, she only received two Constitution-acupuncture treatment sessions at my clinic. It seems as if it's been months.

[Toyang Case 2] Hands Are Itchy

* Patient: Ms. J, 29 years old at the time of visit
* Chief complaints: Skin hives during seasonal changes, herpes on the hands

The patient typically experienced hives on her skin whenever the seasons changed, particularly in spring. However, this time, the issue arose during the transition to fall. She mentioned that her condition began around six years ago after swimming regularly for about a year (Swimming is detrimental to individuals with Toyang Constitution).

She also frequently developed herpes on her hands, commonly referred to as pompholyx. This skin condition is intensely itchy and highly irritating. Having itchy skin on the hands can be extremely frustrating, as so many daily tasks involve using one's hands. Every movement made with her hands triggered the itching, causing significant distress.

Additionally, she reported a burning, hot sensation in the soles of her feet, for which she used an electric fan to cool them down. While this symptom might seem minor to some, it caused her great discomfort, disrupted her sleep, and affected her overall quality of life. She also mentioned pelvic discomfort.

An unusual aspect of her history is her experience with birth control pills. Previously, when she was traveling and her menstrual period coincided with the trip, she took birth control pills to delay it. Despite taking the pills even three times, they failed to work each time. This is highly unusual, as the contraceptive pills are designed to forcefully alter the menstrual cycle through hormonal regulation. This case highlights the incredible diversity of human physiology, with each person responding differently.

The patient had already been diagnosed with Mogyang Constitution at another Eight-Constitutions Korean Medicine Clinic. This diagnosis was based on her external appearance, as her body type might superficially resemble Mogyang Constitution. However, diagnosing Constitution solely based on appearance is often inaccurate. Some clinics attempt to determine Constitution by measuring body parts and analyzing the ratios. While this may offer some helpful insights, it cannot provide a definitive Constitutional diagnosis. I proceeded with the patient's treatment as outlined below.

August 25, 20XX. To treat the hives, I started with a simple two-stage Formula: R. IX III (42). The Fu-system Inflammation Formula was applied only to the right side.

August 26, 20XX. The previous day, I recommended barley meal, and she reported that she liked it because it was very easy to digest. This is an unusual reaction, as barley is comparatively harder for other Constitutions to digest than rice. She also mentioned sleeping deeply and well, feeling no fatigue despite having two hours less sleep than usual. One remarkable effect of Constitution-acupuncture is its ability to improve sleep quality, demonstrating its powerful impact on treating insomnia.

She decided to stop taking her dermatological medications. Although her hands were slightly itchy in the morning, she expressed confidence in her ability to endure it. This was really a courageous step. Active participation from a patient makes the treatment process more enjoyable for the doctor. A patient's cooperation boosts the likelihood of successful outcomes. Conversely, when a patient fails to follow recommendations, such as not adhering to the Constitutional Diet, the treatment process can become frustrating for the doctor. Cooperation between the doctor and the patient is essential for successfully curing a disease. The prescription was strengthened as follows: R. IX III (42) / L. IX V (51). Zang-system Inflammation Formula was added to the left side of the previous prescription.

August 28, 20XX. She reported less intestinal gas and mentioned eating cold foods—which she had previously avoided, thinking she had Mogyang Constitution—without significant discomfort.

She also noted that her itchiness had decreased, despite discontinuing her dermatological medications. Such medications, commonly prescribed for the allergies like hives, are often antihistamines. Antihistamines work by forcibly blocking histamine, a substance released during immune responses that causes itching. Using antihistamines is akin to temporarily resolving a traffic accident by blocking the road without fixing the underlying poor road conditions. They don't treat the root cause but merely mask the symptoms. Hence, once the medication is stopped, symptoms often reappear.

This patient, however, experienced less itching even after stopping the medication. This demonstrates the powerful efficacy of Constitutional treatment. Often, ceasing Western medications leads to more severe symptoms due to withdrawal effects. In this case, Constitution-acupuncture treatment successfully suppressed the withdrawal phenomenon, marking a significant win in her recovery.

Aug 29, 20XX. The patient reported experiencing sudden itching the night before. Fluctuations in symptoms are common during a treatment; it is rare for conditions to improve all at once. The Constitution-acupuncture prescription remained the same, and Constitutional decoction for treating allergies was added.

Aug 30, 20XX. The patient mentioned itching at night, a typical issue for skin diseases that often worsen during sleep. During the day, people can consciously resist the itching, but at night, when the unconsciousness takes over, scratching becomes easier. The Constitution-acupuncture prescription was adjusted as follows: R. IX III (44) / L. IV X IV' III V (44444). The right side remains the same with only the number of repetitions adjusted, while the left side is changed to a prescription for allergies.

Sep 4, 20XX. The blisters on her hands had improved significantly, but other areas of her body were still very itchy, particularly her calves. She also reported constipation. The prescription remained unchanged.

Sep 6, 20XX. The patient said the itching had reduced, and the blisters on her hands were almost gone, an important sign of healing. However, severe constipation and poor digestion with frequent burping were reported. The same prescription was continued.

Sep 8, 20XX. The skin itchiness had subsided, but the patient reported feeling unwell and experiencing diarrhea over the past two days. Since the primary focus was on treating her skin, I interpreted this as the treatment progressing in the right direction. Diarrhea is preferable to constipation because retained stool can release toxins interiorly into the body. The prescription was slightly modified: R. IX III III' (444) / L. IV X IV' III V (44444). The prescription on the right was adjusted to the ulcer Formula for the treatment of the digestive issue.

Sep 9, 20XX. The patient reported feeling increasingly comfortable in her skin. That morning, her stool was soft but no longer classified as diarrhea, indicating improvements in the digestive system. The prescription was upgraded further while maintaining allergy-focused treatment on the left side. R. X IV IV' VIII (4444) / L. IV X IV' III V (44444). On the right, the so-called "Mucous Membrane Ulcer Formula", which is Fu-system 4-stage Formula, was applied. On the left, the allergy prescription was continued.

Sep 11, 20XX. She reported a fresh bowel movements that morning, which indicated steady progress as planned. However, she mentioned ongoing discomfort in her stomach. The previous prescription was continued.

Sep 13, 20XX. The patient noted significant improvement in her stomach, though her stool remained somewhat soft. Her skin continued to improve, but she scratched herself a few times at night. Interestingly, she felt noticeably better after receiving acupuncture treatment. The prescription remained the same.

Sep 15, 20XX. Both her stomach and intestines had improved considerably. However, after exercising in the evening, her feet became hot, prompting her to wake up from sleep and scratch her skin at night. She also noticed some symptoms on her hands, which she attributed to consuming tomato sauce and pepper at lunch. Maintaining the Constitutional Diet is undoubtedly challenging. With so many delicious foods in the world, abstaining can be difficult. The prescription remained unchanged.

Sep 18, 20XX. Her skin showed mild improvement, and she reported good digestion and bowel movements. From my perspective, the treatment seemed to be on track. The same prescription was administered.

Sep 25, 20XX. After a week-long gap between visits, the patient returned. This extended interval indicated she could manage without frequent treatment. Her skin condition had improved so much that she no longer woke up at night. However, spicy foods still triggered symptoms. If spicy foods were removed from Korean cuisine, many people would likely become healthier, but protests from angry individuals would probably ensue. "I want my red pepper back! (just joking)" So, there's no way spicy food consumption will decrease, and the number of people suffering from health problems because of it will only increase... Oh my goodness! I can't help it, either. As a doctor, how can I take responsibility for the food industry? The same prescription was continued.

Sep 30, 20XX. The patient reported almost no itchy skin, though mild itching occasionally occurred. Her digestion and bowel movements were consistently good. I thought to myself, "We're truly on track!" The treatment remained unchanged.

Dec 5, 20XX. More than a month has passed since the last treatment. The patient stated that her skin symptoms had completely resolved. However, when she strayed from the Constitutional Diet, she experienced indigestion, throat pain from reflux esophagitis, and morning diarrhea. Strict adherence to the Constitutional Diet is almost akin to achieving sainthood—an unattainable goal for most people. The prescription was slightly adjusted to: R. IX III III' (444) / L. IV X IV' III V (44444).

The patient continued visiting my clinic every few days until the end of the year but stopped visiting since the New Year began. The desired treatment outcomes, I think, were achieved for her. She was an exemplary patient, diligently attending the treatment sessions and following recommendations. In fact, she was among the best.

It is rare for patients to explicitly declare that they no longer need treatment. Likewise, doctors rarely state that patients can stop visiting. Both doctors and patients know that the body is always susceptible to illness.

Medical care doesn't have a definitive ending. Treatment is an ongoing process, as the body constantly changes, and its future state is unpredictable. The open end? Yes! The body, therefore, is in endless changes. There is no conclusive end, only a continuous journey. The end always finishes unfinished!

[Toyang Case 3] Can't Stand Anger

* Patient: Ms. C, 32 years old at the time of visit
* Chief complaints: lethargy, muscle stiffness, indigestion

This is the case of a patient who traveled from a distant city in Gyeonggi Province to visit my clinic. Her case was unique and stood out in my clinical experience.

When she visited, she reported severe lethargy, but the cause was unusual. About a year and a half prior, she had received a massage at an illegal sports massage parlor. Afterward, her health significantly deteriorated. While a poorly executed massage can occasionally cause discomfort or muscle pain due to excessive force, such symptoms typically subside within a few days. In her case, however, her overall condition worsened dramatically. She described a persistent lack of energy and feeling perpetually fatigued.

Another notable symptom was dizziness during sexual intercourse. In the Zang-Fu structure of Toyang Constitution—"Pancreas-Stomach Heart-Small Intestine Liver-Gallbladder Lungs-Large Intestine Kidneys-Bladder"—the outermost Zang-Fu organ of the Yin Field is the Kidneys-Bladder. A significant imbalance in the Kidneys-Bladder often correlates with diminished reproductive function. Dizziness during intercourse can raise questions about her excessive sexual activity. Interestingly, individuals with Toyang Constitution generally exhibit a lower interest in sexual matters. Many of them with this Constitution are associated with professions such as clergy or individuals leading single, celibate lives, compared to other Constitutions. Her dizziness during intercourse indicated possible reproductive dysfunction due to a weakened Kidneys-Bladder function.

What stood out was her strong interest in sex, which seemed uncharacteristic of her Constitution. Her condition of "cold sweats" suggested Yin deficiency, leading to an excess of internal heat. The Kidneys-Bladder, being the primary Yin organs that generate Water Qi, appeared severely decreased in their potential. In the classic of Oriental medicine, there's a concept known as *Yin-xu-huo-dong* (陰虛火動), where Yin deficiency results in an overactive Fire Qi. This condition can manifest as "empty heat," often dissipated through cold sweats. This imbalance can also be transformed into heightened sexual impulses. Her strong sexual desire seemed to reflect such aspect of her illness.

She also suffered from severe muscle stiffness, particularly in the neck, shoulders, and abdomen. During her sexual intercourse, she reported abdominal muscle tightening, suggesting symptoms like muscle spasms or cramping. These are often linked to poor blood circulation, electrolyte imbalances, or nutritional deficiencies, pointing to her inadequate dietary habits.

Frequent indigestion was another prominent issue. She regularly experienced nausea and abdominal pain, often accompanied by the aforementioned muscle tightness. Additionally, she suffered from severe constipation, further highlighting her Yin deficiency, which was also reflected in her intestinal function.

The Toyang Constitution is prone to hyperactivity in the Pancreas-Stomach and Heart-Small Intestine, leading to anger or feverishness. This can result in headaches or dizziness. Alcohol, which exacerbates Fire Qi, is particularly harmful for individuals with Toyang Constitution. Many people with this Constitution dislike alcohol or cannot tolerate it well (though exceptions exist). Interestingly, she enjoyed drinking and did so regularly, though she didn't seem to be a heavy drinker.

With her complex medical history and unique presentation, I began her treatment journey.

Dec 24, 20XX. The patient reported difficulty with digestion and a hardened stomach. Additionally, she experienced back pain and poor blood circulation. She said that the back of the neck felt tight, and the swelling was severe after childbirth. The swelling persisted even after taking anti-inflammatory or digestive medications. A two-stage Formulae was administered as follows: R. IX V (51) / L. IX III (42). Zang-system Inflammation Formula was used on the right, and Fu-system Inflammation Formula was used on the left.

Feb 7, 20XX. The following year, she visited my clinic in February. Due to living far away, her visits to the Joowonjang Clinic were infrequent. She only sought my treatment when her health worsened significantly. She complained of back pain as well as pain in her pelvis and buttocks, adding that her left lower abdomen also hurt. A unique feature of this patient's condition was that multiple areas of her body would hurt simultaneously during flare-ups. For her musculoskeletal pain, the prescription was adjusted as follows: R. IX V III' (51) / L. IX III (42). The so-called "Disc Formula" was applied to the right, while the Fu-system Inflammation Formula was applied to the left.

Feb 19, 20XX. She visited my clinic again with similar symptoms of back pain and abdominal muscle pain. The same prescription as before was used.

March 6, 20XX. The patient reported that her back and abdominal muscles tightened whenever she applied pressure during sexual intercourse, which also made digestion nearly impossible afterward. The same prescription was administered. One notable aspect of this patient was that despite feeling severe symptoms as if she was on the verge of collapse, she responded exceptionally well to Constitution-acupuncture. After treatment, her condition would improve quickly, with the improvement lasting from a few days to several weeks or even months.

March 10, 20XX. & Mar 15, 20XX. She returned to my clinic with similar symptoms and received the same treatment on both occasions.

March 18, 20XX. The patient reported extreme fatigue and edema throughout her body due to poor blood circulation. She experienced abdominal tightness, stiff shoulders, and arm discomfort. A few days earlier, she had consumed a significant amount of alcohol due to stress caused by her mother-in-law. She added that she usually did not sleep much, but had to sleep a lot lately because of exhaustion. It became evident that much of her illness was rooted in Heart-fire disorders. From her personal accounts, it appeared that her marriage was in crisis. The same prescription was continued.

May 12, 20XX. She returned almost in 2 months. She shared that she had decided to divorce her husband. She had many conflicts with her mother-in-law, but her husband sided with his mother and turned against her. This typical mother-in-law conflict ultimately resulted in the breakdown of her marriage. However, her husband refused to grant her a divorce and instead filed a lawsuit demanding tens of millions of won in child support and alimony from her. The stress had reached a peak, exacerbating her symptoms. She experienced stiffness in her shoulders and lower abdomen, along with persistent back pain. Her menstruation had stopped for two months. The root cause of her health issues was diagnosed as "Hwabyeong" (Heart-fire illness). A two-stage Formula was administered as follows: R. IX V (51) / L. IX III (42). This combination, targeting Zang-system Inflammation on the right and Fu-system Inflammation on the left, served as a detoxification and gastrointestinal treatment.

May 17, 20XX. The patient visited my clinic with similar symptoms. This time, the prescription was slightly adjusted to: R. IX V (51) / L. IX VI (42). Zang-system Inflammation Formula was applied to the right side, and Vitality Formula was applied to the left.

June 14, 20XX. The patient reported that she drank a large amount of Soju (a kind of Korean liquer) and got into a fight with someone at the nearby table. Following this incident, her health significantly worsened, with symptoms of chest tightness, stomach cramps, and extreme fatigue. The same treatment as before was administered. It might seem puzzling why she continues to endure long journeys to receive treatment from me despite recurring health issues. For her, Joowonjang Clinic appears to be the one and only haven where she can alleviate her physical pain, temporarily though. Western medications prescribed by local clinics haven't been effective for her and have often caused side effects instead. Even treatments at local traditional Korean medicine clinics have proven ineffective or worsened her condition. As a result, she had to travel a long distance to my clinic as her last resort.

June 17, 20XX. The patient noted some improvement after her last Constitution-acupuncture session. No matter how severe her symptoms, Constitution-acupuncture at my clinic seems to provide temporary relief, allowing her to live pain-free for a few days, weeks, or even months. I find this fascinating—how can such minimal acupuncture treatment, seemingly so slight and light, produce such a powerful therapeutic effect? For her, Constitution-acupuncture serves as a pain reliever more potent than any pharmaceutical products. It's a magic! The same treatment was administered.

Aug 1, 20XX. The patient reported using a massage device at work a few days prior, which worsened her symptoms. She complained of poor blood circulation, stomach tightness, back pain, indigestion, and a stiff neck. This echoed her initial complaint upon visiting the clinic: feeling unwell after receiving a sports massage. Even though massage devices are designed to promote circulation, relax muscles, and, at most, temporarily improve physical condition, her health deteriorated further, which remains a mystery. The prescription was adjusted as follows: R. IX V III' (551) / L. IX VI (42). The Disc Formula was applied to the right side, and Vitality Formula was applied to the left.

Sep 24, 20XX. After almost two months, the patient returned to my clinic with similar symptoms: indigestion, abdominal pain, and back pain.

She also described new symptoms, including heart palpitations following conventional acupuncture, physical therapy, and cupping therapy at a local Korean Medicine clinic. It seemed clear that my clinic was her only option. The prescription was modified as follows: R. IX III III' (444) / L. X IV IV' (444). On the right side, the gastric ulcer Formula was used, while on the left side, my own Formula was used. The repetition count was modified from the usual 442 to 444, too.

Oct 2, 20XX. She reported that her body hurt all over after receiving a massage the day before. I marveled at the paradox of human behavior—despite experiencing pain after every massage, why does she continue to get it? To me, it seems like nothing more than an endless cycle of self-inflicted harm. Her usual symptoms consistently recurred: lower abdominal pain, back pain, indigestion, and constipation. At times like this, I feel disheartened. Treatment looks futile when patients fail to manage their health properly, undoing any progress made. Health ultimately requires one's discipline and effort. Without a consistent commitment to the discipline, one inevitably succumbs to illness. This reminds me so strongly of the teachings in the *Daehakjanggu* (*The Great Learning*), which emphasizes that the discipline of the body is a fundamental duty for everyone, from emperors to commoners.

The patient continued visiting my clinic regularly with similar symptoms. One time, after drinking, she got into an argument again with a woman at a nearby table, which escalated into a physical violence. The patient reportedly struck the woman with a bottle of soju, after which the woman grabbed her hair and retaliated by beating her severely. The fight left the other woman with significant injuries to her eye, so she filed a lawsuit against the patient for the damage to her eye. The story felt like something out of an action movie, yet for this patient, it seemed like just another day in her daily life. The most I could do was advise her to live more responsibly, and what I could do was continue providing Constitution-acupuncture to ease her pain, even though the relief was merely temporary. "It's just how the life goes on, ain't it?" I muttered to myself, brushing it off as just another episode in the life's ongoing drama.

Toeum Constitution's Clinical Cases

[Toeum Case 1] Man Confined in A Narrow Tube

* Patient: Mr. C, office worker, 38 years old at the time of visit
* Chief Complaints: Dry eye syndrome, muscae volitantes (floaters).[119]

The patient presented with an eye condition, retinitis pigmentosa, which had significantly reduced his vision. He reported no visibility above his line of sight, causing him to frequently bump into objects while walking. His visual field was approximately 60 degrees horizontally and 130 degrees vertically (a condition often referred to as "tunnel vision," where the patient perceives the world as if looking through a narrow tube). A visual field test conducted at the end of the previous year confirmed a near-total loss of peripheral vision, though his central vision remained clear. As a hereditary disease that eventually leads to blindness, it posed a serious concern for the future of this young man with much of his life ahead of him. Yet, his attitude toward the condition was calm, almost as if he were prepared to accept the eventuality of losing his sight.

There was a family history suggesting the hereditary nature of the condition. Both his mother and maternal grandfather experienced night blindness, and the patient himself also suffered from it—a common initial symptom of retinitis pigmentosa.

At the time of visit, the patient had been battling a cold for about five days, presenting with a runny nose, sneezing, and swollen tonsils.

He was taking ginkgo biloba extract, a medication aimed at improving blood circulation in the hope of delaying the progression of the retinal disease. However, this meant the absence of a definitive cure in Western medicine, as the medication served merely as an adjunct without directly preventing the degeneration of retinal pigment cells. I approached the treatment with a somewhat heavy heart, aware of the challenges ahead.

---

[119] A condition where small dots or thread-like shapes appear to float within the field of vision. It can result from degeneration of the vitreous body or the retina.

Jan 27, 20XX. The initial treatment focused on addressing the cold, as treating other illnesses is challenging when a cold persists. The prescribed two-stage Formulae were as follows:

R. V I (42) / L. V IX (51).

Fu-system Inflammation Formula was applied to the right side, and Zang-system Inflammation Formula to the left. A Constitutional decoction was also prescribed simultaneously.

Feb 12, 20XX. The patient returned to my clinic after approximately 15 days, reporting general improvement. Notably, the floaters in his vision had decreased. This outcome suggests that both the Constitution-acupuncture and Constitutional decoction were effective, which is a very encouraging response. When retinal diseases are accompanied by floaters, the reduction of floaters indicates the effectiveness of Eight-Constitution Medicine.

However, the cold had not fully resolved, as the patient still experienced a runny nose, occasional coughing, and fatigue. The prescription for the right side remained the same, while the left side was adjusted to a higher step: R. V I (42) / L. VI II IV' X VIII (55555). This formula is often used for severe colds or flu, including allergies.

Feb 19, 20XX. The cold had resolved, and floaters had significantly decreased, further confirming the efficacy of Constitutional treatment. However, a rash had appeared on the patient's face over the past 3–4 days. The prescription was modified as follows: R. V I (42) / L. II VI IV' I IX (55555). The right side remained unchanged, while the left side targeted allergies and the rash.

Feb 27, 20XX. Although the cold had previously resolved, the patient felt as if another cold might develop. The prescription reverted to the cold formula: R. V I (42) / L. VI II IV' X VIII (55555).

March 5, 20XX. The floaters had almost disappeared, and no new cold symptoms had developed. This reinforced the effectiveness of Constitutional treatment for this patient's conditions. The same prescription was maintained.

April 2, 20XX. The patient returned after about a month and reported feeling well. The same prescription was continued.

April 10, 20XX. The patient noted significant improvement in eye comfort but mentioned feeling tired due to seasonal weather changes. The prescription remained the same, but the repetition count was adjusted as follows: R. V I (42) / L. VI II IV' X VIII (44444).

Following these improvements in his eye health, the patient stopped visiting my clinic. He returned 7 months later.

Nov 25, 20XX. The patient reported significant deterioration in his eyesight, with symptoms including dry eyes, blurry vision, and heightened sensitivity to light. He also admitted to heavy drinking over the past two weeks. Considering the importance of eye health, I emphasized the need to quit alcohol completely and adhere strictly to the Constitutional Diet. Constitution-acupuncture treatment was administered: R. V I (44) / L. VI II IV' X VIII (44444). The prescription remained the same as before, but the frequency was synchronized to four times.

Nov 27, 20XX. The patient said his eyes felt cool after receiving the acupuncture, stayed comfortable until the next day. I whispered to myself, "Surely, Constitution-acupuncture treatment works that well, doesn't it? In cases like this, you really need to come and get acupuncture every day. You, at the brink of the optic death, have to try all your best to cure such a fatal disease. It is a matter of whether 'your eyes' would diminish or 'you yourself' would perish." But I thought he had been too complacent about it. For some people, when their eyes fail, it feels as if their entire life has ended. I reminded him how precious his eyes were, and must come and get treated regularly. The treatment remained the same as before.

Dec 3, 20XX. He noted that his eyes feel dry. In the morning, he said, when clearing the throat, there was a brief flash of light in the eyes, like lightning. Somehow, human diseases often present with mysterious symptoms that defy reasonable understanding. When this happens, patients often ask their doctors why it occurred. But in reality, in most cases, doctors themselves don't know much about it, either. If doctors aren't God, how can they possibly know everything? They simply rely on vague medical jargon, offering an explanation that is not really an explanation. Patients take comfort in the illusion that their question has been answered, as if the mystery has been resolved. The prescription was adjusted as follows: L. V IX (55) / R. VI II IV' X VIII (44444). The left side was treated for Zang-system Inflammation, while the right side for allergies. Constitutional decoction was also prescribed.

Dec 4, 20XX. The patient reported seeing floating objects in his vision. The same prescription was repeated.

Dec 9, 20XX. No significant changes were noted. The prescription was modified as follows: L. V IX (55) / R. VII IX III' I VI (55555). The right side was treated with the Formula commonly used for severe liver conditions, as the liver and eyes are closely connected in Oriental medicine.

Dec 16, 20XX. The patient still noted no changes. The prescription was adjusted further as follows: L. V IX III' (555) / R. VII IX III' I VI (55555).

Jan 1, 20XX. The patient returned after three weeks in the new year, reporting that his eyes felt similar as before. He also mentioned enjoying a recent trip to Angkor Wat in Cambodia. Treatment continued as follows: L. V IX III' (555) / R. VI II IV' X VIII (55555).

Jan 13, 20XX. The patient reported a reduced light sensitivity and an increased comfort in his eyes—a sign of gradual improvement. The same treatment was maintained.

Jan 15, 20XX. The patient noted further improvement, with his eyes feeling more comfortable. After about a month and a half of consistent treatments, his eye condition finally stabilized.

After this, the patient began spacing out his visits, sometimes coming once or twice a month, or every few months. He typically returned when neglecting the Constitutional regimen led to a recurrence of the symptoms. The true leadership in medicine lies with the patients, not with the doctors. Illness is ultimately self-inflicted, and the patients hold the reins of the treatment.

[Toeum Case 2] Man Whose Body Was Purified

* Patient: Mr. Y, office worker, 32 years old at the time of visit
* Chief complaints: allergic rhinitis, flat warts

The patient was primarily an office worker who worked from home. He had chronic allergic rhinitis and recently developed shingles, attributed to the weakened immune system caused by excessive alcohol consumption. After recovering from shingles last year, he noticed the appearance of flat warts.

Despite being relatively young, the patient was highly interested in health and had a history of consuming various health supplements. He reported that taking ginseng caused him to experience heart palpitations and chest tightness. This reaction is an important clue in diagnosing his Constitutional type. While his exact Constitution cannot yet be determined, it is clear that he does not fall under the Suyang Constitution or Sueum Constitution. In other words, these Constitutions can be ruled out as a possibility. A similar observation was made regarding his reaction to honey, which caused him stomach discomfort, providing further evidence to exclude those Constitutions from consideration.

He also reported experiencing diarrhea after drinking excessively. However, this symptom is not particularly helpful in diagnosing Constitution, as individuals of nearly every Constitution can exhibit this reaction. That said, alcohol does not suit any Constitution well.

The patient also shared that an overall vegetarian diet, particularly one rich in greens, felt light on his body and helped improve his bowel movements. This, too, is a significant clue for determining his Constitution, suggesting that Mogyang Constitution or Mogeum Constitution are unlikely possibilities.

Seemingly minor details shared by the patient, such as his dietary preferences and reactions, surprisingly provide valuable insights into diagnosing his Constitutional type. A doctor specializing in Constitutional Medicine must approach every piece of patient's information with a discerning eye, much like Sherlock Holmes, to uncover these subtle but crucial clues for the exact diagnosis of Constitution.

March 17, 20XX. The first treatment started at the low level of Formulae: R. V IX (51) / L. V I (42).

Mar 21, 20XX. The patient visited another Eight-Constitution Clinic near his home and received Geumyang Constitution-acupuncture twice. However, he felt very unwell because of headache and indigestion. He also mentioned persistent intestinal issues, including excessive gas and flatulence. He was doubtful about the Toeum Constitution diagnosis I provided, as it was statistically considered very unlikely and rare. That's why he sought to confirm his Constitution elsewhere.

From a doctor's perspective, while the patient's deviation from the diagnosed Constitution is not ideal, his disclosure helps rule out the Geumyang Constitution, which is sometimes valuable in itself. The Constitution-acupuncture prescription was adjusted as follows: R. V I (42) / L. II VI IV' I IX (44444). Treatment targeted Fu-system Inflammation on the right side and allergy on the left side.

March 22, 20XX. After receiving the previous acupuncture treatment, the patient reported that his stomach discomfort and chest tightness had nearly disappeared. He expressed noticeable improvements, confirming the effectiveness of Constitution-acupuncture. The prescription remained unchanged.

March 24, 20XX. The patient reported no side effects from acupuncture, reduced fatigue, and an absence of morning urine foam, which had been present before. I continued the treatment with the same prescription.

March 25, 20XX. The patient noted improved energy levels and ease in waking up in the mornings, which had previously been difficult. Treatment was repeated with the same prescription.

March 26, 20XX. The patient mentioned a tightness in his right chest lasting 1–2 hours after the acupuncture treatment the previous day, but this had resolved. Treatment continued with the same prescription.

March 27, 20XX. After eating "Dogani soup" (soup of beef knee joint cartilage) and grilled pork for dinner, the patient experienced significant itching on his scalp and anus. While pork suited him well, Dogani soup, made from beef, is unsuitable for Toeum Constitution. Treatment was administered with the same prescription.

March 28, 20XX. The itching had decreased slightly. The patient reported regular bowel movements (1–2 times daily), which were slightly watery but otherwise normal. The prescription remained unchanged.

March 31, 20XX. The patient noted that keeping the Constitutional food rule appropriately eliminated itchiness. However, after consuming a tangerine, he felt unwell, a reaction he had never experienced before. This reaction was explained as a typical response to Constitutional treatment, during which the body's balance improves, toxins are removed, and, as a result of being cleansed, the patient becomes more sensitive to harmful foods. The principle is akin to the difference between dumping waste into a heavily polluted river, where the impact is negligible, and dumping it into a clean, pristine river, where even a small pollutant has an immediate effect. This immediate response to unsuitable foods is a clear indication of the body achieving optimal health. Treatment continued with the same prescription.

The patient returned to my clinic after about two and a half years, reporting remarkable improvements in his health. He shared that he had diligently followed the Constitutional Diet. He proudly stated that his allergies, flat warts, and headaches had completely disappeared since his visit to Joowonjang Clinic. I confirmed his progress and praised his dedication. After receiving Constitution-acupuncture for a few additional days, the patient noted further improvements and smiled as he shared his enhanced condition. Through Eight-Constitution Medicine, this patient has undergone a true transformation, achieving a state of optimal health.

[Toeum Case 3] Fart Captain

* Ms. G, 47 years old at the time of visit
* Chief complaints: Excessive gas in the stomach and intestines, resulting in constant burping and farting.

The patient had chronic issues with excessive gas in her gastrointestinal tract, experiencing constant burping and farting throughout the day. Because of this, she earned the nickname "Fart Captain Poongpoong" during her youth, a title that caused significant challenges in her daily life. Uniquely, as soon as food entered her mouth, burping and farting would immediately follow, indicating that her gastrointestinal tract was already full of gas. The intake of food seemingly triggered the release of this gas due to increased pressure.

Despite these issues, she grew to a height of 167 cm, which is quite tall for a Korean woman. This suggests that her overall nutrition was unexpectedly worked not that bad. However, one might wonder: if her digestive health had been optimal, couldn't she have grown well over 180 cm and perhaps pursued a career as a national basketball player?

In addition to her gas-related problems, she experienced blurred vision, mental fog, and chronic fatigue. Her eyes always felt dim, and her brain was unclear. These symptoms were likely tied to the gas in her digestive system. Gastric gas is a hallmark of "empty heat"—a condition of incomplete digestion. When food is digested properly, the nutrients are efficiently absorbed with minimal byproducts like gas. However, incomplete digestion leads to the production of "hot exhaust gases," often described as the "empty heat" in traditional Oriental medicine. This constant state of inefficiency left her eyes feeling dry and irritated, as if filled with sand, while her head felt oppressively hot, much like a tropical night.

Her lack of energy was also a direct consequence of her digestive problems. Poor digestion led to incomplete energy production, similar to a car running on low-quality fuel and achieving suboptimal performance.

Moreover, the patient exhibited intense and unusual reactions to foods and supplements. For example, after consuming a health supplement containing cultured wild ginseng for just 15 days, she felt such intense anger that she wanted to murder someone. The burning sensation from her body's reaction must have been overwhelming. What a respectful persistence that she continued taking it for that long despite such adverse effects! Most people would have stopped immediately upon experiencing discomfort.

She also reported that nutritional supplements were poorly tolerated, even those suited for her Toeum Constitution. For example, despite vitamin E being appropriate for her Constitution, it caused digestive upset. When she took vitamin C for two months, even a slight breeze through a window caused severe shoulder pain and made all her body feel battered, as if it had been physically struck hard. One might wonder whether such claims were exaggerated.

The patient also sought Eight-Constitutions diagnoses at various clinics, each leading to disappointing outcomes. After receiving Geumyang Constitution treatment at one clinic, she experienced severe flatulence with an unbearable odor. Treatments for Toyang and Sueum Constitution also yielded poor results. More recently, she received treatment for Mogyang Constitution, which caused nausea and a bitter taste in her mouth.

Her dietary restrictions were extreme: she could not eat apples or tangerines under any circumstances. Even foods typically considered gentle on the stomach, like sweet potatoes, potatoes, and pumpkin, were intolerable. Yellow pumpkin was especially problematic. Her extensive list of abnormal reactions to foods and treatments is extraordinary and would be enormously challenging to catalog it fully.

It is easy to question whether all of her reported experiences were accurate, but the severity and consistency of her symptoms left no room for doubt. She presented me with a truly one-of-a-kind case.

March 29, 20XX. As usual, the first treatment began lightly. Prescription: R. V IX (51) / L. V I (42). This involved Fu-system Inflammation Formula on the right and Zang-system Inflammation Formula on the left.

July 19, 20XX. The patient returned to my clinic nearly four months after the initial treatment. She reported feeling comfortable after receiving Constitution-acupuncture last time. During this period, she quit drinking coffee and eating spicy foods. While she had been doing well, she began feeling weak and experiencing leg fatigue starting in June. The same prescription was administered as before.

July 21, 20XX. She returned two days later and mentioned that after receiving the acupuncture treatment, she felt drowsy early in the evening. This is a general "Myeonghyeon reaction" (a healing response feeling like side effects) associated with Constitution-acupuncture. Some patients have reported feeling so drowsy after the Constitution-acupuncture treatment that they had to pull over and nap for 30 minutes or something before continuing their drive home. Patients with insomnia often report improved sleep following Constitution-acupuncture. The prescription remained the same, but the frequency of treatment was adjusted as follows: R. V IX (55) / L. V I (44).

July 25, 20XX. Four days later, the patient noted feeling somewhat more energized. However, numbness in her legs and arms while sleeping persisted. She also shared that after eating spicy peppers the previous day, she experienced severe diarrhea. The same prescription was used: L. V IX (55) / R. V I (44).

August 1, 20XX. A week later, the patient mentioned that she was waking up more easily in the mornings, which had previously been difficult for her. She shared that she injured her hand last week and took antibiotics, which caused severe side effects. She experienced extreme nausea and broke into a cold sweat. While it is well-known that individuals with Toeum Constitution are very sensitive to antibiotics, the severity of her reaction was surprising.

She also recounted an incident in the past when, after fasting for a day, she developed hypoglycemia and began sweating profusely, as if she had just taken a shower. The side effects of antibiotics seemed to mirror a hypoglycemic shock episode. Although low blood sugar may appear less critical than high blood sugar, it is, in fact, more dangerous. While fainting due to high blood sugar is rare, fainting due to low blood sugar is common. When the body's "battery" drains, it leads to an immediate shutdown, much like a car stalling without power. The same prescription was repeated for treatment.

Sep 8, 20XX. About three weeks later, she came back. The patient reported that due to personal circumstances, she had been eating chicken frequently. She explained that she had little choice but to work part-time to help an acquaintance open a fried chicken restaurant. As a result, she experienced severe bloating, foul-smelling flatulence, constipation, a hot sensation in her mouth, extreme thirst, bad breath, and discomfort in the mornings. The same prescription was administered.

Sep 10, 20XX. She reported experiencing some stomach cramps the previous day, along with a significant amount of diarrhea—about five times her usual stool volume. The same prescription was used, with frequencies adjusted to 5:1 on the left and 4:2 on the right.

Dec 26, 20XX. The patient returned after more than three months. She reported having a cold for the past three weeks, so even the slightest contact with water caused her stomach to feel cold. She also felt extremely chill on her back and shoulders during the winter. However, intestinal gas, which had been a previous issue, had decreased significantly. She mentioned difficulty waking up in the mornings. The prescription remained unchanged.

Dec 28, 20XX. Her cold improved significantly. The same prescription was continued.

Jan 2, 20XX. On the second day of the new year, the patient visited my clinic. Although her cold had almost resolved, she still had nasal congestion and a light cough. She reported burping and discomfort around the pit of the stomach. Before arriving at the clinic, she had eaten oyster soup at a nearby restaurant, which left her stomach feeling strange. According to her, this was likely due to chemical seasonings. Additionally, her shoulders felt stiff after sleeping. The same prescription was used, with frequencies adjusted to 5:5 on the left and 4:4 on the right.

Jan 3, 20XX. On the day she received the acupuncture treatment, the patient experienced extreme drowsiness while driving home. She had to stop mid-journey to rest before finally arriving home, where she slept again. The following morning, she felt heart palpitations similar to arrhythmia. The same prescription was continued, with frequencies adjusted to 5:1 on the left and 4:2 on the right.

Jan 5, 20XX. The patient reported an overall increase in energy. However, she experienced back soreness in the mornings, similar to being beaten, and had difficulty urinating. The prescription remained the same.

Jan 9, 20XX. Four days later, she complained of shoulder pain. The same prescription was continued.

Jan 13, 20XX. Another four days later, the patient noted she was waking up earlier in the mornings and felt less tired overall. She was eating and digesting food well. Her urine volume increased, and its color became clearer. However, she experienced difficulty with bowel movements, and her tongue felt stiff at the root, affecting her pronunciation. The same prescription was maintained.

Jan 16, 20XX. She reported persistent shoulder pain. She mentioned taking probiotics the previous Friday, which caused indigestion and discomfort over the weekend. She also experienced significant backaches. The same prescription was used, but the left and right sides were switched: R. V IX (51) / L. V I (42).

Jan 17, 20XX. The next day, the patient reported feeling more comfortable in her stomach, experiencing reduced headaches, and noticing an improved complexion in the mornings. The same prescription was administered.

The patient continued visiting Joowonjang Clinic at intervals of about two to three days, addressing her discomfort and illnesses with Constitution-acupuncture. She has since stopped visiting my clinic and is now managing her health through the Constitutional Diet and exercise.

In truth, such cases as hers represent highly challenging ones. These are the individuals who cannot be treated with Western medicine for sure. This patient is a testament to the efficacy of Eight-Constitution Medicine, which stands as the only path to recovery in such instances.

Mogyang Constitution's Clinical Cases

[Mogyang Case 1] Treating Mental Illness Without Labeling It as Mental Illness

* Patient: Mr. G, office worker, 26 years old at the time of visit
* Chief complaints: Eye strain and difficulty seeing in the dark

The patient reported constant eye strain and soreness, which had been troubling him throughout the day. He explained that it had started two years ago (more than 22 years ago from the present) as a result of severe stress. He was an office worker in the IT industry, primarily handling website programming and system management. Although this has become a common profession today, at the time, his vocation was seen as a rising job in an exciting and rapidly growing field. Overall, he seemingly was an innocent and honest young man.

As is often the case in this field, his work stress was intense. His job required long hours of coding while staring at a computer monitor—a demanding and dehumanizing task. Once he began working, he would lose himself in the endless string of codes, often working 10 to 20 hours straight, completely unaware of time passing. It was as if his soul left his body and hovered above, while his physical self became a mechanical entity tapping away at the keyboard.

The intense focus on the monitor left his eyes feeling scorched and parched, resembling the fields cracked by drought. He was plagued by a sensation like grains of sand scratching his cornea and a stiffness in his eyes, akin to the rigid steering wheel of an old car. His eyes were strained, bloodshot, and swollen. Brain fog often left him in a trance, forcing him to guzzle cans of coke for relief. His desk was cluttered with empty cans—a visual testament to his daily routine.

His eyes were perpetually dim, and his body constantly fatigued. Dark circles like those of a panda shadowed his eyes, and traces of hard life were etched all over his body.

People with Mogyang Constitution often have muscular, robust physiques, and this young man was no exception. Yet, his strong frame seemed deflated, like cabbage wilted by salt. The sight of him, crushed under the weight of life's demands at such a young age, evoked a sense of sadness in me—a situation clearly in need of salvation.

Jan 7, 20XX. I immediately began treatment to alleviate the patient's fatigue. The prescription for Constitution-acupuncture was as follows: R. I VII (55) / L. I V (44). Zang-system Inflammation Formula on the right and Fu-system Inflammation Formula on the left. The repetition counts, as 5:5 and 4:4, were devised by me. Additionally, Constitutional decoction targeting chronic fatigue and eye health was prescribed.

Jan 11, 20XX. Four days later, the patient reported difficulty focusing on distant objects. The prescription was escalated to 5-stage Formula. The right-side Formula remained the same, while the left one was adjusted to IX VII III' VI II (55555), a Formula typically applied to liver-related conditions like cirrhosis or liver cancer. According to Oriental medicine, the eyes are closely related to Liver, as stated in classical texts: "The Liver governs the eyes."

Jan 14, 20XX. The patient noted slight improvement in his vision. The same prescription was maintained.

Jan 16, 20XX. and Jan 18, 20XX. The condition was reported as similar or slightly improved. The same prescription continued.

Jan 21, 20XX. The patient reported significant improvement in his vision, expressing amazement at the efficacy of Constitutional treatment. Indeed, Eight-Constitution Medicine is a remarkable therapeutic approach. The treatment remained the same.

Jan 25, 20XX. The patient enthusiastically shared that his vision had substantially improved. Hearing such feedback from patients is incredibly rewarding. The prescription remained unchanged.

After just the eight sessions of treatment, the patient experienced significant improvement in his eye condition and decided to focus on self-care without further treatment. He revisited my clinic in April, nearly three months later, as spring was in full bloom.

April 12, 20XX. The patient reported difficulty focusing his eyes and mentioned an unusual symptom: peeling of his tongue. I inquired about the cause. He explained that during this period, he had taken medication prescribed by a local neuropsychiatrist. While the psychiatric medication initially alleviated some symptoms, it caused his thinking to slow drastically. He described his days as feeling like watching a slow-motion video, leaving him deeply bored. Suddenly, his tongue began peeling. This led to a complete loss of appetite.

Psychiatric medications often strongly suppress the central nervous system, causing dazed and sluggish feelings. The patient stopped taking the medication to avoid those side effects but found himself so mentally and physically exhausted that when he resumed taking the medication, his anxiety subsided, only for the tongue peeling to return. This cycle led him to revisit my clinic. He speculated that his symptoms resembled panic disorder and described himself as feeling depressed.

I sighed inwardly. "How can this be approached as a mental illness?" When someone is highly stressed and physically exhausted, anxiety is a natural response. This condition can often be effectively managed by resting, recovering from fatigue, and relieving tension through supportive interactions with friends and family. Alternatively, Constitution-acupuncture treatment, such as that provided at Joowonjang Clinic, can improve symptoms in a short time.

However, forcibly suppressing the central nervous system with tranquilizers may temporarily relieve anxiety but is unlikely to restore true health. The fact that the patient's tongue was peeling demonstrates the intensity of the medication.

Peeling of the tongue signifies the loss of the tongue's protective coating—its epithelial cells. These cells serve as the body's first line of defense and are crucial immune organs. Severe loss of epithelial cells, like that seen in burn victims, allows bacteria and viruses to invade freely, leading to widespread inflammation throughout the body. The peeling of epithelial cells is a profound event, indicating that the very foundation of the patient's physical health is being compromised.

Among my long-time patients, there is one with Geumeum Constitution. In her youth, she suffered from a severe skin disease and was treated at the hospital with a chemotherapy drug containing arsenic (As). Using anticancer drugs for skin diseases is highly unusual. In some cases, treatments that deviate from standard protocols are administered in hopes of achieving temporary effects. Moreover, this particular medication was difficult to obtain at the time, so her father resorted to using connections to secure it through a U.S. military hospital based in Seoul. This story dates back several decades.

However, after taking the medication, her skin began peeling extensively, as if her entire body were shedding its outer layer. This condition, called exfoliative dermatitis, left her in immense distress. Alarmed by the worsening symptoms, she asked the doctor if the reaction could be a side effect of the medication. The doctor, dismissing her concerns, insisted it was unrelated and instead doubled the dosage. At that time, doctors wielded God-like authority. This particular physician, a prominent figure frequently featured in the media, was highly regarded. Trusting his words completely, she continued taking the medication, believing it to be part of the healing process. Instead, her skin deteriorated further, the peeling worsened, and her skin's natural defense system was utterly destroyed. Even decades later, her body remains covered in scars resembling the cracked and blistered surface throughout the body.

In this male patient's case, a similar phenomenon occurred internally rather than externally. The peeling of his tongue signified a severe blow to his gastrointestinal system. The tongue, esophagus, and stomach are all lined with epithelial cells that form a continuous protective layer. The psychiatric medications he had been prescribed likely caused extensive damage, stripping the epithelial lining from his esophagus and stomach, too. Under such conditions, it is no wonder that he lost his appetite. The psychiatric medication he had been taking was no different from an anticancer drug in its harsh effects. I strongly advised him to discontinue the medication, warning him of potentially dire consequences.

The prescription for Constitution-acupuncture was as follows: R. I VII (55) / L. II VI IV' X VIII (44444). The right side targeted the Zang-system Inflammation, while the left focused on the so-called Dysautonomia Formula.

The autonomic nervous system, which governs the internal organs, blood vessels, sweat glands, and more, operates independently of conscious control and is distinct from the motor nervous system responsible for voluntary muscle movement. This prescription is designed to balance the Five Zangs and Five Fus, promoting relaxation of both body and mind. Additionally, I prescribed Constitutional decoction to help ease his mental distress.

April 18, 20XX. The patient self-investigated and concluded that he had developed panic disorder as a side effect of psychiatric medication. Initially prescribed to relieve mild anxiety, the medication ironically caused a serious illness—panic disorder—as a side effect. It seemed like a losing exchange of bad for worse. The acupuncture prescription was slightly adjusted as follows: R. I VII III' (555) / L. II VI IV' X VIII (44444). On the right side, Disc Formula was used, while Dysautonomia Formula was applied to the left. The Disc Formula is not only used for herniated discs but also for musculoskeletal issues and brain issues such as headache and brain fog.

April 22, 20XX. Since discontinuing psychiatric medication, the side effect of feeling dazed had decreased. The patient appeared to have been taking antidepressants, which commonly cause a sensation of mental fog as a side effect due to excessive suppression on the central nervous system. Frequent hot water baths, known to be beneficial for individuals with Mogyang Constitution, were recommended. The prescription remained unchanged.

April 26, 20XX. The patient reported some improvement, noting that the hot baths seemed effective. He visited my clinic for several days afterward with similar symptoms and continued receiving the same treatment.

May 4, 20XX. Following the discontinuation of psychiatric medication, the patient reported experiencing brief, sudden electric shock-like sensations in the brain, which disturbed his sleep and caused restlessness. He also mentioned that while on psychiatric medication, he had difficulty with bowel movements and experienced weakened urination. He, again, emphasized that his panic disorder was not an inherent condition but rather a side effect of the medication. The acupuncture prescription was adjusted as follows: R. I V III' (444) / L. I V III' VII IX (55555). On the right, the Formula targeting high blood pressure was used to reduce intracranial pressure, while on the left, the Formula typically used for liver cirrhosis was applied to alleviate fatigue.

May 10, 20XX. The patient reported slight improvement. He admitted to taking psychiatric medication once due to restlessness and insomnia, emphasizing that it was just a one-time occurrence. His determination to avoid dependence on psychiatric drugs was commendable, as breaking free from such dependency is extremely challenging. The same acupuncture prescription was continued.

May 12, 20XX. The patient noted significant improvement. He also mentioned that prolonged use of his smart phone caused difficulty focusing on the surroundings when he looked away. He also experienced nasal congestion in the mornings. Treatment by the same prescription was continued as before.

May 19 and 26, 20XX. The patient reported further significant improvement. The same treatment was administered during these visits.

The patient's symptoms improved considerably, prompting a pause in his visits to my clinic. After about three months, he returned for additional treatment.

Aug 25, 20XX. The patient reported feeling dazed and depressed, with a lingering sense of heaviness in his body. He mentioned that people often commented on his lack of facial expressions. His memory had deteriorated significantly, and he was convinced that these were side effects of the psychiatric medication. Additionally, his younger sister had remarked on the unusual trembling in his hands. My prescription was as follows: R. I VII III' (555) / L. II VI IV' X VIII (44444). Disc Formula was used on the right and Dysautonomia Formula on the left. Constitutional decoction was also prescribed.

Sep 2, 20XX. The patient reported that his headaches had somewhat subsided. For me, a doctor practicing Eight-Constitution Medicine, he was an excellent patient, responding well to the constitutional treatment. The same prescription was continued.

Sep 9, Sep 15, Sep 27, Oct 2, Oct 6, Oct 14, 20XX. As his health improved, the patient was visiting my clinic approximately once a week. His condition remained stable with consistent treatment. The same acupuncture treatment was preformed, and an additional Constitutional decoction was provided.

Oct 21, 20XX. The patient mentioned that the feeling of dullness had disappeared. He shared that, during his youth while serving in the military, he was struck on the left side of his head with a rifle butt, resulting in a severe injury with significant bleeding. What a sad story! This traumatic experience, like many others from that era, could have left lingering effects on his mental and physical health. The treatment remained unchanged.

Oct 28, 20XX. The patient reported that his eyes felt tense the previous day due to his strabismus. This suggested he was under considerable stress at work. He was treated with the same prescription.

Nov 4, 20XX. The patient noted that much of the tense in his eyes had eased. Constitution-acupuncture proved highly effective. Reflecting on how a psychiatrist might have treated the issue, one could assume that antidepressants would have been prescribed, merely suppressing the symptoms. Treatment continued with the same regimen.

Nov 11, 20XX. The stiffness in his eyes had significantly eased. The same prescription was administered.

Nov 18, 20XX. The patient reported substantial improvement, saying that he might only need one more session next week. Treatment was continued with the same prescription.

Nov 25, 20XX. The patient reported feeling fine. However, his colleagues remarked that his expressionless face was unsettling. He shared that, while he was once motivated and energetic, lethargy and frustration had eventually taken hold, leaving him in a constant state of depression. Treatment continued as before.

Dec 2 ~ Dec 16, 20XX. The patient visited my clinic three times at weekly intervals, reporting consistent improvement. The same prescription was maintained.

Dec 23, 20XX. The patient returned after three weeks, sharing that he had an important client meeting three days prior. During the presentation, he became so nervous that his judgment was impaired, leading to awkward speech out of turn. The prescription was adjusted as follows: R. I V III' VII IX (44444) / L. II VI IV' VIII X (44444). On the right, 5-stage Zang-system Formula was administered, and on the left, 5-stage Fu-system Formula was administered. This unique method aimed to balance both Zang-system and Fu-system.

Dec 30, 20XX. The patient reported feeling much better. The same prescription was continued.

Jan 6, 20XX. A week after the new year began, the patient visited my clinic and reported significant improvement in his condition. He shared that he had started practicing hot yoga, which made him feel better as he began sweating regularly. He also mentioned the plans to begin CrossFit and weight training in about four months. CrossFit, known for its high-intensity interval training, combines various exercise elements to enhance physical fitness in a short amount of time. I commended him for starting on such exercises. For individuals with Mogyang Constitution, actively engaging in sweat-inducing activities like hot yoga or weight training is highly beneficial for their health. Treatment continued with the same prescription.

Jan 13, 20XX. The patient reported feeling well. The same prescription was administered.

Jan 20, 20XX. The patient noted that his tinnitus had almost disappeared last Sunday and that the peeling on his tongue had decreased and eventually stopped. Treatment continued with the same prescription, and Constitutional decoction was added.

Jan 27, 20XX. The patient again reported feeling well. I was pleased to see consistent improvement. The same Constitution-acupuncture prescription was applied.

Afterward, the patient continued to visit my clinic approximately once a week for the next six months, completing his treatment. Although his case was not easy, his diligent adherence to the treatment plan led to highly positive outcomes.

Psychiatric disorders are notoriously challenging to treat. It is common for patients to show improvement only to relapse suddenly, as stressors that trigger anxiety are pervasive. For this patient, work stress was a primary factor, compounded by family conflicts and personal issues.

Interestingly, individuals with Mogyang Constitution often experience psychiatric challenges. Anxiety, depression, and panic disorders are not uncommon, and even rarer conditions like obsessive-compulsive disorder or auditory hallucinations can occur, too. While these individuals may appear physically robust and muscular, they often have personalities that are surprisingly sensitive and delicate. The key to maintaining a healthy Mogyang Constitution lies in consuming foods suited to the Constitution and engaging in regular sweat-inducing exercise.

[Mogyang Case 2] Gentleman (君子)'s Tao Begins with Husband-Wife Relationship[120]

* Patient: Ms. Z, 55 years old at the time of visit
* Chief complaints: Numbness in hands and feet after thyroid cancer surgery

The patient developed numbness in her hands and feet after undergoing surgery for thyroid adenocarcinoma five years ago. She has since been taking Synthyroxine,[121] a thyroid hormone medication. Fortunately, her parathyroid gland was not affected during the surgery. She also mentioned a nodule in her lungs, which has been monitored regularly for any changes. Fortunately, her annual follow-ups have shown no significant changes. She previously took medication for high blood pressure but has discontinued it, noting that although her blood pressure was high, she did not experience any noticeable symptoms.

---

[120] The quoted text is from Chapter 12 of *The Doctrine of the Mean* (*Zhongyong*, 『中庸』): "The way of the gentleman begins with the couple. When it reaches its utmost fulfillment, it aligns with and reflects the workings of heaven and earth." (君子之道, 造端乎夫婦, 及其至也, 察乎天地.)

[121] Refers to Synthyroxine tablets. The active ingredient is levothyroxine sodium, a medication used to replace thyroid hormone (thyroxine) following thyroid surgery or to treat hypothyroidism.

The patient visited my clinic accompanied by her husband, who suffered from fibromyalgia, a condition causing widespread pain. Her husband's constant complaints about his pain seemed to burden her significantly. Observing their interaction, it became apparent to me that her husband was the primary source of her stress and subsequent illnesses. He was highly temperamental, easily frustrated by his condition, and quick to anger—a textbook example of "hot-tempered" personality.

She spent most of her time tending on her husband's needs, living under constant stress. In such circumstances, it would be unusual not to fall ill. Despite this, she maintained a kind demeanor, always wearing a smile, which clearly required immense emotional effort. Her smile seemed more like a survival mechanism than a genuine expression, encapsulated by the saying, "I'm laughing, but I'm not really laughing!" If someone else were in her shoes, the person might have pursued a divorce long ago—a sentiment that readers would likely empathize with. However, as a traditionally minded woman who treated her husband with great deference, divorce was an unthinkable option for her.

In such cases, treatment is inherently challenging. The root cause of the illness—chronic stress from her husband—remains ever-present. Even if the treatment improves her condition temporarily, the same stressors are likely to trigger a relapse. Nevertheless, I began her treatment journey, hoping to provide relief amidst her challenging circumstances.

Oct 2, 20XX. Treatment began with a prescription commonly used for degenerative joint issues: R. VIII X IV' II VI (44444) / L. I VII III' VIII (4444). Degenerative arthritis Formula on the right and Disc Formula on the left were administered. Being of Mogyang Constitution, I recommended incorporating meat, wheat, and dairy foods into her diet. While Mogyang Constitution's individuals typically don't have strict dietary preferences, she was accustomed to a more traditional diet, favoring kimchi and vegetables over meat. Implementing these changes would likely be a challenge for her.

Oct 4, 20XX. Two days later, she reported positive effects from the treatment. Despite suffering from allergic rhinitis, which usually impaired her sense of smell, she said she could smell faintly, and her body felt lighter overall. Numbness in her hands and feet had lessened, although she still felt tired around 2 pm. Encouraged by these positive signs, I maintained the same prescription but increased the repetitions on the left side: R. VIII X IV' II VI (44444) / L. I VII III' VIII (5555).

Oct 7, 20XX. Three days later, she reported continued improvement, though her nose remained somewhat stuffy. Occasionally, she could smell things, confirming the effectiveness of Constitution-acupuncture. The same prescription was repeated.

Oct 8, 20XX. She mentioned her nose felt clearer, with only slight numbness in her hands and feet. The speed of her progress exceeded my expectations. The same prescription was continued.

Oct 11, 20XX. Her overall condition improved. One thing special is she experienced an intense episode of numbness about an hour after the previous treatment, followed by relief. The prescription was adjusted to R. I VIII (42) / L. I VII III' VIII (4444).

Oct 14, 20XX. Although she felt well, her blood pressure spiked up to 190 due to the stress caused by her husband. She mentioned a past reliance on blood pressure medication, but was not currently taking it. The treatment remained the same, but the left and right sides were swapped: L. I VIII (42) / R. I VII III' VIII (4444).

Oct 16, 20XX. She felt comfortable, a sign that the ongoing treatment was taking effect. The same prescription was used, with the right side treated at a 5:5:5:5 ratio.

Oct 18, 20XX. She continued to feel comfortable. The same prescription was administered.

Oct 21, Oct 23, 20XX. 10. Although she reported slight numbness, her condition was good overall. The same prescription was applied with the reduced frequency of 4:4:4:4 on the right.

Oct 28, 20XX. After a week, she mentioned postnasal drip and a sore neck after hiking. Blood pressure was recorded at 175/111 with a heart rate of 75. The prescription was updated to R. I VIII III' (551) / L. II VI IV' X VIII (44444), with Disc Formula on the right and Dysautonomia Formula on the left.

Oct 30, 20XX. Her nose felt clearer, though she experienced sporadic stiffness in her fingers. These episodes, sometimes while intense like storm, were brief. The prescription was modified to R. I VIII III' VIII (5555) / L. I VIII (42), using an applied form of Disc Formula on the right and Vitality Formula on the left.

Nov 1, 20XX. She noted that stiffness was manageable. She found it a bit difficult to go about her day on the day of the acupuncture treatment, but felt better afterward. Since the acupuncture somewhat seemed to strain her body, the prescription was reduced to a simpler level: R. I VII (51) / L. I V (42).

Nev 4, 20XX. She reported no significant issues, except for mild pain in her right thumb. Bowel movements were well-regulated, and she appeared to be following the Constitutional Diet effectively. The same prescription was continued.

Nov 6, 20XX. The pain in her thumb had mostly subsided. The same prescription was maintained.

Nov 8, 20XX. The thumb pain occurred only occasionally and was almost negligible. She noted that her eyes no longer hurt when looking at a computer monitor. Since introducing meat into her diet, she felt fuller than before, and consumed less food overall. In the past, she would keep eating to feel full because she was constantly hungry. The same prescription was continued.

By following Constitutional Diet and undergoing Constitution-acupuncture regularly, she experienced a markedly better quality of life than at any point in her marriage. Although her health fluctuated depending on her husband's temperament and stress levels, her overall well-being improved significantly.

She continued to visit Joowonjang Clinic regularly for acupuncture and took Constitutional decoction when needed. Through the consistent treatments, she achieved a more peaceful and balanced life.

[Mogyang Case 3] Sleepless Nights Due to Weight Gain

* Patient: Mr. B, 42 years old at the time of visit
* Chief complaints: Insomnia

Originally, the patient visited my clinic several years ago with a symptom categorized as auditory hallucinations. He described hearing constant sounds—voices of people he knew, his family, and music, particularly popular songs. Initially, he believed the sounds were real. However, a doctor later informed him that these were auditory hallucinations, a symptom of mental illness.

The patient explained that his mental illness developed from guilty consciousness after his father's passing. He blamed himself for disobeying his father and leading a self-indulgent life, which he believed contributed to his father's suffering and early death from illness. Despite his large, imposing physique—which might give the impression of being rough or even gangster-like—he was, in reality, a soft-hearted person.

The patient had a typical Mogyang Constitution's body shape. Standing 180 cm tall and weighing 95 kg, his physique was ideal for an athlete such as a wrestler. For individuals with such energy-rich bodies, the ideal lifestyle would be to find a sport that suits their abilities and pursue a career as a professional athlete. I believe that confining such a dynamic body to desk jobs or sedentary work could be akin to committing a sin against one's physical nature. When there is a mismatch between a person's physical Constitution and occupation, not only physical deterioration but mental exhaustion may become inevitable. Suppressing such irresistible energy could definitely make the body sick.

The patient initially tried to address his auditory hallucinations through psychiatric medication, but it was ineffective. He eventually turned to Joowonjang Clinic, where he received Constitution-acupuncture treatments and Constitutional decoction. His condition improved to some degree, but not to a completely satisfactory level. He would visit my clinic intermittently—when his symptoms worsened—and then stop once he felt better. After a few years of absence, he reappeared at my clinic.

When he returned, I was shocked at his appearance. He had gained a huge amount of weight. Although he had always been a big man, he had never appeared as swollen and overweight as he did at that time. When I inquired about his situation, he explained that his persistent mental illness led him to withdraw from social life and stay home. During this time, he let himself go, allowing his belly to grow like a mountain, which I felt was too excessive.

The reason for his return to my clinic was his severe obesity, which had led to insomnia. He complained that his excessive weight gain was making it impossible to sleep. One might wonder how weight gain affects sleep. In his case, the poor blood circulation caused by the excessive weight made him wake up feeling numb. Additionally, when lying down, the abdominal pressure from his enlarged stomach pushed against the diaphragm, which then exerted pressure on the thoracic cavity. This reduced lung capacity, making breathing difficult and disturbing his sleep, too.

His appearance evoked a memory of Charlie, the protagonist in the critically acclaimed film *The Whale*, which earned the Best Actor Award at the 95th Academy Awards in 2022. Charlie, an extremely obese professor weighing 600 pounds (272 kg), despised his own massive, mountain-like body. Overcome by self-loathing, he isolated himself from the world, conducting online writing classes for his students from a small house while confined to a wheelchair. Brendan Fraser (born in 1968), who portrayed Charlie, underwent extensive special makeup to transform into the character's enormous physique, a transformation that also won the Academy Award for Best Makeup. Although much of it was achieved through special makeup, it was also startling to see Fraser—a once sleek and dashing actor who rose to fame in the 1990s and early 2000s with *The Mummy* series—reappear heavier and almost unrecognizable in real life. That shock mirrored the feeling I experienced upon seeing this patient.

Mental illness not only destroys the mind but also wreaks havoc on the body. The patient seemed to have made considerable efforts to escape his situation. He had participated in Buddhist monk Beomryun's *Jeongtohoe* program (a Buddhistic society of mental discipline), engaged in volunteer work, practiced meditation, and let go of his greed. His visit to Joowonjang

Clinic was, in itself, a testament to his determination and effort. My clinical experience repeatedly shows that conventional advice offers little help to those suffering from mental illness. Common suggestions like, "Don't just stay at home—go see a movie or travel!" may sound reasonable but are meaningless to them. For someone with this kind of mental disorder, even taking one step outside the front door can feel as daunting as climbing Mount Everest. The treatment process was as follows.

Nov 25, 20XX. The patient reported gaining approximately 30 kilograms of weight compared to his original weight. He experienced frequent numbness in his feet while sleeping, likely due to poor blood circulation caused by the heavy weight. The initial Constitution-acupuncture prescription was as follows: R. I VII III' VIII (5555) / L. I VIII (44). Disc Formula was applied to the right and Vitality Formula to the left. I started the treatment with a basic prescription approach.

Nov 26, 20XX. The patient reported reduced tingling in his feet after the previous day's treatment. The same prescription was continued.

Nov 30, 20XX. The condition remained stable. The treatment plan was upgraded to a five-stage Formula, akin to shifting a car from second to third gear: R. VIII X IV' II VI (33333) / L. I V III' VI VIII (33333). Degenerative Arthritis Formula applied to the right, and Edema Formula to the left. This prescription is typically effective for musculoskeletal disorders.

Dec 1, 20XX. The patient reported a significant reduction in the tingling sensation in his feet. The same prescription was maintained.

After his symptoms improved, the patient discontinued getting the treatment and stopped visiting my clinic. However, about five months later, he returned with similar symptoms. Once again, Constitution-acupuncture was applied with the similar prescription, effectively resolving his sleep issues. Following his recovery, he disappeared from my clinic again.

Mogeum Constitution's Clinical Cases

[Mogeum Case 1] Cold Abdomen Makes the Body Sick All Over

* Patient: Ms Z, 25 years old at the time of visit
* Chief complaints: Irritable Bowel Syndrome

The patient had a condition characterized by heightened intestinal sensitivity, namely irritable bowel syndrome (IBS). Additionally, experiencing severe coldness in the abdomen was also difficult to endure. The patient often had back pain, commonly associated with poor intestinal health. Misdiagnosing this as a sort of muscle pain or spinal condition such as disc disease, and treating it with orthopedic interventions would not provide any relief. The patient also reported pain in the lower extremities, describing it as an unpleasant sensation even with light touch.

The patient suffered from reflux esophagitis, which flared up during periods of severe stress or in enclosed spaces, further indicating a highly sensitive personality. Sweating was another prominent symptom, particularly in the hands and armpits, which worsened when the patient felt nervous.

Interestingly, there were no issues with consuming meat or milk, but eating fish, especially raw fish, often caused diarrhea or stomach discomfort. A diet primarily composed of vegetables, fish, and seafoods also seemed to deteriorate the patient's overall health. Drinking coffee triggered hand tremors and a racing heart, highlighting that coffee may not suit everyone with Mogeum Constitution. In medicine, exceptions are so prevalent that absolutes are rare.

The patient reported generally having regular bowel movements but found even a single day without one to be very painful—another hallmark of Mogeum Constitution. If her lower abdomen became cold, diarrhea would immediately occur, which is also a typical symptom of this constitution. Treatment was administered to address the intestinal issues.

April 30, 20XX. The patient reported being diagnosed with this Constitution the previous year and had been doing well while following the Constitutional Diet. However, recently, she developed a digestive disorder. Even drinking water caused intestinal gas and diarrhea, leading to dozens of trips to the bathroom daily, along with common symptoms of enteritis. Additional complaints included nasal bleeding, numbness in the hands and feet, and overall body fatigue. The patient also experienced immediate diarrhea after consuming even small amounts of cold-temperature food. Constitution-acupuncture was initiated with the following prescription: R. VII I (51) / L. VII III (42). The treatment began with 2-stage basic prescriptions.

May 1, 20XX. The patient reported significant improvement since the previous day. Drinking water and eating cold food no longer caused issues. It's a reminder of how forgetful humans can be—despite having severe diarrhea just the day before, the patient now felt better, and without hesitation, began eating foods that previously caused harm. Treatment continued with the same prescription.

May 4, 20XX. The patient's condition initially improved after the acupuncture treatment but worsened the following day, likely due to experiencing significant stress at work. Numbness in the hands and feet persisted. The treatment continued with the same prescription.

May 8, 20XX. Intestinal gas had decreased significantly, but frequent bowel movements remained an issue. Even small snacks caused the patient to pass large stools, leaving him constantly hungry. The same treatment was maintained.

May 11, 20XX. Post-acupuncture, gas and hunger were greatly reduced. Despite being a low-level prescription, its effectiveness surpassed that of high-level ones, demonstrating that higher-level prescriptions are not always the solution. Treatment continued with the same prescription.

May 18, 20XX. Gas generation was nearly gone, and the frequency of bowel movements immediately after eating had decreased. Fatigue was also reduced. While many consider frequent post-meal bowel movements normal for individuals with Mogeum Constitution, I hold a different perspective. When the body is fully normalized, bowel movements should reduce significantly to around once per day. This observation, confirmed through other patients with Mogeum Constitution, supports my belief that frequent bowel movements of Mogeum Constitution are not a physiological trait but rather a pathological symptom. Treatment remained unchanged.

May 25, 20XX. The patient experienced leg cramps after eating cabbage and fish and reported immediate bowel movements after eating. This indicated a return of discomfort. Treatment was continued with the same prescription.

May 29, 20XX. Gas was significantly reduced compared to previous levels. Previously, any food triggered a bathroom trip within 5 minutes, but this was no longer the case. Fatigue also decreased. Treatment continued as before.

June 8, 20XX. The patient reported that chest tightness had improved after Constitution-acupuncture. However, frequent bowel movements persisted, though gas had further reduced. Reflux esophagitis worsened on weekends, which the patient attributed to not consuming yogurt during that time. The same treatment was maintained.

June 12, 20XX. The patient drank whiskey on Friday and felt very unwell afterward, experiencing body aches, mental fog, and an inability to work. Enteritis symptoms worsened significantly, leading to dozens of bowel movements per day, along with excessive gas and diarrhea. In addition to Constitution-acupuncture with the same prescription, Constitutional decoction targeting the stomach and intestines was introduced.

Initially, the patient visited my clinic frequently and received periodic treatments. Once her condition improved, she shifted to visiting only when feeling unwell, relying on Constitution-acupuncture and Constitutional decoction to maintain her health.

While frequent visits may be ideal for treatment, most people face limitations due to work or household responsibilities. The key is to get Constitutional treatment to restore the body to a manageable state. From that point on, individuals can maintain their health independently. In cases of illness or discomfort, revisiting the clinic for Constitutional treatment will help restore balance. As previously stated, health is an eternal process.

[Mogeum Case 2] The World Suddenly Becomes Quiet

* Patient: Ms. S, 54 years old at the time of visit, office worker
* Chief complaints: Sudden hearing loss

The patient was diagnosed with the Mogeum Constitution at Doh-ol Clinic a long time ago and was aware of her Constitution. Following the diagnosis, she adhered to Constitutional Diet, becoming so healthy that she no longer needed to visit this clinic. The patient initially had hepatitis B, but after undergoing Constitutional treatment, she developed antibodies. This demonstrates that Eight-Constitution Medicine has a significant effect on boosting immunity.

The patient reported having bowel movements once or twice a day. This observation challenges the notion that Mogeum Constitution inherently has frequent bowel movements immediately after eating. A healthy and balanced Mogeum Constitution aligns with having bowel movements once or twice a day, similar to the average person.

The patient also noted that stress caused her abdomen to feel cold. This aligns with a typical characteristic of Mogeum Constitution: feeling the abdomen cold when the body is unwell or becoming unwell when the abdomen feels cold. She reported no issues with consuming meat or milk, but felt uncomfortable after eating fish, which is consistent with her Constitutional characteristics.

The patient mentioned experiencing significant discomfort if unable to have a bowel movements for even just one day, a trait commonly observed in those with Mogeum Constitution. Treatment was administered accordingly.

July 24, 20XX. Approximately four days before visit, the patient was diagnosed with sudden hearing loss in the left ear at a local clinic. She reported having worked on computer processing at a pharmacy for about six months, often listening to loud music. It was her first time in such a role, requiring significant mental focus. The patient had already received three steroid injections and was on a prescribed medication. The initial Constitution-acupuncture prescription was as follows: R. VIII IV IV' II X (55555) / L. VII III III' II X (55555). The right-side targeted infectious diseases (e.g., flu), while the left-side addressed autoimmune diseases (e.g., rheumatism). Additionally, Constitutional decoction was prescribed to replenish energy.

July 27, 20XX. The patient reported significant improvement, stating that her ear discomfort had eased. This progress highlighted the effectiveness of Constitutional therapy. Sudden hearing loss is notoriously challenging to treat with Western medicine, often relying solely on steroids or blood circulators. Many patients with severe sudden hearing loss seek Oriental medicine after failing to achieve results in otolaryngology (ENT) clinics or general hospitals, frequently missing the "golden time" for treatment, leading to irreversible auditory nerve damage.

Fortunately, this patient sought treatment early within four days, benefiting from Constitutional therapy. While her hearing improved, she reported severe dark circles under her eyes due to physical strain. The same acupuncture prescription was continued.

July 31, 20XX. The patient continued to report improvement, saying her ears felt fine. However, she mentioned experiencing pain in the right calf after physical exertion. The prescription was adjusted to the following: R. and L. VIII IV IV' II X (55555). Treatment was administered symmetrically on both the left and right sides.

Aug 3, 20XX. The patient reported that her ears felt fine and that they were overall in good condition. Treatment continued with the same prescription.

Aug 7 – Sep 4, 20XX. The patient visited my clinic regularly, approximately every three days, to receive Constitution-acupuncture treatment. Symptoms such as deafness and stuffy feeling in the ear caused by the sudden hearing loss were almost resolved. Although her hearing was slightly diminished compared to pre-onset levels, it did not significantly impact her daily life.

Following this treatment period, the patient continued to maintain her health by visiting my clinic for follow-ups and taking Constitutional decoction to support overall well-being.

The case illustrates the potential of Eight-Constitution Medicine in effectively managing sudden hearing loss, particularly when treatment is initiated early. The combination of Constitution-acupuncture and Constitutional herbal medicine not only addressed the acute symptoms but also supported the patient's general health recovery.

[Mogeum Case 3] Can't Stand Anger 2

* Patient: Mr. Y, 70 years old at the time of visit
* Chief complaints: Chest pain caused by angina pectoris

The patient had a history of myocardial infarction surgery. However, two months ago, he was diagnosed with angina pectoris again at a local general hospital. Despite diligently taking the prescribed medications, his chest pain recurred. As his heart condition worsened, his trust in the hospital collapsed. The hospital recommended another surgery, but the patient stated that he feared the surgery more than death itself. After extensive research, he and his son traveled from Gyeonggido Province to seek treatment at my clinic.

The patient had been taking medications for angina pectoris for seven years prior to this recurrence. He worked as a security guard, a job with irregular and demanding hours, which seemed to have contributed to his declining health. Even before his myocardial infarction surgery, he experienced daily chest pain in the mornings. The hospital dismissed this as psychogenic, attributing it to worry and stress, and only prescribed painkillers. The patient accepted this explanation at the time because his chest pain was usually linked to feelings of anxiety or being in a bad mood. His son supported this view, noting that the patient was highly sensitive to mental and emotional influences.

The patient had a very impatient and fiery personality. He described himself as someone who "exploded like a volcano" when angry, unable to suppress his emotions. He also mentioned suffering from calcific tendonitis in his shoulder, which he suspected was caused by taking Western medicine.

While the timeline of events seemed to align with this theory, the causal relationship could not be confirmed.

He was very susceptible to cold weather. He said that when the temperature drops, his hands get very cold. This means that blood circulation is not good.

His stool wasn't coming out well either. He felt very frustrated when he was constipated. He says that it does not come out well at first and then becomes a little watery in the end. He says that when he goes to bathroom, it's normal for him to move the bowel for 30 minutes.

The Zang-Fu Structure of Mogeum Constitution is "Liver-Gallbladder Heart-Small intestine Pancreas-Stomach Kidneys-Bladder Lungs-Large intestine", and the Large intestine of the Yin Field belongs to the outermost organs. Just opposite to Geumeum Constitution, this Constitution has the shortest large intestine. Therefore, if you, with Mogeum Constitution, are in a situation where stool does not come out properly, you may face quite a serious problem. This is because the capacity to store feces is less than that of other Constitutions. This is why the patient feels very frustrated when he has difficulty passing stool. This is absolutely due to the physical conditions of the large intestine's lack of space.

So, it is very important for Mogeum Constitution to somehow pass the stool. For this reason, people with Mogeum Constitution often have frequent bowel movements. They go to bathroom after breakfast, go to bathroom after lunch, and go to bathroom after dinner. During a baseball game, when the pitcher has trouble controlling the ball with all the bases loaded, the batter and runner are forced to walk, resulting in a situation where the runners on the bases are pushed out to the base ahead. Each runner advances a base for free, so the runner on third base can effortlessly walk in and step on the home base. Frequent bowel movements for people with Mogeum Constitution is like being pushed out.

However, there are often cases where frequent bowel movements are normal for someone with Mogeum Constitution. This is because the stool sack of Mogeum Constitution is physiologically small, not because there is a disease or problem with the digestive tract (at this time, the general stool condition of the one with Mogeum Constitution can be said to be normal or a little watery). Even so, there is a problem with doing it too often. As mentioned earlier, this is because people with normal Mogeum Constitution state do not defecate that too often.

However, the fact that this person has to struggle for 30 minutes to defecate means that he is constipated. It is not a good situation for a person with angina pectoris to have constipation. Unexpected emergencies may occur. If you exert too much force during bowel movements, your blood pressure may rise, putting a strain on your heart.

May 6, 20XX. The first treatment was performed with the following prescription: R. VII I III' (551) / L. VIII IV IV' X II (44424). On the right side, Disc Formula was used to treat shoulder pain, and on the left side, Dysautonomia Formula was applied as a Upper Burner treatment. Due to the patient's tendency to become mentally excited easily, Dysautonomia Formula was administered. This approach was chosen because the main triggers for angina pectoris include mental factors such as tension, anger, and excitement. It was emphasized that the patient must avoid anger.

May 7, 20XX. The patient reported no chest pain and felt at ease. He also mentioned that he had stopped taking cholesterol medication on his own, feeling confident that he could manage it through Constitutional Diet control. The same prescription was used for the treatment.

May 8, 20XX. The patient continued to feel comfortable and reported no pain. The same Constitution-acupuncture prescription was applied, and a Constitutional herbal medication beneficial for angina pectoris and blood circulation was prescribed.

May 9, 20XX. The patient expressed difficulty visiting my clinic daily due to the 4-hour round trip. He mentioned eating bread and drinking a beverage, such as soda, at 4 PM the previous day and experiencing some chest pain after waking up at 5 AM. Meanwhile, his accompanying son noted a visible improvement in his father's appearance, particularly in his eyes, which had previously been yellow and cloudy but were now clearer. The same acupuncture prescription was used.

May 10, 20XX. The patient reported improvements in bowel movements.

Previously, his stool was hard at the beginning, requiring considerable effort to pass, and only softened after significant straining. Now, the stool was consistently soft throughout, and the feeling of a lump in the abdomen had disappeared, which was a proof of normalized intestinal motility. The patient smiled, expressing satisfaction with the improvement. Healthy bowel movements is a critical marker of health together with urine and a sign of successful treatment. I recommended him vitamin A to his question about vitamin. The same acupuncture prescription was continued.

May 11 ~ May 16, 20XX. The patient visited my clinic almost daily, receiving Constitution-acupuncture. He reported no chest pain and easier bowel movements. The same prescription was used.

May 20 ~ June 3, 20XX. Due to the difficulty of daily visits, the patient started visiting my clinic every 2 to 3 days. While he occasionally felt short of breath, his overall condition was good. The prescription remained the same.

June 5, 20XX. The patient caught a cold after being exposed to strong air conditioning in the subway train. Symptoms included a runny nose, cough, hoarseness, and headache. Exposure to air conditioning adversely affected his Constitution, as the Lungs, along with the Large intestine, are among the lowest Zang-Fu potential in his Constitution. The prescription was adjusted as follows: R. VIII IV IV' X II (44444) / L. VII III III' I IX (44444). Dysautonomia Formula was used on the right to support the nervous system, while Zang-system 5-stage Formula was applied to the left to boost immunity.

June 7, 20XX. The patient reported that his cold persisted and that he experienced shortness of breath while walking. The cold pathogen of the air conditioner emerged as an "ambush" that disrupted the progress of treatment progressing well. The same prescription was used.

June 10 ~ June 14, 20XX. The patient reported improvements in his overall condition, with the cold symptoms largely resolved. The same prescription was continued.

The patient successfully managed angina pectoris by visiting my clinic regularly every 2–3 days for treatment. However, chest pain occasionally recurred during stressful situations. One day, he arrived at my clinic with a frowning countenance, a clear sign of chest pain. Upon inquiry, he revealed that the pain began after watching a soccer match a few days ago. The incident occurred during the World Youth Soccer Championship semifinals against Colombia, which ended in a tense penalty shootout. The anxiety and excitement of watching the penalty shootout strained his heart, resulting in chest pain.

"You should watch it calmly and enjoy it. What good does it do to get so nervous?" I joked with him.

"I wasn't going to watch it because I knew this symptom might recur, but I was so curious that I couldn't help myself!" he replied, scratching his head and making excuses.

For a heart disease patient like him, watching an exhilarating national soccer game can genuinely be life-threatening. It's essential for him to manage both his body and mind carefully, avoiding stressors that could overly stimulate the heart. Constitution-acupuncture was administered, and the chest pain subsided right away.

"As long as I stay calm, I feel fine!" the patient remarked. However, stressful events can significantly strain his heart over again.

On one occasion, there was a commotion in the waiting room. When I opened the door, I found him angrily yelling at the nurse. He was upset because the nurse had allowed a patient who arrived after him to enter the treatment room before him. This incident clearly showed how emotional triggers contribute to angina episodes.

"Just let it go! Is this really worth getting so angry over?" I said with a smile, encouraging him to calm down.

This patient struggles to control his anger when things don't go his way. After receiving Constitution-acupuncture, the chest pain was relieved.

He was visiting an ophthalmologist for an eye infection that persisted despite the treatments there. I treated him for his eyes with Constitution-acupuncture. He returned to my clinic a few days later and reported that his eyes had softened and completely healed the day after his last Constitution-acupuncture session. He was amazed that his eye condition, which hadn't improved after nearly two months of treatments at the ophthalmologist, was completely resolved with just one session of Constitution-acupuncture.

This case highlights a key distinction between Western and Oriental medicine. There is a saying: while Western medicine often provides immediate relief by directly treating symptoms, it may not address the root cause of the disease; In contrast, Oriental medicine, though sometimes slower to act, aims to address the underlying cause, providing fundamental healing. However, in this patient's case, Constitution-acupuncture demonstrated both immediate and fundamental effectiveness, offering quick relief while treating the root of the problem.

Suyang Constitution's Clinical Cases

[Suyang Case 1] Living Life Without Energy All Life Long

* Patient: Ms. Y, 50 years old at the time of visit
* Chief complaints: chronic fatigue, edema, menopausal syndrome

The patient had been suffering from chronic fatigue since her teens. Recently, it has worsened to the point where even daily routine of life has become difficult. The Suyang Constitution is structured with "Kidneys-Bladder Lungs-Large intestine Liver-Gallbladder Heart-Small intestine Pancreas-Stomach." Since the outermost Zang-Fu of the Yin Field in this Constitution is the Pancreas-Stomach, a significant imbalance can cause a rapid decline in the Zang-Fu potential of the Pancreas-Stomach, resulting in decreased digestive power and insufficient nutrient absorption. As these issues accumulate, the body becomes severely depleted of Qi. Qi is the body's vital energy. If it diminishes, it leads to constant fatigue and lethargy.

Edema is said to occur easily in such individuals, which is also attributed to decreased Pancreas-Stomach function. A weak Pancreas-Stomach hampers digestion and energy production, causing poor blood circulation and impaired water metabolism, which results in swelling. Although edema is often associated with kidney issues, in Suyang Constitutions, Pancreas-Stomach dysfunction is usually the main cause.

The patient mentioned finding it difficult to mentally focus on things deep, resulting in feeling overwhelmingly frustrated, which a hallmark trait of Suyang Constitution. In classical Oriental medicine, there is a phrase: "Deep thoughts and excessive contemplation may harm the Pancreas (思慮傷脾)." This means excessive or troublesome thoughts can weaken the Pancreas. These thoughts refer to negative or stress-inducing concerns rather than positive ideas. While stress is harmful to all Constitutions, it is particularly detrimental to Suyang Constitution.

In *Donguisusebowon*, Je-ma Lee discusses the theory of disease in relation to the Soeumin (to which the Suyang Constitution belongs) and presents a clinical case of an 11-year-old child with a serious illness called "Mangyang disease (亡陽病)." The illness was caused by "Lao-xin-jiao-si (勞心焦思)," referring to anxiety and stress. This child, Constitutionally prone to a weak stomach, became extremely anxious about chronic diarrhea, which was accumulating severe stress. This led to acute symptoms, including profuse sweating on his face, headaches, fever, cold sweats, and fecal obstruction.[122]

For individuals with Suyang Constitution, it is crucial to avoid stress-inducing emotions such as worry, excessive sadness, and anger. These emotions can severely aggravate their health, due to making mental and emotional balance fail.

The patient who visited my clinic for this case was prone to conditions affecting her five sensory organs. Her tongue was constantly sore, and her eyes were often heavily clogged with mucus. These are common symptoms that arise when immunity is low.

There were many instances when she still felt hungry even right after eating. In those moments, if she consumed beef, her hunger would disappear, and she would feel significantly better. For someone with Suyang Constitution, beef serves as the primary source of energy. This Constitution struggles to digest oil efficiently, so lean meats with minimal fat are preferable. Chicken is also beneficial, but fried chicken is particularly harmful. Instead, boiled or grilled chicken is recommended.

When she felt unwell, eating anything often led to diarrhea. This is similar to the child previously mentioned, who suffered from "Mangyang disease," as featured in Je-ma Lee's *Donguisusebowon*. The child experienced severe diarrhea as well. How could energy be replenished when nutrients were not being absorbed but entirely lost through diarrhea?

There were significant issues with her reproductive organs as well, leading

---

[122] "I once treated an 11-year-old Soeumin child for a disease (a condition causing excessive sweating and significant energy loss), and I was concerned that the child might develop diarrhea. The child was so distressed that sweat poured down his face every time he ate. Then, one day, he suddenly experienced a headache, developed a fever, broke out in a cold sweat, and his stool became impacted, resulting in constipation." Je-ma Lee, *Donguisusebowon* (Seoul: Haenglim Publishing, 1993), p. 34.

to a hysterectomy. At the time of visit, the patient was menopausal, her body was swollen, and she sweated profusely, akin to rain. She said that in such cases, drinking Gorosoe water (water extracted from Korean maple tree) could help reduce swelling. However, excessive sweating in someone with Suyang Constitution is a critical concern. For individuals with normal Suyang Constitution, their pores should be so tightly sealed that not a single drop of sweat would emerge, even when climbing a high mountain under the scorching summer sun. For those with Suyang Constitution, sweating leads to loss of Qi, making it difficult to recover. In fact, this patient, like the child with Mangyang disease, could fall into a critical condition any time.

Additionally, the patient reported constant soreness in the ankles. This could indicate fluid retention in the ankles due to poor blood circulation. In such cases, the ankle joints become swollen and throbbing, causing pain with every step.

The patient experienced numerous side effects from food. She mentioned that eating Korean cabbage kimchi caused diarrhea, as did consuming leafy vegetables or salads. Although Korean cabbage kimchi is a staple food for Koreans, it is not suitable for this Constitutional type. While kimchi is an excellent fermented food, if it does not align with one's Constitution, it becomes ineffective, or worse, because it can cause diarrhea and harm the body. Leafy vegetables are generally detrimental to those with Suyang Constitution.

Years ago, an artist who painted Buddhist artworks visited my clinic. At the time of visit, her health was in a very poor state. During the consultation, it was revealed that she often worked sitting on her knees on the floor and frequently used "Jusa" (a pigment made from cinnabar, or mercury). Having Suyang Constitution, the regular use of Jusa, a very toxic substance for this Constitution, is a major issue. Jusa, made from mercury, is commonly used to depict red color in Buddhist paintings. In Constitutional Medicine, Jusa belongs to Toyang or Toeum Constitution, but it is rarely used due to its toxicity as the poison from Jusa can seep into the body unknowingly (I have never used it before; most illnesses can be adequately treated with other herbal medicines without resorting to such rare and toxic substances).

It was not feasible for her to stop painting, which presented a paradoxical challenge. I recommended that she wear a mask while painting and avoid inhaling harmful substances whenever possible.

Another issue she faced was her diet. Being a Buddhist, she primarily followed a vegetarian diet. The problem lay in leafy vegetables, such as cabbage, kale, and various wild greens. Leafy vegetables are unsuitable for individuals with Suyang Constitution (or Sueum Constitution). I advised her to eat only root vegetables such as radish, bellflower root, lotus root, and burdock. Shortly after following this advice, the patient reported significant improvements in her health by adopting a vegetarian diet focused solely on root vegetables.

Let's return to the patient of this clinical case with Suyang Constitution who visited my clinic. This patient also experienced diarrhea after drinking milk. While beef is beneficial for those with Suyang Constitution, milk is paradoxically categorized as a harmful food. Although it was initially difficult for me to accept due to its discrepancy, it became irrefutable after repeated confirmation in my clinical cases. You can't deny the clinically proven fact. Constitutional Dietary recommendations must be understood through the lens of statistical analysis rather than that of abstract principles.

The patient also mentioned that taking herbal medicines with a strong foul smell or high concentration made her feel unwell. This can be described as a typical symptom of having a "weak Pancreas-Stomach," as commonly expressed. Among high concentrated herbal medicines, a representative example is "Shudihuang" (熟地黃, Prepared Rehmannia Root), which, according to Je-ma Lee, is a herbal medicine for Soyangin (Toyang Constitution or Toeum Constitution). In other words, it is a medicinal herb for those with opposite Constitutions to Suyang Constitution.

For Suyang Constitution, the representative herb is ginseng, a symbol of Qi replenisher. No matter how much ginseng is added or how long it is boiled, the resulting decoction remains clear and transparent. Herbal medicines for Suyang Constitution or Sueum Constitution are primarily designed to restore Qi, so they tend to be light and clear rather than thick and dense. This patient's aversion to herbal medicine can be understood as a dislike for medicines that do not align with her Constitution. If the herbal medicine had suited her Constitution, such adverse reactions would have rarely occurred.

This sensitivity extended beyond herbal medicines to health supplements as well. The patient mentioned being highly averse to unpleasant smells, which scared her off from trying certain substances.

The patient also experienced many side effects from nutrient injections. She mentioned trying these injections to combat fatigue but never completing a course because the pain and discomfort outweighed the benefits. She must have been told multiple times that she seemed excessively nervous.

Additionally, the patient could not eat glucose candies, as they caused headaches. While glucose candies are beneficial for individuals with Geumyang or Geumeum Constitution, they proved unsuitable for this Constitution. Is there anything this patient can eat, then? Yes, there is. Although not much.

Despite the challenges, there are certain foods that align with this patient's Constitution. For example, she found relief from the summer heat by consuming lacquered chicken. Lacquer is a thermogenic medicine that improves blood circulation and relieves stagnant blood, while chicken is an excellent protein source for individuals with Suyang Constitution. Chicken, in particular, is known to replenish Pancreas-Stomach Qi, making lacquered chicken a perfect health food for individuals with Suyang Constitution whose Qi has been depleted by extreme summer heat.

The patient also reported significant benefits from taking wild "Jangnoe ginseng" (a type of ginseng artificially grown in mountain). As previously mentioned, ginseng is highly suitable for the individuals with Suyang Constitution. Jangnoe ginseng, in particular, can be roughly compared to wild ginseng and is considered a powerful energy-boosting herb.

Interestingly, the patient mentioned feeling less fatigued after being treated with bee acupuncture. Bee acupuncture, along with honey or pollen, is known to be a beneficial treatment for individuals with Suyang Constitution (and Sueum Constitution).

The patient noted that she felt an improvement in her condition after receiving placenta injections. Placenta, known as Zi-he-che (紫河車) in traditional medicine, pharmacologically replenishes both Qi and Xue (blood) at the same time. This treatment was likely effective because the patient was suffering from severe Qi-Xue depletion at the time. The fact that this highly sensitive patient benefited from Zi-he-che suggests that it is a suitable herbal medicine for individuals with Suyang Constitution. Zi-he-che is commonly applied to conditions such as tidal fever, night sweats, tachycardia, and forgetfulness caused by Qi and blood deficiencies.

For patients as sensitive as this one, determining the Constitutional suitability of foods, medicines, health foods, and supplements is crucial. Most people do not experience immediate side effects from consuming substances that are not suitable for their constitutions, thanks to the human body's adaptive mechanisms. However, prolonged consumption of harmful substances can eventually overwhelm the body, leading to severe illness. For sensitive individuals like this patient, their immediate reactions to foods and supplements provide valuable insights into their Constitutional compatibility. Due to her heightened sensitivity, this patient is considered highly valuable in the study of Constitutional Medicine. Treatment began with careful attention to her Constitution.

Aug 24, 20XX. The first treatment began with my proprietary prescription: R. IX V (51) / L. IX III (42).

Sep 4, 20XX. The patient returned to my clinic after 11 days and reported that her facial complexion had improved. Although she had previously struggled even with 500g weight loss, she experienced no issues after losing approximately 1kg following her Constitutional Diet. The patient mentioned that this improvement allowed her to visit Joowonjang Clinic on her own, something she had previously considered unimaginable due to her lack of vitality. Listening to the patient, I found it difficult to imagine the hardships the patient had endured. This was undoubtedly a positive sign of recovery, which uplifted my feelings. A doctor's emotions often tend to synchronize with those of the patient. Treatment continued with the same prescription.

Because this patient lived in a district area, regular visits to Joowonjang Clinic for ongoing treatment were not feasible. It seems she is managing her condition cautiously, much like walking on thin ice, by adhering to the Constitutional regimens that have worked for her so far.

In any case, with the guiding compass of health provided by the Suyang Constitution, I hope the patient reaps the rewards by overcoming the hardships of life through the faithful practice of appropriate health methods.

[Suyang Case 2] Depression

* Patient: Ms J, 35 years old at the time of visit
* Chief complaints: depression, chronic fatigue, allergic skin, reflux esophagitis

The patient was quite obese for someone with a Suyang Constitution, especially compared to others with the same Constitution. At the time of visit, she was 162 cm tall, weighed 80 kg, and had a BMI of 30.5. Outwardly, she had a voluptuous physique that appeared robust and healthy, which contrasted with the general tendency of individuals with a Suyang Constitution to have an average, slim, or even very thin body type. Nevertheless, she exhibited many characteristic traits of Suyang Constitution.

She was extremely sensitive to cold and had to sleep under a thick blanket even during the summer to avoid catching a cold in the morning. She reported that eating red bean Kalguksu (Korean wheat noodle soup with red beans) caused stomach rumbling, cucumbers made her vomit foam, and frozen blueberries made her stomach stopped. These are typical digestive issues experienced by individuals with Suyang Constitution (or Sueum Constitution) when consuming cold-natured or cold-temperature foods.

Most herbal medicines also caused her digestive problems. When she received a glucose injection, her body swelled, and it had to be stopped midway. This repeatedly confirmed that glucose is unsuitable for those with Suyang Constitution.

She mentioned that she required less energy for physical activities after eating meat; however, this specifically applied to beef or chicken, excluding pork.

Finely ground potatoes or corn were good to her, which are also recommended as good foods for this Constitution.

She noted that consuming deer antler significantly lifted her mood and gave her energy. Deer antler is considered an excellent tonic for individuals with Suyang Constitution.

As a child, she felt extremely unwell and lacked energy when her diet consisted mainly of vegetables or seafood. She explained that avoiding vegetables these days helped her avoid diarrhea. However, eating fried chicken, beer, and squid together made her feel ill and caused headaches. While chicken is generally a good food for her Constitution, fried chicken is not. Instead, grilled or boiled chicken is better.

She also mentioned getting a stye when eating chicken, but it was likely due to consuming fried chicken rather than other preparations.

The patient suffered from severe depression and was taking psychiatric medication, including drugs that regulate serotonin and dopamine. Without dopamine-regulating medication, she felt completely drained of energy.

Chronic fatigue was a persistent symptom that never left her. She constantly felt weak and lethargic due to a lack of energy.

She also had chronic reflux esophagitis, which often caused nausea or a sensation of a foreign body in her throat.

Frequent coughing was another issue, and when she became tired, her throat would often swell, and she frequently developed a low-grade fever.

Allergies often resulted in acne in affected areas, leading to recurring skin problems.

She originally had low blood pressure, which made her body feel lethargic and caused significant difficulty in carrying out her daily routine. However, since starting psychiatric medication about two months ago, her blood pressure had risen, and her energy levels had improved.

To address these symptoms comprehensively, I began Constitution-acupuncture treatment.

Dec 11, 20XX. The initial treatment began with the following basic prescription: R. IX V (51) / L. IX III (42).

Dec 14, 20XX. The patient reported feeling fine after Constitution-acupuncture treatment and noted some weight loss. Rather than actual weight loss, it seemed that swelling in the body had subsided. The patient experienced frequent burping, which is often a sign of improved stomach activity and digestion. If burping occurs when there was none before, it typically indicates improved digestive function. However, excessive burping beyond the usual frequency could indicate worsening digestion.

The patient also mentioned eye pain after drinking a cold beverage. For individuals with Suyang Constitution, substances in cold temperature are like poison and must be avoided. I advised careful adherence to Constitutional Diet. Acne had decreased significantly after my treatment, indicating the elimination of toxins from the body. As a first treatment, the results were encouraging. Treatment continued with the same prescription.

Dec 16, 20XX. The patient felt sick after consuming something cold, suggesting a lack of understanding or adherence to the Constitutional Diet, or possibly an inability to commit to it fully. She vomited due to stomach acid reflux but noted that the vomit did not taste sour, which suggests insufficient gastric acid production. Normally, vomit would have a sour taste if gastric acid levels were normal.

The patient explained that she frequently vomited foam without a sour taste after eating cucumbers, cold foods, or taking digestive medicine. This is another indicator of low stomach acid. She had eaten Nuroongji (scorched rice soup) the previous day, which caused stomach pain and repeated vomiting until early in the morning. Vomiting seemed to have become a daily occurrence for the patient. The prescription was adjusted as follows: R. IX V (55) / L. IX III III' (444).

Dec 18, 20XX. The patient reported that her feet became warm immediately after the last acupuncture session, indicating improved blood circulation. This is a testament to the effectiveness of Constitution-acupuncture. Additionally, the patient noted that her stomach acid production had increased, a positive development for someone with insufficient gastric acid.

Although she now experienced reflux and stomach pain in the mornings, digestion had improved overall, with stomach growling after eating beneficial foods to her Constitution. Previously, her stomach had been inactive and lethargic. The patient also reported improved saliva production, which plays a crucial role in digestion, as saliva itself acts as a digestive agent.

The patient mentioned being allergic to cold air, which used to cause facial breakouts. However, she reported no such reactions now. Her mother also had a cold wind allergy, which might indicate the same Suyang Constitution for her mother. The treatment continued with the same prescription.

Dec 21, 20XX. The patient reported that her feet and body had become warm, which gave her more energy. She mentioned walking for over an hour on Saturday without much difficulty. Her skin had also improved, but her stool became slightly watery. On Friday night, she ate four pieces of fried chicken wings and felt unwell afterward. However, she felt better after consuming a supplement containing dandelion and silymarin. The treatment prescription remained unchanged.

Dec 23, 20XX. The warmth in her feet persisted. The patient mentioned eating red pepper on Monday without experiencing any swelling on Tuesday. This observation reinforced the idea that improving Pancreas-Stomach activity can alleviate edema in individuals with Suyang Constitution. The same prescription was used for treatment.

Dec 26, 20XX. The patient once again reported warm feet and expressed how much better this made her feel each time she visited my clinic. This improvement highlighted how cold and painful her feet had been before. She also noted further improvement in her skin, which repeatedly indicated her becoming healthier overall.

The patient mentioned experiencing a sour taste in her mouth, which was a new sensation for her. However, reflux esophagitis symptoms persisted. She also reported losing a total of 3 kg of body weight since starting Constitution-acupuncture, with swelling decreasing day by day. Additionally, her cold wind allergy disappeared. In the past, moving from a cold place to a warm one would cause skin allergies, but this was no longer an issue.

Dec 28, 20XX. The patient reported getting a headache after eating unsuitable food, which improved after drinking red ginseng tea. She also noted that her face, which used to turn red during exercise, now flushed less and recovered quickly. The cold wind allergy had completely disappeared. The patient mentioned that she was now able to lose weight through exercise, which was previously impossible. This improvement indicated better blood circulation. The treatment prescription remained unchanged.

Dec 30, 20XX. The patient mentioned an increase in appetite. For individuals with Suyang Constitution, developing an appetite signifies the improved Pancreas-Stomach activity, which is a crucial sign of health for Suyang Constitution. The same treatment regimen was continued.

Jan 5, 20XX. The new year began, and this was the patient's first visit of the year. Her appetite remained steady, and reflux esophagitis had improved. However, she sprained her right leg a few days earlier, experienced frequent diarrhea, and needed to use the bathroom often. The prescription was adjusted as follows: R. IX V III' (555) / L. X IV IV' VIII VI (44444). Disc Formula was applied to the right side, and Dysautonomia Formula to the left. Additionally, Constitutional decoction to improve digestion, promote blood circulation, and stabilize the mind and body was prescribed.

Jan 6, 20XX. The patient reported that the symptom of her body trembling when tired had disappeared. While her ankle still hurt, it was functioning better. She ate steamed chicken the previous day, but it was too salty, which caused discomfort. Salty foods are not suitable for individuals with Suyang Constitution, as they overstimulate the Kidneys and Bladder Qi. She also ate strawberries, which caused stomach pain. Strawberries are harmful to Suyang Constitution. Treatment continued with the same prescription.

Jan 8, 20XX. The patient felt better after taking Constitutional decoction. Her appetite increased, and swelling reduced. For the first time, she turned off the electric mat while sleeping, as she felt too warm. This was a remarkable improvement, considering she used to sleep under a thick blanket even during summer. It indicated a significant improvement from her Yang Qi deficiency. After Constitution-acupuncture, itching in the ankles also decreased. While her blood pressure dropped slightly, she experienced mild headaches. The same treatment was continued.

Jan 11, 20XX. The patient experienced constipation, but it improved after drinking plenty of water. Typically, people with Suyang Constitution have cold Pancreas-Stomach and tend to avoid drinking water, but the patient's Pancreas-Stomach activity improved enough to handle larger amounts of water. She reported eating well three times a day but struggled with excessive sleepiness in the mornings. I advised her to be cautious about overeating, despite her good appetite. The patient walked a lot the previous day without pain, but her legs were sore next day, which was normal. Menstrual pain had also decreased.

Significantly, the patient mentioned she was not taking psychiatric medication and that her condition wasn't too bad. Despite the challenge, she was enduring well. Treatment continued unchanged.

Jan 13, 20XX. The nurse working for the psychiatrist hospital advised the patient that stopping psychiatric medication could worsen her condition after three months, so the patient decided to resume taking the medication and was instructed to continue it for a year. I expressed disappointment, as it had been a golden opportunity to break free from the psychiatric drugs. The patient reported feeling anxiety after taking Western medicine the previous day but found some relief with Constitutional decoction. After discussing her anxiety caused by psychiatric medication with her psychiatrist, the medication was changed.

I questioned on her medication, designed to treat anxiety but cause it instead. Concerns were raised about whether the patient would truly be able to stop after a year and how to overcome the inertia of continued use. Despite doubts, the patient had decided, and there was no choice but to respect her decision. The acupuncture prescription remained unchanged.

Jan 15, 20XX. The patient experienced stomach discomfort after eating raw vegetables. Many vegetables are unsuitable for Suyang Constitution, and consuming them raw exacerbates the issue. She was advised to cook and eat root vegetables instead. The same prescription was used for treatment.

Jan 20, 20XX. The patient strayed from her Constitutional Diet while traveling on Monday and experienced headaches the following day. She continued to feel stomach discomfort and nausea caused by foul smells. Consuming flour-based foods, coffee, and other unsuitable items worsened her condition. Constitution-acupuncture was administered with the same prescription, and additional Constitutional decoction was prescribed.

Jan 22, 20XX. The patient reported feeling better after receiving

Constitution-acupuncture treatment, but poor eating habits quickly made her feel unwell again. She expressed a strong aversion to smells like perfume, smoke, alcohol, and fried food, which made her nauseous. The heightened sensitivity to smells, characteristic of Suyang Constitution, seemed particularly severe.

Because the patient lived far away in another province, it became increasingly difficult for her to visit Joowonjang Clinic. She responded well to Constitutional treatment, about which I felt sorry that she could not keep getting my treatment. I hope that the patient continue to follow her Constitutional regimen diligently and regain her health.

[Suyang Case 3] Living with Stomach Stasis

* Patient: Ms G, 31 years old at the time of visit
* Chief complaints: chest pain and nausea due to stomach stasis, migraine

The patient mentioned that she consistently experiences stomach stasis throughout the year. Once she experienced it, each episode seemed to last nearly a month. According to her, the issue is said to have occurred five or six times a month. So, how does that calculation work? Does a year have over 60 months for her? Or is she implying that the issue overlaps repeatedly? It almost feels like there should be a condition called "overlapping stomach stasis syndrome." Either way, she seems to live a life where stomach stasis is part of her daily routine.

In my case, I don't recall ever experiencing a genuine stomach stasis, though occasionally, I feel a sense of heaviness or tightness in my chest after eating foods like boiled sweet potatoes. The patient mentioned she was always carrying a needle and thread in her bag to prick her finger whenever she felt unwell in her stomach.

The patient also reported experiencing chest pain, dizziness, and a migraine on the right side of her head whenever her stomach stasis occurred. In fact, these symptoms often occur together for most people, especially headaches. However, people tend to recognize illnesses as isolated problems rather than understanding them comprehensively. For example, they might think of indigestion and headaches as entirely separate issues. This fragmented perspective is a common mistake, not just among the general public but also among the medical doctors. As a result, patients might visit both a gastroenterologist and a neuropsychiatrist, receiving separate prescriptions for each issue. In reality, there's no need to visit a neuropsychiatrist. The problem arises when the headache worsens and the patient neglects her digestive issues, focusing solely on treating the headache. Taking headache medication alone does not lead to recovery. While painkillers may provide temporary relief from the headache, the pain inevitably returns as the underlying issue remains unresolved. This creates a cycle where patients rely on headache medicine repeatedly, leading to chronic headaches.

The patient also shared that a gynecological exam revealed vaginitis. She was prescribed antibiotics to treat it but ended up with diarrhea. Switching to another medication led to constipation instead. Cases like this highlight how much Western medicine misunderstands the human body. Western medicine often treats symptoms in isolation, leading to a "balloon effect"—pressing one symptom down causes another to pop up elsewhere.

Constitutional Medicine, on the other hand, avoids this "partial medicine" approach and strives for "Wholistic Medicine." It focuses not on curing the disease itself but on correcting the body as a whole.

However, this does not mean that Constitutional Medicine neglects specific symptoms. Every detail is also addressed (as demonstrated in the Compound Formulae introduced earlier). Both the part and the whole must always be considered together to gain "a whole view" of the patient.

Dec 30, 20XX. The first treatment began with my preferred prescription: R. IX V (51) / L. IX III (42).

Dec 31, 20XX. The patient visited my clinic the following day, literally on the last day of the year. She reported having an excellent bowel movements after receiving acupuncture the previous day. People with Suyang Constitution often experience diarrhea when unwell, but are also prone to frequent constipation. Observing the effectiveness of the treatment not only confirms its success but also validates the accuracy of the Constitutional diagnosis. This confirmation allows for greater confidence in treating the patient.

However, the patient mentioned feeling unwell after eating steak and spaghetti the previous day. While steak is beneficial for the Suyang Constitution, spaghetti is not. When consuming both beneficial and harmful foods together, people often rationalize the situation by asking themselves, "Doesn't it balance out?" This reflects a tendency to justify actions, attempting to escape the difficult situation. Humans seem naturally inclined to rationalize their behaviors—perhaps as a survival mechanism to navigate challenges without constant regret.

People are driven by momentary desires, make mistakes, and then seek excuses to justify them. Perhaps, since it was the end of the year, the patient thought, "I've worked hard enough this year; I deserve a reward today!" or "Now that I have Eight-Constitution acupuncture to maintain my health, I can eat whatever I want!" However, the body remains unaffected by such reasoning and adheres strictly to biological principles.

The same prescription was used to treat indigestion, confirming its effectiveness. The ability to alleviate her constipation really is an excellent outcome. In clinical practice, treating constipation is often more challenging than one might expect.

Mar 5, 20XX. Approximately two months into the new year, the patient returned to my clinic. She had visited a gynecologist due to heavy periods and were diagnosed with near symptom of uterine fibroids. This explained the new onset of menstrual cramps, which she hadn't experienced before. Additionally, she was taking medication for vaginitis.

The patient also complained about her needle-like tongue condition of glossitis constantly on and off for no apparent reason. However, such things don't happen without a cause—it was evident she hadn't been following the Constitutional Diet. It's as if the situation is so obvious that no further inquiry is needed. The patient also mentioned discomfort with her stool, a clear indication of dietary misconduct.

Constitutional Medicine provides clear guidelines for treatment. For this patient, addressing digestive system issues was the priority. Without doing so, she would likely need to visit multiple specialists, including oral medicine, gastroenterology, and obstetrics and gynecology. The treatment continued with the same prescription as before.

Mar 6, 20XX. The patient reported that her stomach felt better, and she was in a good mood. As I always say, having good bowel movements is extremely important. When toxins are removed from the body, one feels more comfortable, physically and mentally, and immunity normalizes. The same prescription was continued.

Mar 7, 20XX. The patient reported having good bowel movements again that day. While it's commonly believed that constipation is normal for individuals with Suyang Constitution, this patient demonstrates that this is not necessarily the case. If someone with Suyang Constitution improves one's health, the one will have regular bowel movements every day. The same prescription was continued.

Mar 8, 20XX. The patient reported swollen and painful tonsils. Additionally, she mentioned some slight genital irritation due to vaginitis. However, she also reported having another good bowel movements that day. She was particularly pleased, noting that no residue was left on the toilet paper. Perfect bowel movements mean there's no need for toilet paper—a phenomenon commonly observed in healthy animals like dogs and cats. Have you ever seen a dog or a cat using toilet paper? If they needed it, it would mean they were not healthy. The prescription was adjusted as follows: R. IX V (51) / L. X IV IV' VI VIII (55555). The prescription for cold was applied to the left.

Mar 10, 20XX. The patient reported another bowel movements that day, even though the amount was small. She expressed amazement, saying she had never experienced this consistency before and felt so much better. There is no happiness quite like the daily joy of successful elimination. Additionally, the patient noted that her tonsil swelling had disappeared. The fact that bowel movements are mentioned before the tonsil issue underscores the crucial role of digestion in her overall health. The same prescription was continued.

Mar 11, 20XX. The patient mentioned eating three meals a day. While this may seem unremarkable, for her, it's something she hadn't experienced before. Individuals with Suyang Constitution often lack an appetite, so this indicates her Pancreas-Stomach is functioning well. The same prescription was continued.

Mar 12, 20XX. Excited about her improving condition, the patient is visiting my clinic daily. She reported feeling consistently hungry and said she had rediscovered the joy of eating. Remarkably, this is the first time in her life that she's had regular bowel movements for an entire week. A revolutionary change seems to be occurring in her body. The same prescription was continued.

Mar 13, 20XX. The patient reported having her period without even realizing it. Previously, she experienced extreme irritability and depression in the days leading up to her period, to the extent that her premenstrual symptoms became unbearable. She recounted having major arguments with her family during her period and, at her worst, wandering the streets in silent anger and frustration for no apparent reason. Severe premenstrual syndrome made her life indescribably unbearable.

Although her period came a week earlier than usual this time, she noted that it was on schedule considering it had been a week late the previous month. This indicates that her cycle is stabilizing and returning to its original rhythm. Constitutional treatment seems to have a restorative effect. Treatment was continued with the same regimen.

Mar 14, 20XX. The patient reported feeling fine. She mentioned that she could now sit on the toilet in the morning and strain slightly for easy bowel movements. There's nothing off-limits in the patient-doctor relationship—it almost feels like being a priest hearing confessions. Treatment continued with the same prescription.

Mar 15, 20XX. The patient noted that this was the first time in her life she'd had regular bowel movements for ten consecutive days. She continues to set personal records. The same treatment was administered.

Mar 17, 20XX. The patient reported that menstruation had stopped producing blood and was only discharging a dark brown color for three days, which made her feel irritable. She also mentioned a sore throat due to a cold. Overeating during the weekend caused difficulty passing stool. The body always has a cause-and-effect relationship. The prescription was adjusted as follows: R. IX VIII (42) / L. X IV IV' VIII VI (55555). The left side was changed to Dysautonomia Formula, while the right side used a prescription tailored for intestinal condition.

Mar 18, 20XX. The patient attributed her depression the previous day to menstrual syndrome. She mentioned that it would usually last a day or two, leaving her so overwhelmed that she would cry alone. This experience, while common for women, is difficult for men to understand. How could a male like me understand the estrogen's magic spell, the representative feminine hormone? As Lao Tzu said, "Strong winds do not last all morning, nor do torrential rains fall all day." This too shall pass. The same prescription was continued.

Mar 19, 20XX. The patient said her body felt better. The prescription remained the same, with a 4:4 ratio for the right Formula.

Mar 20, 20XX. The patient mentioned experiencing a stomach stop again. The prescription was adjusted as follows: R. IX III (44) / L. X IV IV' VIII (4444). The right side addressed Fu-system Inflammation, and the left side focused on Mucosal Ulcer Formula.

Mar 21, 20XX. The patient reported the tightness in her chest due to the stomach stop. The prescription was adjusted as follows: R. IX III (44) / L. IX V III' (551). The left Formula was used to manage pain.

Mar 22, 20XX. The patient attended a wedding ceremony the previous day and overeating led to diarrhea in the morning. However, she reported feeling relieved afterward. Treatment continued with the same prescription.

Mar 24, 20XX. The patient experienced diarrhea four or five times from the morning until the afternoon. There have been many cases of diarrhea during her period, and her menstruation really started yesterday. In January, there were a lot of lumps in the menstrual blood, but in February, there were fewer. This month, uterine discharge started two days ago, followed by menstruation. The prescription was adjusted as follows: R. IX III (44) / L. X IV IV' VIII (4444). The right Formula focused on Fu-system Inflammation, while the left addressed Mucosal Ulcer.

Mar 25, 20XX. The patient reported difficulty digesting. Although there was less bubbling in her stomach, the sensation of needing to burp but being unable to was frustrating. She expressed relief at not catching a cold during this seasonal change, a benefit attributed to Constitutional treatment strengthening her immunity. Additionally, she noted that consuming honey was beneficial; drinking hot honey tea calmed her stomach quickly. While tea caused frequent urination, honey tea did not. The prescription was adjusted as follows: R. IX V (51) / L. X IV IV' VIII (4444). The right side focused on Liver support with Zang-system Inflammation Formula, while the left continued addressing Mucosal Ulcer.

Mar 27, 20XX. The patient noted her digestion was fine due to eating lightly the previous day. For those with Suyang Constitution, restraint on meal is key—no matter how strong the appetite, overeating will eventually cause illness to this Constitution. The same prescription was continued.

Mar 28, 20XX. The patient experienced diarrhea after drinking cappuccino, attributing it to the milk. Any milk product, she said, consistently caused diarrhea. The same prescription was continued.

Mar 29, 20XX. The patient fell asleep on the bus home after receiving Constitution-acupuncture and missed her stop. Acupuncture relaxes her body and often induces drowsiness. She noted significantly less acne this month compared to before when she would typically get one or two large pimples during her period. Unlike hormonal acne during puberty, adult acne is often a skin reaction to toxins. This improvement suggests that Constitutional treatment effectively eliminated toxins. The prescription was slightly adjusted as follows: R. IX V (51) / L. X IV IV' VIII VI (44444). The left side was raised to Dysautonomia Formula.

Mar 31, 20XX. The patient ate beef shabu-shabu but reported poor bowel movements afterward. Her bowel issues had persisted since her last irregular movement. The prescription was adjusted as follows: R. Fu-system Inflammation Formula (4:2) / L. Dysautonomia Formula.

April 1, 20XX. The patient reported feeling better, with improved bowel movements. She also mentioned having a cold, with an itchy throat and phlegm. Despite sleeping less, her sleep quality had improved. The right Formula remained the same, while the left was adjusted to treat the cold: R. IX III (42) / L. X IV IV' VI VIII (44444).

The patient continued visiting my clinic and consistently received Constitution-acupuncture treatments, managing her health and addressing occasional symptoms. When she ate unsuitable foods, digestive problems and skin issues inevitably arose. However, Constitutional treatment helped regulate these problems and restore her body to normal.

The patient once mentioned experiencing severe skin issues with cosmetics, particularly those containing BHA or AHA ingredients, which caused skin troubles. She noted that avoiding products with those ingredients prevented further problems. Additionally, she mentioned feeling embarrassed when dead skin cells appeared on her body after showering with warm water. This indicates that, for those with Suyang Constitution, bathing in overly hot water is not beneficial. And excessively cold water may also be unsuitable. Using moderately cool or lukewarm water is recommended.

Previously, it was mentioned that honey tea was good for stomach upsets, and the patient also noted that red pepper and black pepper were effective for indigestion. This suggests that spices with a pungent flavor can aid digestion.

The patient frequently emphasized that her skin condition improved after Constitutional treatments. Skin health is a crucial indicator of overall well-being, as individuals with good skin rarely suffer from illness. Improved skin condition is clear evidence of significant health improvements.

The patient recounted a severe reaction after eating flatfish sashimi. The fish tasted unpleasantly fishy, made her feel nauseous, and caused intense diarrhea. She felt better after consuming tomato paste with red and black pepper. While many people use peppers to mask greasy smells, this patient found them to be an effective remedy for digestive disorders.

One instance involved an upset stomach after eating two slices of watermelon, leading to about 12 trips to the bathroom early in the morning. Despite excessive urination, the patient did not feel thirsty, which she found quite mysterious. However, she did report that watermelon made her abdomen feel very cold—something she had never experienced before. She once experienced severe stomach pain after eating a melon, describing the sensation as if her stomach was being scratched by fingernails. She said she experienced a similar feeling after eating this watermelon.

The patient also visited my clinic with a burn on her philtrum caused by a skin ointment prescribed by a doctor. This was identified as a kind of chemical burn. She was prescribed medications at two hospitals but couldn't use any due to severe side effects. The patient expressed frustration, noting that doctors often lacked knowledge about the medications they prescribed and failed to provide satisfactory answers.

The patient discovered valuable information on a pharmacist's blog about the effects of medications and expressed concern that relying solely on luck when visiting doctors could be life-threatening. According to the blog, antibiotic overuse is rampant for conditions that don't require strong prescriptions. The patient described experiencing severe side effects after taking a new medication prescribed by her doctors, likening the experience to "tasting hell." These reactions highlight the significant side effects Western medications can have on individuals with Suyang Constitution.

Sueum Constitution's Clinical Cases

[Sueum Case 1] All Diseases Lead to the Stomach

* Patient: Ms Y, 30 years old at the time of visit
* Chief complaints: indigestion, dizziness, vomiting, chronic fatigue, allergic rhinitis

The patient continued to feel unwell after eating raw fish at a sushi restaurant. Symptoms include dizziness and vomiting. It had been about a week since the initial discomfort began, but the condition had not improved. The skin on her face had become rough, and acne had appeared persistently on her chin. Due to indigestion, food did not seem to process properly and caused pain as it moved down the pit of the stomach. Breathing exacerbated back pain, and the shoulders felt tight and sore. The patient found it more comfortable to have an empty stomach.

She use to experience dizziness and occasional stomachaches with indigestion, but this time the symptoms were particularly severe. Interestingly, the symptom of vomiting and dizziness would ease after bowel movements.

The patient also reported feeling extremely tired, lacking energy, and experiencing a noticeable loss of vitality. Additionally, she had allergic rhinitis, which developed after eating the raw fish, and allergic conjunctivitis, which had persisted for 3 to 4 days. All these discomforts stemmed from eating the raw fish. Observing the etiologies of various patients revealed patterns that were as complex and varied as a kaleidoscope.

The patient also suffered from severe menstrual irregularities, with a highly inconsistent cycle. Menstrual pain was intense, and she was particularly concerned about this issue due to a family history—specifically, her mother had uterine cancer.

Overeating tended to make her feel unwell easily. She rarely drank water or soup and generally avoided fluids, nor did she consume salty foods. These eating habits reflected the typical characteristics of the Sueum Constitution. Treatment commenced accordingly.

Jan 9, 20XX. Two Formulae were applied simultaneously to treat stomach ulcers: R. V I III' (442) / L. VI II IV' VIII (4444). The right side targeted the ulcer, while the left side focused on the mucosal ulcer.

Jan 31, 20XX. The patient visited my clinic after almost three weeks. After receiving Constitution-acupuncture during her last visit, her digestion improved significantly, confirming the powerful effect of this treatment. However, the patient reported persistent allergic rhinitis, causing severe sneezing. The treatment was adjusted as follows: R. V I (ana 42) / L. II VI IV' I IX (44424). The Fu-system Inflammation Formula for Upper Burner was treated on the right, while allergy Formula for Upper Burner was treated on the left.

July 23, 20XX. Six months after the previous visit, the patient returned. She reported feeling sick for a week and unable to eat anything, a recurring condition that didn't resolve without treatment. Interestingly, even when the symptoms feel unbearable, Constitution-acupuncture quickly alleviates them. For such patients, Eight-Constitution Medicine can be a lifesaver. Treatment included as follows: R. VI II IV' VIII (4444) / L. V I III' (442). The right side targeted the mucosal ulcer, and the left side focused on the ulcer.

July 24, 20XX. The patient reported feeling slightly better the previous night. After eating apple yogurt for breakfast, her body temperature dropped, and she passed a bit of watery stool, which provided some feeling of emptiness. She said that these days, drinking more than one cup of coffee in the morning caused trouble sleeping in the evening. In addition, she experienced difficulty breathing, and discomfort in her back akin to being pricked by a needle. This indicates that the stomach had not fully recovered. Treatment continued with the same prescription, and Constitutional decoction to support digestion was prescribed.

July 25, 20XX. After lunch, the patient felt better, and her heart palpitations subsided. However, she still experienced tightness in her chest and difficulty breathing, a common symptom when stomach issues suppress the lungs. She mentioned that after eating "dakgalbi" (roasted chicken rib with cabbages) yesterday, she felt like it might be difficult to digest, so she took her Constitutional decoction, which helped her digest it well and sleep soundly. The same treatment was administered.

July 26, 20XX. The patient reported further improvement. She had eaten fried chicken donburi (roasted chicken with cabbages and soy sauce on rice) and blueberry latte (milk with crushed blueberry) the previous night, felt sleepy afterward, and worried about digestion. Surprisingly, digestion was fine, but she felt tired the next morning. Treatment continued as before.

Aug 1, 20XX. The patient ate buckwheat noodles, two fried dumplings, and brown rice during the day, but couldn't digest them well. Feeling better often leads people to indulge in foods unsuitable for their Constitution. The same treatment was given.

Aug 6, 20XX. The patient found digestion challenging after overeating, which is strictly prohibited for Sueum Constitution. She also reported blisters on her hands and feet that were itchy and eventually burst. The same treatment was continued.

Sep 23, 20XX. After over a month, the patient returned, reporting illness since eating red bean bread and pumpkin bread two weeks ago, followed by fried chicken a week ago. Allergic rhinitis also flared up, accompanied by one or two pompholyx on her hands. She felt heat in her hands and feet, particularly struggling during summer, and complained of the intense air conditioning in her office. Most of her issues originated and ended with stomach stasis. The same acupuncture treatment and Constitutional decoction were provided.

Sep 24, 20XX. The patient reported feeling fine internally and having regular bowel movements. Treatment continued as before.

Sep 28, 20XX. Digestion improved, but rhinitis persisted, with frequent sneezing. The same treatment was continued.

Oct 7, 20XX. Rhinitis symptoms fluctuated. The patient rested for five days but experienced indigestion, which she described as resembling a "gastroptosis-like" condition. Despite drinking soju and vomiting after the Constitution-acupuncture treatment the other day, she felt surprisingly well the next day. However, she expressed concern about over-reliance on Constitution-acupuncture while indulging in unsuitable habits. The same treatment was provided.

Oct 24, 20XX. The patient caught a cold but reported improvement.

Rhinitis persisted, but she shared a new habit of stopping eating as soon as she felt full, which aided digestion and prevented sickness. This demonstrated a deeper understanding of managing her Sueum Constitution. The prescription was adjusted as follows: R. V I (ana 42) / L. II VI IV' I IX (44424). The Fu-system Inflammation Formula was applied for Upper Burner on the right, and allergy Formula for Upper Burner on the left.

With consistent adherence to the Constitutional Diet and occasional clinic visits, the patient appeared to have mastered managing her Sueum Constitution. By maintaining these habits, she could likely avoid significant illnesses and live a healthier life.

[Sueum Case 2] The Stomach Revived

* Patient: Ms G, 48 years old at the time of visit
* Chief complaints: gastroptosis, indigestion

The patient had gastroptosis, a hallmark condition of Sueum Constitution. While other Constitutions may exhibit mild gastroptosis, this case represented a true and severe sagging of the stomach. The Zang-Fu Structure of Sueum Constitution is as follows: "Kidney-Bladder Liver-Gallbladder Heart-Small Intestine Lungs-Large Intestine Pancreas-Stomach." Among these, the Stomach is positioned at the lowest Zang-Fu Potential. Individuals with this Constitution must navigate life with these structural limitations. However, acknowledging these limitations and following a proper Constitutional regimen allows for a healthy and enviable life. Conversely, ignoring these restrictions makes escaping the cycle of illness impossible. This rule applies universally across all Constitutions due to their inherent Structural constraints.

The patient naturally suffered from frequent indigestion. In cases of gastroptosis, lying down after meals is generally recommended, but this patient found lying down more uncomfortable. Additionally, she suffered from nervous gastritis, experiencing stomach discomfort even with minor stress. When digestion was impaired, nausea ensued, and even drinking water caused unease. The patient noted that drinking water unconsciously when thirsty led to rapid stomach stop and worsened her condition.

Apples were noted as the best food for this patient, as she felt the moved easily through the digestive system when eaten. Interestingly, the patient reported that eating rice seemed to "tighten the throat," possibly due to her weakened stomach despite it being generally suitable for her Constitution. In such cases, glutinous rice could be an alternative. With proper Constitutional treatment, rice consumption should no longer pose an issue. The patient also noted that beef was tolerable. I began treatment.

Mar 29, 20XX. A prescription was applied to treat the stomach: R. V (5) / L. V I (42). Constitutional decoction was also prescribed to regulate the stomach.

Mar 30, 20XX. The patient returned the next day, reporting improvement after taking Constitutional decoction. The same acupuncture prescription was used.

April 4, 20XX. The patient reported symptoms such as bloating, belching, upper abdominal pain, thirst, and loss of appetite, indicating a lack of gastric vitality. The prescription was adjusted as follows: R. V I (44) / L. VI II IV' VIII (4444). The right side targeted Fu-system Inflammation, while the left addressed mucosal ulcer.

April 5, 20XX. The patient noted improved digestion, suggesting the Constitution-acupuncture was taking effect. The same prescription was continued.

April 8, 20XX. The patient reported rising burping and stomach discomfort. Treatment continued with the same prescription.

April 11, 20XX. Occasionally, the patient passed stools that resembled "rabbit droppings." The pit of the stomach felt tight and painful at times, but digestive function had improved with Constitutional decoction. Despite this progress, the patient still felt low energy. Treatment remained the same.

April 14, 20XX. The pain in the pit of the stomach had subsided, and bowel movements were normalizing. Things appeared to be stabilizing. Treatment was continued with the same prescription.

April 18, 20XX. The patient reported feeling well. She mentioned needing to travel to Qingdao, China, at the end of June. She is a Korean-Chinese. Treatment continued as before.

April 19, 20XX. The patient expressed concern that stopping Constitutional decoction might cause a relapse. She was reassured that, with proper treatment and adherence to her Constitutional Diet, she would maintain her health in the future. Treatment was continued as before.

April 24, 20XX. The patient reported having regular bowel movements after breakfast—something unprecedented. This normalization of bowel movements was an encouraging sign of improved biological rhythms. Treatment was continued with the same prescription.

April 25, 20XX. The patient reported feeling completely fine. The same treatment was maintained, and additional Constitutional decoction was prescribed.

April 27, 20XX. The patient visited my clinic one last time before departing for China earlier than planned. She expressed gratitude for the treatment. The same prescription was used for the final session. I wished the patient with the continued health and well-being in China.

[Sueum Case 3] All Is Suffering (一切皆苦, Yi-qie-jie-ku)

* Patient: Ms C, 57 years old at the time of visit
* Chief complaints: bitter taste after meals

Whenever the patient ate something, she experienced a bitter taste in her mouth, especially after dinner. Recently, she has been eating only breakfast and lunch to feel better, as having an empty stomach is more comfortable.

Three years ago, she underwent corrective leg surgery, during which she received painkiller injections and antibiotics. Following this, she suddenly started experiencing sickness and vomiting. Since then, she has consistently suffered from bitter taste and general unwellness.

These days, she mixed raw potato juice with honey and consumed it lukewarm, which she said was soothing and good for her stomach. On the day of her way to my clinic, she ate chicken breast and felt better. She reported that consuming cold food made her insides feel frozen, and her stomach hardens like a freezer. Drinking cold water caused immediate sickness.

She recalled a time when Dr. Sang-gu Lee appeared on TV promoting vegetarianism. After adopting a vegetarian health regimen at the time, she experienced severe health problems. She developed dark blemishes on her face, a stomach ulcer, osteoporosis, and even pernicious anemia. While on a vegetarian diet, she would vomit blood due to bleeding from her stomach ulcer rising up to her throat. Fortunately, her osteoporosis improved after consuming "Chomilan", a health food made by dissolving fertilized eggs in vinegar, then adding honey and pollen. This mixture includes the foods that are all beneficial for those with Sueum Constitution.

The patient mentioned that her health began improving after following Mogyang Constitution's diet. Although her Constitutional diagnosis at the time was incorrect, she experienced "extraordinary luck" because the dietary recommendations for that Constitution also emphasized meat and root vegetables, which align well with her actual Constitution, Sueum. However, since Constitution-acupuncture and decoction differ significantly between the two Constitutions, the treatment effects were limited. Nonetheless, the dietary overlap brought some improvement. She recalled being happy while eating during that time. However, her meal times were very long, often taking an hour, as she needed to chew roasted grains thoroughly.

The patient explained that she had felt unwell if she didn't eat meat, and loved something as sweet as honey so much at that time. She also mentioned that eating charcoal powder had helped her feel better. However, consuming Fuzi (附子) among herbal medicines caused her liver levels to rise. According to Je-ma Lee, Fuzi is used as a medicine for Soeumin, which includes this Constitution. So, the patient's experience of liver damage caused me some confusion. In Je-ma Lee's *Dongeuisusebowon*, Fuzi is frequently mentioned as an ingredient in prescriptions related to Soeumin's theory on disease, symptoms, and treatment protocols.

In fact, I rarely use Fuzi in my clinical practice. There are many alternative prescriptions that do not require such a toxic herb, and the effectiveness of Constitution-acupuncture is so robust that it can address most diseases without the need for high-risk herbs like Fuzi. In baseball, exceptional players make quick, calculated decisions to handle the ball effectively. There is no need to make a high-risk play, such as throwing your whole body to make a sliding catch for an ordinary batted ball, due to slow judgment or poor footwork. Similarly, Constitution-acupuncture operates like a star player, offering efficient and precise treatment without unnecessary risk. Treatment for the patient began.

May 13, 20XX. The first treatment began with my preferred two-stage prescription:

R. V IX (51) / L. V I (42).

May 15, 20XX. The patient reported following a very thorough Constitutional Diet and maintaining a sleep pattern of going to bed around 9 pm and waking up at 4 am. The same Constitution-acupuncture treatment was performed, and Constitutional decoction was added to the prescription.

May 18, 20XX. The patient expressed satisfaction with the Sueum Constitution's diet, noting that it offered a variety of foods. The Seueum Constitution's diet aligns well with modern culinary culture, being compatible with most meats (except pork) and Korean spices like red pepper, garlic, green onion, ginger, pepper, and cinnamon. Root vegetables such as radish, burdock, lotus root, and bellflower root are also beneficial, while caution is required with flour-based foods and leafy vegetables. The same acupuncture prescription was used.

May 22, 20XX. The patient reported responding well to Constitution-acupuncture treatment. She remarked on the relief of the significant symptoms after switching to the Constitutional food chart presented by my clinic, which differs from the other Eight-Constitution clinics. She noted a unique taste in the prescribed Constitutional decoction and said it was the first time she had encountered such a flavor. The patient added that eating mustard greens and chives was easy to digest and felt beneficial. She was pleased with her stool consistency, describing it as similar to "Garaetteok" (a Korean rice cake in round stick form), which is a key indicator of health improvement. Additionally, she found beef seaweed soup very comfortable and nourishing. The same acupuncture prescription was continued.

May 25, 20XX. For the first time in nearly 13 years, the patient ate cooked eggplant for breakfast and reported enjoying it. She also tried mugwort pancakes and noted that red peppers were beneficial. Previously, the patient needed to chew xylitol gum after meals to combat the bitter taste, but reported no longer needing to do so now. She shared that drinking water now feels unnecessary, confessing that it had been stressful to force herself to drink 2 liters daily based on advice from doctors on morning TV shows.

Sueum Constitution has a lot of Water Qi in itself like Suyang Constitution, so water can act as poison. Overconsumption of water may lead to water retention, severe indigestion, and depletion of Yang Qi, causing symptoms like severe coldness and extreme lethargy due to lack of energy. For individuals with these Constitutions, minimal water intake just to quench thirst is sufficient. The prescription level for acupuncture was raised to better balance the patient's Zang-system and Fu-system organs: L. VI II III' X VIII (55555) / R. V I III' IX VII (55555).

May 29, 20XX. The patient expressed happiness, stating that physical discomfort had decreased by 90%. Potatoes were described as excellent, and while sweet potatoes previously caused issues when paired with apples, eating an apple alone now is tolerable. The patient praised eggplants as tasting like meat and shared her joy in eating mugwort for the first time in 20 years, finding its scent delightful. She noted that she no longer felt constant hunger and no longer needed sweets or gum to suppress it. The same acupuncture prescription was continued.

June 1, 20XX. The patient shared concerns about the potential recurrence of previous symptoms after eating. She remarked that the water used for brushing their teeth, previously described as bitter, now tasted sweet. Previously, she had to change toothpaste several times to alleviate the painful bitter taste, but this issue now had resolved.

Nowadays, she said that even if she felt like having just one more spoonful of food, she knew she should boldly put down the spoon. If she feels fully satisfied after a meal, she considers it a failed meal. This mindset is truly akin to that of a Taoist or even a saint. To achieve this level of restraint and wisdom, countless individuals must undergo repeated self-discipline. It's no exaggeration to say that concepts like emptying the mind and letting go of attachments are all aimed at reaching the state this patient has described. The patient has finally reached a high level of personal discipline.

The patient shared that since her early 30s, she had suffered from recurring colds, otitis media, and sinusitis which underwent the surgery three times. Tinnitus was another chronic and incurable condition that had plagued her. Now, she says, is the best time in her life. She also mentioned developing proteinuria from taking excessive sinusitis medications, noting how strong otolaryngology drugs can be. From that point on, she started exploring healthy foods and even tried the vegetarian health method promoted by Dr. Sang-gu Lee, but it only led to numerous illnesses and left her feeling like she was dying. Interestingly, her health improved significantly after abandoning vegetarianism, though she eventually began experiencing bitter-tasty water coming from her mouth.

She joked that after receiving treatment at Joowonjang Clinic and resolving the bitterness, she suddenly felt aimless and mentally empty. The prescription for Constitution-acupuncture remained the same.

June 5, 20XX. The patient reported that the bitterness after meals had become inconsistent—sometimes absent, sometimes present, but disappearing after about an hour when it occurred. That morning, she said she didn't feel any bitterness at all. She described having a good appetite, enjoying food, and feeling great overall. "My husband really likes this new version of me," she remarked (Constitutional Medicine fosters harmony in a married couple's relationship). The same Constitution-acupuncture prescription was continued, along with additional Constitutional decoction.

The patient visited my clinic a few more times, but as the bitterness after meals diminished significantly, she eventually stopped visiting. It is assumed that she is now living well by obeying the Constitutional food chart provided.

There are many strange diseases in the world. Western medicine often overlooks these rare conditions that cause significant suffering because they cannot be detected through tests. Such conditions are labeled as "neurotic." However, Eight-Constitution Medicine regards all symptoms a patient complains of—no matter how trivial they may seem—as legitimate diseases, deserving equal attention and treatment. The distinction between severe and mild illnesses is relative; what may seem minor to one person could be major to another. For this patient, the persistent bitter taste in her mouth was a huge illness that deeply affected her essence of life. Every illness, no matter how small, is important and must be treated with biggest care.

Completing Clinical Cases of the Eight Constitutions

In the clinical cases presented here, you must have appreciated the rich and ever-changing "differences" that unfold as vividly as a rainbow for each Constitution. In this way, every individual is unique. Constitutional Medicine honors these differences. This perspective is deeply rooted in our tradition, which has thrived for thousands of years within a worldview of continuous Yin and Yang, dynamic and ever-evolving changes.[123] After all, the very concept of "Constitution" implies a recognition of diverse individuals, not identical ones.

Constitutional Medicine brings to mind the philosophy of "difference" proposed by French philosopher Gilles Deleuze (1925–1995), who emphasized the primacy of difference over the "sameness" traditionally valued in philosophy. In clinical practice, we observe countless variations among individuals, even within the same Constitutional type. Moreover, within a single individual, differences arise and shift moment by moment. I think this reflects the deeper meaning of "difference" that Deleuze captures in his statement: "Difference resides in repetition" (*La différence réside dans la répétition*).

In observing patients, we frequently encounter the same disease recurring in a single individual. At the same time, we see how the same disease manifests in various forms across different Constitutions. Every scenario has two sides: difference within sameness and sameness within difference. These dual aspects are always interwoven.

A doctor bears the responsibility of employing all available knowledge and skills to treat a patient's illness and fully heal the patient's body and mind. Constitutional Medicine never gives up on its commitment to addressing each patient's unique differences with unwavering dedication until the patient is free from suffering. The journey of Constitutional Medicine will persist, progressing toward its ultimate goal: helping patients of all Constitutions achieve the peace of body and mind.

---

[123] "一陰一陽之謂道." (Once Yin operates, once Yang operates—that is called the Tao.) Tao resides in the Qi that alternates, becoming Yin once and Yang once, ceaselessly interchanging with each other. From Young-oak Kim, *Doh-ol Zhouyi Xici Zhuan* (檮杌 周易 繫辭傳), p. 115. "生生之謂易." (Constantly creating and creating again is called Yi.) Yi refers to the perpetual cycle of creation and recreation. From Young-oak Kim, *Doh-ol Zhouyi Xici Zhuan* (檮杌 周易 繫辭傳), p. 124.

CHAPTER 9

The Theory of Constitutional Diet and New Constitutional Diet Table

CONSTITUTIONAL DIET REFERS TO FOOD THAT YOUR INTESTINES LIKE, NOT WHAT YOUR PALATE LIKES.

CHAPTER 9

The Theory of Constitutional Diet and New Constitutional Diet Table

The Constitutional Diet was originally developed by Master Do-won Kuon and serves as a critical method for treating and preventing diseases in Eight-Constitution Medicine. It represents a unique form of health wisdom that is unparalleled anywhere else in the world. Eight-Constitution Medicine identifies the consumption of foods incompatible with an individual's Constitution as a major factor contributing to disease. Below, I outline the foods that are beneficial and harmful for each Constitution. Beneficial foods help correct Zang-Fu imbalances within each Constitution, promoting a state of dynamic equilibrium, while harmful foods exacerbate Zang-Fu imbalances, leading to a disrupted dynamic equilibrium.

Meaning of Constitutional Diet

Constitutional Diet was first introduced by Do-won Kuon in his thesis in 1974 at Myongji University, titled *"Study on Constitutional Acupuncture Treatment."* This work reflected nearly a decade of extensive clinical experience and statistical analysis tailored to different Constitutions nearly after 10 years since his first thesis.

The Constitutional food chart was also used in a study on the correlation between food and Constitution, conducted with students (124 students from the College of Home Economics) for a master's thesis by Lee Pil-ja in 1985 at the Department of Food and Nutrition, Ewha Womans University.[124]

The food table has continued to evolve, incorporating new informations as clinical experiences with various foods have accumulated. This Constitutional Diet Table is a cornerstone of Eight-Constitution Medicine, representing over 50 years of clinical verification.

The essence of the food table is straightforward: it categorizes foods into those that are beneficial and those that are harmful to each Constitution. Harmful foods can trigger adverse reactions specific to the individual's Constitution, including digestive disturbances such as upset stomach, diarrhea, bloating, or abdominal pain, as well as systemic issues like headaches, insomnia, anxiety, or reduced energy levels. Prolonged consumption of these foods may lead to the development of chronic internal diseases, even if no immediate symptoms are apparent.

Conversely, beneficial foods are those that harmonize with the individual's Constitution, supporting digestive health, enhancing vitality, and promoting overall well-being. These foods play a pivotal role in maintaining and improving the health of individuals when aligned with their Constitutions.

In the following sections, we will delve deeper into the classification of beneficial and harmful foods for each Constitution.

Let's first discuss the Geumyang Constitution as an example. The Zang-Fu Structure of the Geumyang Constitution includes "Lungs-Large intestine Pancreas-Stomach Heart-Small intestine Kidneys-Bladder Liver-Gallbladder." Beneficial foods for the Geumyang Constitution primarily

---

[124] Journal of the Korean Society of Nutrition, Volume 18, No. 2, 1985, Sook-hee Kim, Hwa-young Kim, Pil-ja Lee, Do-won Kuon, Young-oak Kim, *"Study on the Correlation Between Food Preference and Nutritional Status According to the Constitutional Classification Method of Constitutional Medicine"* (pp. 155–166).

This study originates from author Lee's master's thesis in the Department of Food and Nutrition at Ewha Womans University. The students were consuming diets that were not related with their Constitutions before the research. However, the study found that adopting a Constitutionally tailored diet could lead them to beneficial changes in blood composition, highlighting the positive impact of dietary choices aligned with one's Constitution.

enhance Liver-Gallbladder potential and secondarily support Kidney-Bladder potential (i.e., properly boosting the potentials of the Yin Field Zang-Fu organs). On the other hand, harmful foods primarily increase Lung-Large Intestine potential and secondarily elevate Pancreas-Stomach potential (i.e., excessively increasing the potentials of the Yang Field Zang-Fu organs).

The Mogyang Constitution, in contrast, has a completely opposite structure to the Geumyang Constitution. Therefore, the dietary recommendations are also reversed. Foods that benefit the Geumyang Constitution are harmful to the Mogyang Constitution, and foods harmful to the Geumyang Constitution are beneficial to the Mogyang Constitution.

The Geumeum Constitution has Zang-Fu Structure that includes "Lungs-Large intestine Kidneys-Bladder Pancreas-Stomach Heart-Small intestine Liver-Gallbladder." While the Geumyang and Geumeum Constitutions have the same arrangement at both ends of their structure, their in-between Zang-Fu organs differ slightly, leading to subtle variations in dietary needs. The Geumeum Constitution also benefits from foods that enhance the Liver-Gallbladder potential and reduce the Lungs-Large intestine potential, similar to Geumyang Constitution. The differences arise from variations in the arrangement of the three, intermediate Zang-Fu organs except the outermost Zang-Fu of the Yin and Yang Field. Naturally, the dietary recommendations for the Mogeum Constitution are opposite to those for the Geumeum Constitution.

For both the Geumyang and Geumeum Constitution, foods like rice, green vegetables, sea fish, seafood, and shellfish are generally beneficial. On the other hand, foods such as meat, flour-based products, dairy foods, root vegetables, artificial seasonings, and chemicals are harmful. Conversely, for the Mogyang and Mogeum Constitutions, foods like meat, flour-based products, dairy foods, root vegetables, and nuts are beneficial, while sea fish, seafood, and shellfish are considered harmful.

Toyang Constitution has a Zang-Fu Structure consisting of "Pancreas-Stomach Heart-Small intestine Liver-Gallbladder Lungs-Large intestine Kidneys-Bladder." Beneficial foods for this Constitution primarily enhance the Kidneys-Bladder potential and secondarily the Lungs-Large intestine potential. Harmful foods, on the other hand, primarily increase the Pancreas-Stomach potential and secondarily increase the Heart-Small intestine potential. As expected, the Suyang Constitution has the opposite dietary needs.

Toeum Constitution has a Zang-Fu Structure consisting of "Pancreas-Stomach Lungs-Large intestine Heart-Small intestine Liver-Gallbladder Kidneys-Bladder." Since the outermost Zang-Fu is similar to that of the Toyang Constitution, there are shared elements in their dietary requirements. However, the three intermediate Zang-Fu organ arrangement differ, leading to some variations in the specific foods recommended. The dietary recommendations for Sueum Constitution are opposite to those for the Toeum Constitution.

For both the Toyang and Toeum Constitutions, there is an abundance of heat in the Pancreas and Stomach, making cooling foods that replenish the Water Qi of the Kidneys and Bladder highly beneficial. Spicy foods that generate heat or over-stimulate digestion are generally classified as harmful. In general, warm foods traditionally believed to boost Qi in Oriental medicine are also often harmful. Conversely, these same foods tend to benefit those with Suyang or Sueum Constitution.

Loss of Instinct

People often rationalize this line: the food they like is the food that suits them. Alternatively, they may say that the foods they crave are what their body needs to fill its deficiencies, so they should eat whatever they desire. On the surface, this logic appears plausible and persuasive. However, it is fundamentally flawed. This belief is yet another example of false superstitions about food.

This concept can be applied to animals. For pure, natural animals, instinct governs all actions, operating independently of conscious will. However, humans fall into a different category. There is very little about human behavior that can be described as purely natural. Most human actions are shaped and manipulated by the constructs of civilization.

Take the example of sex. Many believe it to be instinct, and while there is some truth to that, human sexual behavior deviates significantly from pure instinct. For humans, sexual activity is more frequently a pursuit of pleasure than a means of reproduction. While offspring may sometimes result from this activity, the act itself is rarely driven by the instinctual urge to reproduce. Some people may choose to have children deliberately, but the majority engage in sexual activity primarily for pleasure.

The same principle applies to human eating habits. If eating were truly instinctive, as the earlier question suggested, all foods consumed would naturally benefit the body. Yet, this is not the case. Humans, for example, enjoy drinking alcohol—a particularly pronounced tendency among Koreans. Observing people working for corporations, it seems many drink two or three times a week, and some even drink daily. Alcohol is said to be highly incompatible with the conditions of human bodily fluids—in essence, it acts as a poison to the human body. If one consumes such a poison several times a week, or even daily, can this really be considered instinctual? Or might it align with what Sigmund Freud (1856–1939) referred to as the death instinct, or Thanatos, a drive toward self-destruction?

Learning the Constitutional Diet Is A Must

We often eat harmful foods even when we know they will cause discomfort or other adverse effects. Inevitably, we end up suffering as a result. This clearly demonstrates that humans are not governed by instinct. Most of our natural instincts have been lost. Instead, what drives human behavior is not instinct, but the human mind—often dominated by greed. This phenomenon can be seen as a consequence of humanity's continual departure from nature in the process of building civilization.

To correct these artificial mistakes, we must learn which foods suit our individual Constitutions and adopt lifestyles aligned with them through intentional education. By doing so, we can bridge the gap created by the loss of instinct. This is where the importance of the Constitutional Diet of Eight Constitutions comes into play. Everyone should learn which foods are beneficial for one's Constitution and cultivate the habit of living accordingly. This practice will naturally lead to better health.

In the next section, I will introduce the Eight-Constitution Diet Table proposed by Master Do-won Kuon, which has been further refined and supplemented through my clinical experience.

Geumyang Constitution's Food Table

[Beneficial Foods]

Vegetables: napa cabbage, water parsley, perilla leaves, bean sprouts, fern, bok choy, lettuce, cucumber, cabbage, eggplant, celery, kale, broccoli, mustard greens, mugwort, cauliflower, asparagus.

Grains: milled rice, buckwheat, mung beans, brown rice, rye, millet, peas.

Meats: almost none.

Fish and Seafood: flounder, croaker, herring, shad, saury, sea bream (red sea bream, parrot sea bream, tile sea bream, striped sea bream), salmon, pufferfish, rockfish, yellowtail, tuna, mullet, anchovies, whitebait, octopus, shellfish (clams, razor clams, scallops), abalone, jellyfish, crabs (blue crab, snow crab, king crab), shrimp, lobster, sea cucumber, sea squirt, crucian carp.

Condiments: persimmon vinegar, glucose powder, brown rice vinegar, balsamic vinegar, onion, mustard, horseradish (wasabi), sea salt, bamboo salt, agave syrup, capers.

Cooking Oils: brown rice oil, flaxseed oil, canola oil, sunflower seed oil.

Fruits: kiwi, banana, strawberry, peach, cherry, persimmon, green grape, plum, blueberry, blackberry, mangosteen, papaya.

Teas and Beverages: cocoa (unsweetened), dark chocolate, quince tea, persimmon leaf tea, buckwheat tea, plum tea, pine needle tea, citron tea, chamomile, rooibos tea, brown rice tea.

[Harmful Foods]

Vegetables: radish, carrot, potato, sweet potato, red pepper, red pepper leaf, pumpkin, lotus root, burdock, mushroom, green pepper, paprika.

Grains: all flour-based foods (bread, cold noodles, ramen, kalguksu, jajangmyeon, udon, noodles, spaghetti, pizza, biscuits), corn, sorghum, soybeans, tofu.

Meats: pork, beef, chicken, lamb, all dairy products (milk, cheese, butter, yogurt, low-fat milk, non-fat milk, ice cream, cake), processed meats (ham, sausage, hot dogs, hamburgers).

Fish and Seafood: catfish, snakehead, freshwater shrimp, seaweeds (seaweed, kelp).

Condiments: garlic, red pepper, sugar, chemical seasonings, apple cider vinegar, pepper, curry, chili sauce, honey, corn syrup, soy sauce, mayonnaise.

Cooking Oils: soybean cooking oil, corn oil, pumpkin seed oil, margarine.

Fruits: apple, pear, chestnut, melon, tangerine, orange, watermelon, nuts, mango, longan, apricot.

Teas and Beverages: coffee, green tea, ginseng tea, coix seed tea, corn tea, processed beverages, ionic beverages, chrysanthemum tea, black tea, arrowroot tea.

Geumeum Constitution's Food Table

[Beneficial Foods]

Vegetables: napa cabbage, water parsley, perilla leaves, bean sprouts, fern, pak choy, lettuce, cucumber, cabbage, eggplant, celery, kale, broccoli, mustard greens, mugwort, cauliflower, asparagus.

Grains: milled rice, buckwheat, mung beans, glutinous rice, rye, millet, peas.

Meats: almost none.

Fish and Seafood: flounder, croaker, sea bream (red sea bream, parrot sea bream, tile bream, striped sea bream, etc.), puffer fish, rockfish, yellowtail, tuna, mackerel, anchovies, whitebait, saury, herring, shad, pollack, shellfish (clams, tympanum clams, scallops), abalone, jellyfish, crabs (blue crab, snow crab, king crab), lobster, conch, crucian carp.

Condiments: mustard, ginger, onion, wasabi, sea salt, bamboo salt, glucose powder, white balsamic vinegar, red balsamic vinegar, agave syrup, lemon, capers.

Cooking Oils: grape seed oil, flaxseed oil, canola oil, sunflower seed oil.

Fruits: grapes, peaches, cherries, pineapple, strawberries, plums, kiwis.

Teas and Beverages: buckwheat tea, ginger tea, quince tea, plum tea, citron tea, chamomile tea, rooibos tea, lemon tea.

[Harmful Foods]

Vegetables: radishes, carrots, potatoes, sweet potatoes, red peppers, red pepper leaves, pumpkin, lotus root, burdock, mushrooms, paprika.

Grains: all flour-based products (bread, cold noodles, ramen, kalguksu, sujebi, Jajangmyeon, udon, noodles, spaghetti, pizza, biscuits, etc.), corn, sorghum, soybeans, tofu, barley, glutinous barley, red beans.

Meats: pork, beef, chicken, lamb, all dairy products (milk, cheese, butter, yogurt, low-fat milk, non-fat milk, ice cream, cake); processed meats (ham, sausage, hot dogs, hamburgers, etc.).

Fish and Seafood: eel, catfish, snakehead, freshwater shrimp, oysters, seaweed.

Condiments: garlic, sugar, red pepper, chili sauce, black pepper, white pepper, soy sauce, honey, corn syrup, apple cider vinegar, mayonnaise.

Cooking Oils: soybean oil, pumpkin seed oil, corn oil, margarine.

Fruits: pear, apple, melon, chestnut, watermelon, nuts, orange, tangerine, longan, apricot.

Teas and Beverages: coffee, green tea, coix seed tea, ionic beverages, processed beverages, black tea, chrysanthemum tea, ginseng tea, arrowroot tea, fennel root tea, peppermint tea, corn tea, snail tea.

Toyang Constitution's Food Table

[Beneficial Foods]

Vegetables: napa cabbage, cucumber, carrot, pumpkin, burdock, bok choy, mallow, bean sprouts, chicory, kale, celery, broccoli, cauliflower, fern, water parsley, sweet potato, mung bean sprouts.

Grains: milled rice, barley, beans (black beans, soybeans, kidney beans, peas, tofu), red beans, noodles (kalguksu, sujebi, udon, etc.), glutinous barley, mung beans, oats, buckwheat.

Meats: pork, beef, milk, cheese, yogurt.

Fish and Seafood: flounder, croaker, puffer fish, eel, mackerel, cod, flatfish, yellowtail, mullet, sea bream (red sea bream, parrot sea bream, tile sea bream, striped sea bream, etc.), monkfish, rockfish, loach, whitebait, shrimp, crab (blue crab, snow crab, king crab), lobster, shellfish (clams, mussels, razor clams, scallops), conch, jellyfish.

Condiments: persimmon vinegar, soybean paste, Korean traditional soy sauce, Japanese soy sauce, sea salt, bamboo salt, onion, maple syrup, agave syrup, capers, lemon, mint.

Cooking Oils: soybean oil, pumpkin seed oil, olive oil, flaxseed oil, sunflower seed oil, canola oil.

Fruits: Persimmon, banana, pear, melon, watermelon, strawberry, nuts (walnuts, almonds, pistachios, macadamias, cashews, acorns, chestnuts), blackberries, blueberries, mangosteen, papaya, longan.

Teas and Beverages: barley tea, persimmon leaf tea, goji berry tea, ionic beverages, chive tea, chrysanthemum tea, white lotus tea, rooibos tea, jasmine tea, chicory tea, Korean blackberry juice.

[Harmful Foods]

Vegetables: potatoes, peppers, lettuce, red pepper leaves, chives, green peppers, paprika, mustard greens, mugwort.

Grains: brown rice, glutinous rice, scorched rice, sesame seeds, corn, sorghum, flour-based foods (bread, ramen, jajangmyeon).

Meats: chicken, goat meat, eggs, lamb, duck.

Fish and Seafood: seaweed (kelp, laver), mackerel, skate.

Condiments: red pepper, black pepper, ginger, green onion, curry, mustard, honey, cinnamon, apple cider vinegar, brown rice vinegar, mayonnaise, corn syrup, wasabi, chili sauce, sugar.

Cooking Oils: sesame oil, grape seed oil, brown rice oil, corn oil, margarine.

Fruits: apple, tangerine, orange, mango, tomato, grape, peach, kiwi, peanut.

Teas and Beverages: ginseng tea, honey tea, jujube tea, ginger tea, cinnamon tea, carbonated drinks, arrowroot tea, corn tea, quince tea, chestnut tea, pine needle tea, green tea, black tea.

Toeum Constitution's Food Table

[Beneficial Foods]

Vegetables: napa cabbage, cucumber, pumpkin, burdock, bok choy, mallow, bean sprouts, kale, celery, broccoli, cauliflower, fern, water parsley, sweet potato, mung bean sprouts.

Grains: milled rice, barley, beans, red beans, glutinous barley, mung beans, oats, rye, buckwheat.

Meats: pork.

Fish and Seafood: flounder, croaker, puffer fish, eel, tuna, yellowtail, salmon, mullet, mackerel, cod, whitebait, sea bream (red sea bream, parrot sea bream, tile sea bream, striped sea bream, etc.), monkfish, rockfish, shellfish (clams, mussels, razor clams, scallops), crab (blue crab, snow crab, king crab), shrimp, squid, octopus, oyster, abalone, lobster.

Condiments: Korean traditional soy sauce, Japanese soy sauce, soybean paste, sea salt, bamboo salt, onion, glucose powder, agave syrup, persimmon vinegar, balsamic vinegar, capers, mint.

Cooking Oils: soybean oil, pumpkin seed oil, grape seed oil, flaxseed oil.

Fruits: persimmon, pear, melon, strawberry, banana, grapes, watermelon, peaches, blueberries, blackberries, mangosteen, peanuts, papaya, longan.

Teas and Beverages: barley tea, persimmon leaf tea, dark chocolate, unsweetened cocoa, ionic beverages, goji berry tea, chive tea, citron tea, white lotus tea, rooibos tea, Korean blackberry juice.

[Harmful Foods]

Vegetables: potatoes, peppers, lettuce, red pepper leaves, chives, green peppers, paprika, mustard greens, mugwort.

Grains: brown rice, glutinous rice, scorched rice, corn, sorghum, sesame seeds, flour-based foods.

Meats: chicken, goat meat, egg, lamb, duck, beef, processed meats (ham, sausage, hot dogs, hamburgers), most dairy products (milk, cheese, butter, yogurt, ice cream).

Fish and Seafood: seaweed (kelp, laver), mackerel, saury, skate.

Condiments: red pepper, black pepper, ginger, green onion, curry, mustard, cinnamon, brown rice vinegar, apple cider vinegar, honey, garlic, wasabi, chili sauce, sugar, corn syrup, mayonnaise.

Cooking Oils: sesame oil, brown rice oil, corn oil.

Fruits: apple, tangerine, orange, mango, tomato, melon, nuts, kiwi.

Teas and Beverages: ginseng tea, jujube tea, honey tea, cinnamon tea, ginger tea, carbonated drinks, coffee, green tea, black tea, cassia seed tea, corn tea, chrysanthemum tea, quince tea, arrowroot tea, pine needle tea, chamomile.

Mogyang Constitution's Food Table

[Beneficial Foods]

Vegetables: radish, potato, sweet potato, carrot, lotus root, burdock, mushrooms, pepper, pumpkin, red pepper leaves, bean sprouts, paprika, shepherd's purse, chives.

Grains: flour-based foods (bread, kalguksu, sujebi, udon, noodles), milled rice, soybeans, other beans, tofu, sorghum, corn, sesame seeds.

Meats: pork, beef, chicken, lamb, milk, cheese, butter, yogurt.

Fish and Seafood: freshwater eel, loach, catfish, seaweed (kelp, laver, green seaweed), croaker, oysters.

Condiments: garlic, sugar, red pepper, ginger, pepper, curry, chili sauce, Korean traditional soy sauce, Japanese soy sauce, soybean paste, honey.

Cooking Oils: soybean oil, pumpkin seed oil, corn oil, olive oil, sesame oil, margarine.

Fruits: pear, watermelon, apple, nuts (walnuts, almonds, pistachios, macadamias, cashews, chestnuts), orange, tomato, mango, melon, longan, apricot.

Teas and Beverages: coffee, ionic beverages, chrysanthemum tea, arrowroot tea, coix tea, ginseng tea, corn tea, coriander tea, green tea, black tea, puerh tea.

[Harmful Foods]

Vegetables: napa cabbage, lettuce, cucumber, perilla leaves, bok choy, fern, water parsley, kale, Swiss chard, celery, broccoli, mustard greens, eggplant, cauliflower.

Grains: buckwheat, barley, glutinous barley, mung beans, red beans, rye, brown rice.

Meats: almost none

Fish and Seafood: flounder, croaker, mackerel, saury, tuna, yellowtail, mullet, salmon, whitebait, sea bream, puffer fish, rockfish, octopus, sea urchin roe, jellyfish, crabs (blue crab, snow crab, king crab), lobster, shellfish, abalone, conch, sea squirt, sea cucumber, carp.

Condiments: persimmon vinegar, mustard, horseradish (wasabi), sea salt, bamboo salt, glucose powder, brown rice vinegar, balsamic vinegar, mayonnaise, capers, agave syrup, lemon.

Cooking Oils: grape seed oil, brown rice oil, flaxseed oil, sunflower seed oil, canola oil.

Fruits: persimmon, cherry, green grape, grape, banana, strawberry, kiwi, peach, plum, blackberry, blueberry, mangosteen, papaya.

Teas and Beverages: cocoa, chocolate, quince tea, persimmon leaf tea, carbonated drinks, buckwheat tea, plum tea, pine needle tea, goji berry tea, rooibos tea, chamomile.

Mogeum Constitution's Food Table

[Beneficial Foods]

Vegetables: radish, potato, sweet potato, carrot, lotus root, burdock, mushrooms, pepper, pumpkin, red pepper leaves, bean sprouts, paprika, wild chives, shepherd's purse.

Grains: flour-based foods (bread, kalguksu, sujebi, udon, noodles), soybeans, other beans, tofu, sorghum, corn, sesame seeds, barley, glutinous barley.

Meats: pork, beef, lamb, milk, cheese, butter, yogurt.

Fish and Seafood: freshwater eel, loach, catfish, seaweed (kelp, laver, green seaweed), croaker, oysters, shrimp.

Condiments: garlic, sugar, soybean paste, red pepper, chili sauce, Korean traditional soy sauce, Japanese soy sauce, starch syrup, mayonnaise.

Cooking Oils: soybean oil, pumpkin seed oil, corn oil, olive oil, sesame oil, margarine.

Fruits: chestnut, pear, melon, apple, watermelon, orange, tangerine, nuts (walnuts, almonds, pistachios, macadamias, cashews, acorns), longan, apricots.

Teas and Beverages: coffee, coix tea, ionic beverages, chrysanthemum tea, arrowroot tea, corn tea, green tea, black tea, puerh tea, round root tea.

[Harmful Foods]

Vegetables: napa cabbage, lettuce, cucumber, perilla leaf, bok choy, fern, water parsley, kale, Swiss chard, celery, broccoli, mustard greens, eggplant, cauliflower.

Grains: buckwheat, mung beans, rye.

Meats: almost none.

Fish and Seafood: flounder, croaker, mackerel, saury, tuna, yellowtail, mullet, salmon, whitebait, sea bream, puffer fish, rockfish, pollack, octopus, sea urchin roe, jellyfish, crabs (blue crab, snow crab, king crab), lobster, shellfish, abalone, conch, crucian carp.

Condiments: persimmon vinegar, ginger, cinnamon, mustard, wasabi, bamboo salt, agave syrup, glucose powder, balsamic vinegar, lemon, capers.

Cooking Oils: grape seed oil, canola oil, flaxseed oil, sunflower seed oil.

Fruits: grapes, green grapes, cherries, persimmons, peaches, banana, strawberry, kiwi, blackberry, blueberry, mangosteen, papaya, plum, tomato, mango.

Teas and Beverages: cocoa, chocolate, quince tea, carbonated drinks, persimmon leaf tea, buckwheat tea, goji berry tea, plum tea, rooibos tea, chamomile.

Suyang Constitution's Food Table

[Beneficial Foods]

Vegetables: radish, potato, lettuce, peppers, red pepper leaves, wild chives, shepherd's purse, chives, ginger, green pepper, paprika, mustard greens, eggplant, mushrooms, burdock, bellflower root, mugwort.

Grains: milled rice, brown rice, glutinous rice, sesame seeds, corn.

Meats: chicken, beef, lamb, goat, duck, eggs.

Fish and Seafood: seaweed (kelp, laver, green seaweed), croaker.

Condiments: red pepper, pepper, green onion, curry, ginger, cinnamon, mustard, honey, chili sauce, wasabi, paprika, sugar, corn syrup, rice syrup, glucose powder, apple cider vinegar, brown rice vinegar, balsamic vinegar.

Cooking Oils: sesame oil, brown rice oil, corn oil, grape seed oil.

Fruits: apple, orange, tomato, mango, tangerine, grape, peach.

Teas and Beverages: ginseng tea, cinnamon tea, ginger tea, honey tea, jujube tea, corn tea, brown rice tea, black tea.

[Harmful Foods]

Vegetables: cucumber, cabbage, bean sprouts, water parsley, fern, kale, bok choy, pumpkin, broccoli, cauliflower.

Grains: barley, red beans, glutinous barley, mung beans, flour-based foods (bread, kalguksu, sujebi, udon, noodles, ramen, jajangmyeon).

Meats: pork, processed pork (ham, sausage, hot dog).

Fish and Seafood: flounder, croaker, puffer fish, eel, mackerel, tuna, yellowtail, salmon, cod, crab, sea bream, monkfish, rockfish, squid, octopus, shellfish (clams, mussels, razor clams, scallops, etc.), crabs (blue crab, snow crab, king crab), shrimp, lobster, oysters, abalone, conch, jellyfish.

Condiments: persimmon vinegar, soy sauce, sea salt, bamboo salt, mint.

Cooking Oils: flaxseed oil, sunflower seed oil, canola oil, pumpkin seed oil, margarine.

Fruits: persimmon, melon, watermelon, banana, strawberry, pear, plum, kiwi, cherry, grape, papaya, blueberry, blackberry, nuts.

Teas and Beverages: barley tea, goji berry tea, ionic beverages, persimmon leaf tea, coffee, chrysanthemum tea, cocoa, chocolate, Korean black raspberry tea, pine needle tea, arrowroot tea, quince tea, chamomile, rooibos tea.

Sueum Constitution's Food Table

[Beneficial Foods]

Vegetables: radish, potato, lettuce, pepper, red pepper leaves, wild chives, shepherd's purse, chives, ginger, bell pepper, paprika, mustard greens, eggplants, mushrooms, bellflower root, mugwort.

Grains: milled rice, brown rice, glutinous rice, sesame seeds, corn.

Meats: chicken, beef, lamb, goat, duck, eggs, milk, cheese, butter, yogurt.

Fish and Seafood: seaweed (kelp, laver, green seaweed), loach, croaker.

Condiments: red pepper, pepper, green onion, curry, ginger, cinnamon, honey, garlic, chili sauce, mustard, wasabi, paprika, sugar, rice syrup, corn syrup, apple cider vinegar, brown rice vinegar, mayonnaise.

Cooking Oils: sesame oil, brown rice oil, corn oil, margarine.

Fruits: apples, tangerine, orange, tomato, mango, chestnut.

Teas and Beverages: ginseng tea, cinnamon tea, ginger tea, jujube tea, honey tea, corn tea, brown rice tea, chamomile.

[Harmful Foods]

Vegetables: cucumber, cabbage, bean sprouts, water parsley, fern, kale, bok choy, pumpkin, broccoli, cauliflower.

Grains: barley, red beans, glutinous barley, mung beans, flour-based foods (bread, kalguksu, sujebi, udon, noodles, ramen, jajangmyeon).

Meats: pork, processed pork (ham, sausage, hot dog).

Fish and Seafood: flounder, croaker, puffer fish, eel, mackerel, salmon, yellowtail, cod, crab, sea bream, monkfish, rockfish, squid, octopus, shellfish (clams, mussels, razor clams, scallops, etc.), crabs (blue crab, snow crab, king crab), shrimp, lobster, oysters, abalone, conch, jellyfish.

Condiments: persimmon vinegar, sea salt, bamboo salt, soy sauce, mint.

Cooking Oils: grape seed oil, pumpkin seed oil, flaxseed oil, sunflower seed oil, canola oil.

Fruits: persimmon, melon, banana, strawberry, grape, green grape, kiwi, peach, plum, cherry, watermelon, pear, nuts, papaya, blueberry, blackberry.

Teas and Beverages: barley tea, chocolate, cocoa, ionic beverages, persimmon leaf tea, pine needle tea, goji berry tea, quince tea, arrowroot tea, green tea.

APPENDIX

Characteristics of Eight Constitutions

Characteristics of 8 Constitutions

Summary of the Key Characteristics of Each Constitution

The following provides a concise summary of the main characteristics of each Constitution. By keeping this general outline in mind while examining the details of each Constitution, you will gain a clearer understanding of Eight-Constitution Medicine.

First, when discussing the characteristics of Constitutions broadly, there are general similarities between the two groups:

Geumyang Constitution and Geumeum Constitution (collectively referred to as Geum-Constitution) share similar traits; Toyang Constitution and Toeum Constitution (To-Constitution) also align in characteristics; Mogyang Constitution and Mogeum Constitution (Mog-Constitution) are similar; Lastly, Suyang Constitution and Sueum Constitution (Su-Constitution) share similarities.[125] With these relationships in mind, proceed carefully to understand the distinct characteristics of each Constitution described below.

[125] In Korean, "Geum" means Metal, "To" means Earth, "Mog" means Wood, and "Su" means Water.

Important Considerations About Food and Constitution

There are some misconceptions about the relationship between Constitution and food that must be addressed.

Food Preferences and Constitution

Many believe that people naturally prefer foods that suit their Constitution and reject those that do not. However, this is not the case. In reality, people's food preferences often have little to do with their Constitution. People may prefer certain foods simply because they enjoy the taste, not because the food is inherently suitable for their Constitution. While it is possible that someone may instinctively like food that happens to suit their Constitution, this is not a universal rule. Therefore, you should set aside the assumption that you will automatically like a food simply because it aligns with your Constitution.

Immediate Reactions to Unsuitable Foods

A common belief is that eating foods unsuitable for your Constitution will inevitably lead to digestive problems or discomfort, such as indigestion, abdominal pain, diarrhea, bloating, or constipation. While this seems logical in theory, it is not always true in practice. For some, consuming unsuitable foods might indeed cause immediate discomfort or gastrointestinal symptoms. However, most people do not experience any noticeable issues. On the contrary, they may enjoy the food or even feel psychologically energized by it, leading to a false sense of compatibility. Therefore, just because you feel good after eating a particular food does not mean it is suitable for your Constitution.

Long-Term Effects of Unsuitable Foods

Even if unsuitable foods do not cause immediate symptoms or discomfort, this does not mean they are safe to consume over time. The absence of symptoms simply means there is no immediate reaction at that moment. From a long-term health perspective, it is essential to avoid foods unsuitable for your Constitution as much as possible, even if no discomfort is initially evident. Adopting this mindset will contribute to better health and well-being in the long run.

Geumyang Constitution's Characteristics

Zang-Fu Structure

(Yang Field)		|	(Yin Field)	
LU·LI	PA·ST	HT·SI	KI·BL	**LR·GB**

(LU: Lung, LI: Large intestine, PA: Pancreas, ST: Stomach, HT: Heart, SI: Small intestine, KI: Kidneys, BL: Bladder, LR: Liver, GB: Gallbladder. This abbreviation rule holds true to all Constitutions in this appendix.)

Characteristics Related to Food

Rice, leafy vegetables, fish, and seafood are suitable for this Constitution, while flour-based foods, meat, dairy products, and spicy foods are unsuitable. This conclusion comes from Constitutional Diet developed by Master Do-won Kuon. However, many people do not enjoy vegetables, fish, and seafood—foods beneficial for this Constitution—but instead prefer meat and flour-based foods, which are harmful. This demonstrates the common belief that people naturally prefer the foods that suit their constitution is not always true.

The Impact of Beneficial and Harmful Foods

Health problems are more likely to arise when beneficial foods are underconsumed, and harmful foods are overconsumed. If the harmful foods were indigestible and the beneficial foods were easily digestible, adherence to the Constitutional Diet would come naturally. However, in reality, these dietary effects do not always align with theoretical expectations, leading to various diseases and health issues over time.

Specific Food Preferences and Reactions

* **Meat:** Meat is one of the most challenging foods for Geumyang Constitution. Many people enjoy eating meat even though it does not suit their Constitution. Among them, some experience digestive issues or discomfort, while others do not exhibit such symptoms.

Sensitive individuals may often get upset stomach after eating meat and consume little or only lean meat. Some even avoid meat entirely since young because they find the smell repellent. However, a surprising number of Geumyang individuals have no immediate problems with eating meat and may even prefer it to vegetarian or fish-based diets.

Despite the absence of short-term effects, long-term consumption of meat can lead to severe health issues, such as cerebrovascular diseases (e.g., stroke), cardiovascular problems (e.g., myocardial infarction), allergies, and other organ-specific diseases. Hence, it is best to avoid meat whenever possible. Among Geumyang individuals who enjoy meat, hyperlipidemia, high blood pressure, and diabetes are common conditions.

* **Fried and Fatty Foods:** Many individuals with this Constitution experience digestive discomfort from fried or fatty foods, such as fried chicken or greasy Chinese dishes, which often lead to indigestion.

* **Flour-Based Foods:** Flour-based foods, such as bread or noodles, often cause bloating or discomfort in some individuals. However, there are those who prefer flour-based foods to rice and digest them without an issue. As they age, it is common for people to feel an increased burden of indigestion from consuming flour-based foods.

* **Milk:** Compared to other Constitutions, people with this Constitution are more likely to experience stomach discomfort or diarrhea after consuming milk. Nevertheless, some individuals have no problem with milk and may drink several liters daily.

* **Vegetables:** Vegetables, particularly green leafy ones, are highly beneficial for Geumyang Constitution, which is common among strict vegetarians. However, vegetarians with this Constitution should be cautious about yogurt, cheese, beans, mushrooms, and certain fruits they consume as meat substitutes, as these are unsuitable.

Interestingly, some people dislike vegetables despite being well-suited for them. This tendency is more common among younger generation and more prevalent in men than women. This reiterates that there is no natural law dictating that people would like what suits their Constitution. Humans, as beings with free will, frequently act against what might seem natural or beneficial.

* **Fruits:** Many individuals with this Constitution enjoy fruits. Unfortunately, common fruits—such as apple, tangerine, orange, pear, and watermelon—are unsuitable for this Constitution. It is unfortunate that the most widely available fruits fall into the harmful category.

Additionally, some individuals are allergic to certain fruits (e.g., kiwi, peach) classified as suitable for this Constitution. This may lead to confusion about whether their diagnosed Constitution is correct. However, allergies to these fruits can be resolved through Constitutional treatment, such as Constitution-acupuncture or Constitutional decoction, enabling individuals to enjoy these fruits later.

* **Fish and Seafood:** In general, many people enjoy fish and seafood, but quite many dislike them due to the smell or other reasons. Some people say they hate cooked fish but enjoy raw fish. Raw fish is also a preferred food for this Constitution, though not a few often dislike it. Surprisingly, there are more people than expected who experience stomach discomfort from oily fish like mackerel. This is a common issue among those with a weaker ability to digest fats. Similarly, stomach discomfort caused by shellfish such as clams is not uncommon. Among these, grilled clams are the most likely to cause such symptoms. However, when cooked in a stew or soup, clams usually do not lead to such problems.

* **Crustaceans:** Raw oysters are another typical food that can cause digestive issues such as severe stomachache and diarrhea. However, when properly cooked, these problems can be avoided. Allergic reactions to crustaceans like shrimp and crabs are also common. Such allergies can often be mitigated with the treatments like Constitution-acupuncture or Constitutional decoction.

* **Alcohol:** There are many people who generally dislike alcohol, find it difficult to drink even small amounts, or cannot drink at all. On the other hand, it is surprisingly common for others to enjoy alcohol and drink more than the average. Among these drinkers, alcohol addiction is not uncommon, and excessive drinking significantly increases the risk of developing alcoholic cirrhosis or liver cancer.

Diseases When the Constitutional Diet is Violated

Allergies

This Constitution is prone to various allergic diseases, which are common and characteristic. Many individuals suffer from allergic skin conditions such as urticaria, unexplained itching, contact dermatitis, metal allergies, and dermographism. Food allergies often lead to hives, and in severe cases, swelling of the respiratory tract can cause breathing difficulties, sometimes necessitating emergency medical care. Early stages of allergies often manifest in people with dry skin.

Respiratory allergies are also prevalent, including allergic rhinitis and asthma. While pollen, animal hair, dust, mites, and cold air are commonly cited as causes, the more fundamental trigger lies in foods and diets incompatible with the Constitution.

Lung Disease

The Lungs and respiratory tract, being the outermost Zang-Fu organs of the Yang Field, often become the primary route of disease. Many individuals experience prolonged coughing or chronic lung conditions following a severe cold or during the periods of weakened immunity. This pattern has become more frequent since the COVID-19 pandemic.

Chronic obstructive pulmonary diseases (COPD), characterized by persistent phlegm, coughing, and shortness of breath during exercise, are not uncommon in this Constitution. Examples include chronic bronchitis, pneumonia, and emphysema, which involve the partial obstruction of the respiratory tract, from the nasal cavity to the trachea, bronchi, and alveoli. People with a history of pulmonary tuberculosis often exhibit a high likelihood of having this Constitution.

Digestive Diseases

When the Pancreas-Stomach digestive system in the Yang Field becomes the primary disease route, people may experience bloating, abdominal distension, heartburn, reflux esophagitis, constipation, and diarrhea. These issues often arise in those who fail to maintain this Constitutional Diet.

Metabolic Diseases or Lifestyle Diseases

Diabetes frequently occurs in individuals who neglect this Constitutional Diet. Similarly, stagnated blood can result in poor circulation, leading to conditions such as high blood pressure and hyperlipidemia.

Immune System Diseases

Prolonged neglect of Constitutional regimen can lead to diseases rooted in immune system dysfunction. A key example is atopic dermatitis, an autoimmune condition characterized by severe itching, keratinization, lichenification, inflammation, and fever on the skin. From the Constitutional perspective, unsuitable foods or stress are considered primary factors.

Rheumatoid arthritis (RA) is another common immune disease. This Constitution has the higher prevalence of autoimmune and rare diseases, compared to other Constitutions.

Hepatobiliary Diseases

Diseases affecting the Liver and Gallbladder, part of the Yin Field, are also prevalent. Reduced liver detoxification capacity can lead to chronic fatigue and, in severe cases, progress to conditions such as hepatitis, cirrhosis, and liver cancer. The gallbladder, closely related to the liver, is susceptible to the conditions like cholecystitis, gallstones, and gallbladder cancer.

Genitourinary Diseases

The Kidneys-Bladder in the Yin Field is often affected, resulting in frequent urination, cystitis, and nephritis. Women are prone to uterine and ovarian diseases, including infertility, while men may experience early signs of reduced sexual function, such as premature ejaculation or erectile dysfunction.

Neurosis

Individuals with this Constitution are often emotionally and psychologically sensitive, making them prone to neuropsychiatric conditions like anxiety, insomnia, depression, and panic disorder. This emotional sensitivity frequently leads to nervousness and, in some cases, hyperhidrosis of the hands, feet, or head.

Excessive sweating is often misunderstood in Constitutional diagnosis. Many assume it indicates the Taeeumin (Mogyang or Mogeum Constitution), but it is often associated with the opposite Constitutions (Geumyang or Geumeum Constitution). From Constitutional perspective, the former is physiological sweat, while the latter is pathological. It is crucial to distinguish between the two when evaluating the sweating patterns.

Other Considerations

Due to low liver detoxification capacity in the Yin Field, individuals with this Constitution are more prone to side effects from chemical drugs like antibiotics, painkillers, and hormones. Some even experience life-threatening reactions to anesthesia or contrast agents. This Constitution requires extreme caution for drug use.

Geumeum Constitution's Characteristics

Zang-Fu Structure

(Yang Field)		|	(Yin Field)	
LU·LI	KI·BL	PA·ST	HT·SI	**LR·GB**

Characteristics Related to Food

Similar to the Geumyang Constitution, vegetables, fish, and seafood are well-suited for this Constitution. However, it is not uncommon for individuals to dislike or rarely eat these foods, instead favoring meat, flour-based foods, and dairy products, which they consume frequently without apparent issues. (Note: This does not mean these foods are inherently safe. Over time, a diet incompatible with one's Constitution can lead to the accumulation of toxins and result in serious illnesses.)

Specific Food Preferences and Reactions

* **Meat and Flour-Based Foods:** In general, a characteristic of this Constitution is a tendency to experience digestive problems when consuming meat or flour-based foods. However, some people enjoy these foods and consume them without experiencing any apparent issues.

* **Oily Foods:** Many individuals with this Constitution can experience digestive discomfort from fried or fatty foods. Representative examples include fried chicken and oily Chinese cuisine, both of which are unsuitable for this Constitution.

* **Dairy Products:** Many people feel unwell or experience diarrhea after consuming milk. However, some individuals can consume large quantities of milk without issues.[126] (Again, this does not mean it is safe or advisable to consume these products.)

* **Spicy Foods:** Spicy foods often cause stomach discomfort or diarrhea for many people with this Constitution. However, a small number of people enjoy spicy foods without manifesting any discomfort.

* **Vegetarian Diet, Fish, and Seafood:** Typically, individuals with this Constitution enjoy a vegetarian diet, fish, and seafood. When their diet aligns with their Constitution, their stool is thick and abundantly produced, and their bowel movements are smooth and quick, resulting in a dramatically pleasant experience. This is considered the ideal indicator of good health for this Constitution.

However, some people may experience stomach discomfort after consuming oily fish like mackerel, indicating difficulty in digesting fatty foods. Others may experience stomach discomfort or diarrhea after eating crustaceans or shellfish, particularly shrimp and raw oysters, which are unsuitable for this Constitution.

While many people enjoy vegetables and fruits, some dislike them or struggle with digesting them.

* **Alcohol:** Most individuals with this Constitution are weak drinkers and dislike alcohol. However, some enjoy alcohol and can drink heavily, which may predispose them to alcoholism.

---

[126] There are unexamined myths about dairy products. One common belief is that milk is a "complete food," leading some people to feel compelled to consume it even when it does not suit their Constitution. This trend is especially noticeable in growing children, who are often encouraged to consume milk for its calcium content, and in middle-aged or elderly individuals who fear osteoporosis. However, milk is not a complete food, nor is it essential to consume. There are plenty of foods more suited to your Constitution that can replace dairy products. Simply focus on eating those foods instead.

Diseases When the Constitutional Diet Is Violated

Digestive Disease

When consuming foods unsuitable for their Constitution or under high stress, individuals may experience diarrhea or thin stools, often diagnosed as irritable bowel syndrome (IBS). Common symptoms include a cold sensation in the lower abdomen and lower abdominal pain (requiring differential diagnosis, as these symptoms are similar to those of Mogyang or Mogeum Constitution).

Eating excessive amounts of meat, flour, or soy-based foods can lead to gas accumulation in the intestines, resulting in frequent flatulence. Other symptoms may include chest tightness, nausea, loose stools, or frequent bowel movements. A characteristic symptom of this Constitution is "difficulty passing stool," where the stool is thin or soft yet difficult to pass. In such cases, diarrhea often leads to a noticeable loss of energy.

Reactions to incompatible foods can also manifest as skin or respiratory allergic symptoms, but they more commonly appear as digestive system issues.

Neurosis

Occasionally or periodically, individuals may feel an indescribable discomfort in the chest, leading to anxiety about potential heart problems. However, this is often a type of referred pain related to the stomach. This excessive worrying about the symptom frequently leads to hypochondria in this Constitution.

Lifestyle Diseases

A diet inconsistent with this Constitution can result in blood issues like poor circulation, high blood pressure, and hyperlipidemia.

Hepatobiliary Disease

With reduced ability of liver detoxification, individuals with this Constitution are more prone to hepatitis, cirrhosis, and liver cancer. Diseases of the gallbladder, such as gallstones, cholecystitis, and gallbladder cancer, are also more frequent than in other Constitutions.

Allergies

There is a higher prevalence of allergic reactions to foods or medications in this Constitution. Common symptoms include allergic rhinitis, skin dryness, itching, and allergies to metals or sunlight.

Skin Diseases

Many individuals with psoriasis have this Constitution. Psoriasis is a chronic inflammatory skin condition characterized by red papules or plaques of varying sizes with well-defined borders, covered with silvery-white scales. These lesions often appear on the elbows, knees, buttocks, scalp, hands, and feet.

In severe cases, psoriasis may cause itching, though significant itching is generally uncommon. It differs from atopic dermatitis in that it more frequently occurs on the outer protrusions, such as the elbows or knees, rather than the inner folds.

In colder weather, the skin near the fingertips of this Constitution may crack, sometimes leading to bleeding and pain—symptoms resembling eczema. Individuals with skin conditions similar to atopic dermatitis are also frequently observed.

Myoneural System Diseases

Excessive stress and frequent consumption of unsuitable foods can lead to myoneural disorders and incurable diseases such as myasthenia gravis, Lou Gehrig's disease, Parkinson's disease, and muscular dystrophy.

* **Myasthenia Gravis:** A progressive and incurable disease where limb weakness, often triggered by severe stress or intense anger, is a hallmark symptom. Prodromal signs may include extreme fatigue before the disease fully develops. Historical references to "Jieyuzheng (解㑊證)" in Je-ma Lee's *Donguisusebowon* are believed to describe myasthenia gravis or Lou Gehrig's disease.

* **Lou Gehrig's Disease:** Known for its association with the legendary American baseball player Lou Gehrig, this fatal condition causes muscle atrophy and paralysis. Renowned physicist Dr. Stephen Hawking (1942-2018) also suffered from this disease.

* **Parkinson's Disease:** A progressive condition characterized by tremors and muscle stiffness. For example, heavyweight boxing legend Muhammad Ali (1942–2016) suffered from this disease.

* **Alzheimer's Disease:** Often observed in those with the Geumeum Constitution, this degenerative central nervous system disease (commonly known as senile dementia) was experienced, for instance, by former U.S. President Ronald Reagan (1911–2004).

From the Constitutional perspective, these diseases often stem from long-term consumption of unsuitable foods (such as meat) or cumulative effects of repeated intense anger.

Other

Individuals with Geumeum Constitution are more prone to side effects from Western medicine. This includes heightened sensitivity to drugs and potential adverse reactions.

Toyang Constitution's Characteristics

Zang-Fu Structure

(Yang Field)		|		(Yin Field)
PA·ST	HT·SI	LR·GB	LU·LI	**KI·BL**

Characteristics Related to Food

In general, many individuals with this Constitution have a good appetite and enjoy eating a wide variety of foods. However, there are rare cases where individuals eat only small amounts. While they tend to eat most types of food, some dislike meat and rarely consume it. They often follow a vegetarian diet but may become very tired and lethargic as a result. (However, exceptions exist. For example, a patient at Joowonjang Clinic, a famous TV drama actress with a Toyang Constitution, was significantly overweight. She adopted an extreme vegetarian diet, successfully lost weight, and greatly improved her health.)

Specific Food Preferences and Reactions

* **Meat Consumption:** Many individuals with a Toyang Constitution enjoy eating meat and find it difficult to maintain their energy levels without it. They typically consume various types of meat, such as beef, pork, and chicken. However, chicken is one of the most harmful foods for this Constitution, and some individuals often fall ill after eating it.

* **Fish and Seafood:** Generally, fish and seafood are well-liked and enjoyed. However, individuals who are sensitive to smells may dislike fish and seafood and avoid eating them usually.

* **Vegetables:** Most people with this Constitution enjoy vegetables and eat them well. However, there are some who strongly dislike vegetables, and this tendency is more common in younger individuals.

* **Fruits:** Many people like fruits and eat them well, though there are rare exceptions of individuals who dislike fruits.

* **Spicy Food:** Spicy food is very harmful to this Constitution. While some individuals can consume spicy food without any issues, many others typically experience stomach upset or diarrhea. In severe cases, they may be unable to eat spicy food at all due to frequent diarrhea. Before such symptoms become pronounced, many people in this group, who constitutionally have robust digestion and strong stomach walls, are able to enjoy extremely spicy foods like Cheongyang pepper.[127] However, prolonged consumption of spicy food often leads to serious stomach problems for this Constitution.

* **Cold Food:** People with this Constitution typically enjoy cold foods and beverages, such as ice, shaved ice, or icy cold water, and they rarely experience any adverse effects from consuming them. However, there are rare cases where individuals dislike cold food and feel unwell after eating it.

* **Raw Food:** Many people with this Constitution enjoy raw foods such as raw fish or raw meat, which they can digest easily.

* **Alcohol:** Most individuals with this Constitution dislike alcohol and avoid it. However, there are exceptions where some people enjoy drinking alcohol and tolerate it well.

---

[127] Cheongyang pepper is a type of chili pepper native to South Korea, renowned for its intense spiciness. It is a hybrid of a local Korean chili pepper and a Thai chili, combining the unique flavor of Korean peppers with the intense heat of Thai chili. The pepper is named after the Cheongyang region, although it is now cultivated widely across the country.

Diseases When the Constitutional Diet Is Violated

Digestive Diseases

Enjoying spicy foods can lead to discomfort, gastritis, or peptic ulcers. Gastric cancer is also relatively more common in individuals with this Constitution.

If overeating and neglecting exercise, obesity can easily develop. For individuals with this Constitution, losing weight after gaining it is comparatively much more difficult. Some individuals, despite eating little and exercising frequently, find their weight remains constant and cannot lose it.

Regularly consuming foods unsuitable for the Constitution can impair kidney function, leading to easy swelling (edema). In many cases, this persistent edema progresses to obesity.

Lifestyle Diseases

Diabetes is relatively common as a result of weight gain.

A lack of proper Constitutional dietary habits can lead individuals with this Constitution to experience poor blood circulation, high blood pressure, hyperlipidemia, and related conditions.

Urogenital Diseases

Kidney function is weaker compared to other Constitutions, making the body prone to swelling and frequent urination.

In women, reproductive diseases such as ovarian cysts, uterine fibroids, and tumors are more prevalent. Infertility is also more common than in other Constitutions, although pregnancy itself generally poses no problems in most Toyang Constitution.

Sexual interest is relatively low, leading to a higher prevalence of single individuals in celibacy or those with religious vocations such as priests, nuns, and monks.

Neurosis

The heart in this Constitution is easily excited, causing palpitations and anxiety. Long-term stress or family discord often leads to mental issues such as depression or Xinhuobing (心火病).

Hyperhidrosis (excessive sweating) is common. While some individuals experience it on their hands and feet, others sweat profusely in their upper body, particularly on the head, when they are tense or focused.

Allergies

Allergic conditions, such as allergic rhinitis, asthma, hives, and hypersensitive skin, are frequent.

Allergic reactions to pollen, animal fur, dust, sunlight, and metals are also common.

Atopic Dermatitis

This condition is often thought to be exclusively associated with the Geumyang Constitution, but it can also occur in individuals with the Toyang Constitution. It manifests in characteristic areas such as the inner folds of the elbows and knees. Even if not diagnosed with atopic dermatitis, many individuals exhibit skin resembling "chicken skin (goose bumps)."

Drug Side Effects

People with this Constitution are prone to numerous drug side effects, especially hypersensitivity to antibiotics. These can result in gastrointestinal disorders, immunological hypersensitivity reactions, and severe issues in sensory organs such as the eyes and ears.

Toeum Constitution's Characteristics

Zang-Fu Structure

(Yang Field)		|		(Yin Field)
PA·ST	LU·LI	HT·SI	LR·GB	**KI·BL**

Characteristics Related to Food

Many people with this Constitution experience digestive problems when consuming meat, flour-based foods, or spicy dishes. Generally, a diet similar to that of the Geum Constitution—emphasizing vegetables, fish, and seafood as beneficial—is well-suited. Pork is considered a beneficial meat option.

* **Meat Consumption:** Digestive issues often arise when eating beef or chicken. Nonetheless, young individuals or those with good digestive function may not encounter any problem. Pork is regarded as the meat with the least side effects for this Constitution. As individuals with this Constitution age, they often develop an aversion to meat, with many transitioning to a vegetarian diet or incorporating mixed grains into their meals. Many individuals naturally prefer vegetarian diets and, even with a plant-based lifestyle, do not experience significant nutritional deficiencies.

* **Spicy Foods:** Spicy foods are particularly harmful to this Constitution, often leading to side effects such as digestive distress, allergic reactions, and skin problems. However, there are individuals who can tolerate spicy foods without issues.

* **Wheat Flour Foods:** Flour-based foods frequently cause digestive problems for this Constitution, especially items like pizza, noodles, jajangmyeon (Korean-style Chinese noodles), and ramen, which often lead to reflux in the throat. However, some people enjoy flour-based foods without notable side effects.

* **Fish and Seafood:** Seafood is generally beneficial for this Constitution. Blue colored fish like mackerel, due to reflux in the throat, are said to be less suitable compared to the fish with white flesh. Most seafood is well-tolerated, except for certain seaweed types, such as "Gim" (dried laver) or "Miyeok" (sea mustard, kelp), which may cause issues.

* **Cold Foods:** Due to their naturally hot and active stomach Constitution, these individuals often enjoy and can tolerate cold foods, such as ice, shaved ice, and cold beverages, without any issues. Rare cases of stomach discomfort from cold foods can occur when gastrointestinal function is severely compromised. Once the stomach recovers, cold foods are usually fine. On the contrary, a preference for hot foods—both in temperature and nature—within this Constitution may lead to inflammation or even esophageal or stomach cancer. Appetite is generally good.

* **Alcohol:** People with this Constitution generally dislike alcohol and have a low tolerance for it.

Diseases When the Constitutional Diet Is Violated

Digestive Diseases

Frequent gastrointestinal conditions such as upset stomach, indigestion, and colon-related diseases like diarrhea, hemorrhoids, bloody stool, and colitis are common. These are often triggered by consuming spicy foods or foods unsuitable for this Constitution, such as meat, flour-based foods, and processed foods.

Allergic Diseases

Skin conditions like hives, itching, contact dermatitis, and other allergies are prevalent. Allergic rhinitis is also a common issue.

Atopic Dermatitis

Atopic dermatitis can manifest in this Constitution. Sometimes, it may be more severe than in those with the Geumyang constitution. My clinical cases occasionally involve individuals with severe atopic dermatitis, with their entire body covered in dead skin cells.

Hyperhidrosis

Excessive sweating in localized areas such as the head, hands, and feet is common, causing significant discomfort in daily life.

Drug Side Effects

People with this Constitution are highly sensitive to antibiotics, with penicillin shock being a typical hypersensitivity reaction. Clinical observations have included cases of coma caused by anesthetic reactions, indicating a high likelihood of side effects from various drugs.

Other Characteristics

The Toeum Constitution shares many physiological and pathological similarities with the Geumyang Constitution. These include experiencing side effects from consuming meat, flour-based foods, dairy products, and spicy foods; the ability to maintain health without eating meat; a tendency toward adverse drug reactions; and a high prevalence of allergic conditions. The occurrence of atopic dermatitis in this Constitution, a condition typically associated with the Geumyang Constitution, further underscores these similarities.

Mogyang Constitution's Characteristics

Zang-Fu Structure

(Yang Field)		|		(Yin Field)
LR·GB	KI·BL	HT·SI	PA·ST	**LU·LI**

Characteristics Related to Food

In general, this Constitution is best suited for a Western diet (focused on meat, flour-based foods, and dairy products), with few side effects from a regular diet. People with this Constitution tend to have a robust appetite and often eat large portions (unfortunately, overeating can lead to indigestion often). Even when unwell in their health, they generally retain their appetite.

* **Meat:** This Constitution requires regular meat consumption to maintain physical strength. A prolonged lack of meat diet can lead to fatigue and poor mental focus. Some individuals report excessive saliva production and drooling when they do not eat meat long. There are cases where people consume meat at every meal or even eat grilled pork belly in the morning. Based on dietary habits, this Constitution can be likened to carnivores in the animal kingdom.

* **Wheat Flour Foods:** Individuals with this Constitution often find flour-based foods more suitable than rice. Most wheat foods, such as bread, noodles, pizza, and spaghetti, are well-suited to this Constitution. Some people can even eat only bread or noodles three times a day.

* **Dairy Products:** Dairy products, including milk, yogurt, cheese, and butter, are generally beneficial for this Constitution. Drinking milk can soothe

an upset stomach, and constipation is often alleviated by consuming milk or yogurt.

* **Leafy Vegetables, Fish, and Seafood:** Many people with this Constitution enjoy leafy vegetables, fish, and seafood, but if they don't eat them frequently, there is little noticeable effect. However, frequent consumption may lead to increased fatigue and changes in stool consistency. Eating large amounts of leafy vegetables or fish can sometimes cause stomach pain, bloating, or a sensation of tightness in the throat, depending on the individual. Such issues are less likely when consuming root vegetables and meat.

* **Alcohol:** There is a wide range of alcohol tolerance among people with this Constitution. While most are strong drinkers, a few are highly sensitive, turning bright red and unable to handle even a single drink.

A Disease When the Constitutional Diet Is Violated

Digestive Diseases

Generally, eating foods unsuitable for this Constitution can lead to gastrointestinal diseases. However, since most modern diets—including meat, flour-based foods, and dairy products—suit this Constitution well, digestive issues are relatively rare. The primary concern for individuals with this Constitution is overeating. Despite having a large appetite, their stomach function is relatively weak, making them prone to bloating or indigestion after overeating.

Due to shorter intestines, some individuals experience frequent bowel movements after eating, and others may suffer from diarrhea when their stomach becomes cold. Keeping the lower abdomen warm is an essential health practice. Consuming warm food and beverage is highly beneficial, while frequent consumption of cold or raw food can lead to stomach upset, coldness in the abdomen, and significant health risks.

Lifestyle Diseases

Neglecting Constitutional Diet and regular exercise can lead to abdominal obesity and metabolic disorders such as diabetes or circulatory diseases, including strokes and heart disease.

Psychiatric Illnesses

Psychiatric conditions such as anxiety, auditory hallucinations, and obsessive-compulsive disorder may arise from psychological trauma. Auditory hallucinations are particularly characteristic of the Mogyang Constitution. This Constitution unexpectedly often exhibits timid or cautious tendencies in their behavior.

Lung Diseases

Due to the Lungs being at their lowest potential, the respiratory system is often weak. Common symptoms include cough, phlegm, asthma, and increased susceptibility to colds during seasonal changes. Despite having a strong, muscular appearance, individuals may struggle with long-distance running due to respiratory limitations.

Typical symptoms of lung diseases in this Constitution include severe coughing, phlegm, fever, and difficulty breathing. In severe cases, asthma may develop. Unlike the Geum-Constitution, where heightened Lung sensitivity leads to allergic respiratory diseases, Lung issues in the Mog-Constitution result from the lowered Lung potential.

Immune System Diseases

While autoimmune and other rare immune disorders are uncommon, failure to adhere to Constitutional Diet can increase the frequency of immune-related diseases.

Allergies

Allergic rhinitis is occasionally observed, but the current dietary trend of meat and flour-based foods generally benefits this Constitution, making allergic diseases less common. However, individuals with sensitive body who deviate from their Constitutional Diet may develop immune hypersensitivity symptoms, such as itchy skin or respiratory allergies.

Blood Pressure

High blood pressure is Constitutionally common in this group. However, individuals with low blood pressure are also frequently observed, highlighting variability within the Constitution.

Other Symptoms

People with Mogyang Constitution tend to sweat a lot when healthy. However, in clinical practice, excessive sweating is not always observed in this Constitution. In fact, individuals with this Constitution who visit medical facilities often experience reduced sweating due to poor physical condition.

When health deteriorates, people with Mogyang Constitution may experience very little sweating. This lack of sweating is a potential red flag and should be addressed immediately. Conversely, in the case of healthy Mogyang individuals, excessive sweating—though a sign of good health—can be bothersome and may be mistaken for hyperhidrosis.

For Constitutions like Geum-Constitution or Su-Constitution, the pattern is the opposite—sweating increases as health worsens. These variations in sweating patterns based on health status are critical to note. For individuals with Mogyang Constitution, a lack of regular sweating, even in the absence of overt illness, should prompt suspicion of underlying health issues. Therefore, taking appropriate action is vital to maintaining health.

Mogeum Constitution's Characteristics

Zang-Fu Structure

(Yang Field)		|		(Yin Field)
LR·GB	HT·SI	PA·ST	KI·BL	**LU·LI**

Characteristics Related to Food

This Constitution enjoys not only meat and flour-based foods but also vegetarian dishes, fish, and seafood. While this Constitution, like the **Mogyang Constitution**, typically favors meat, unexpectedly, there are individuals within this Constitution who do not enjoy it. However, flour-based foods are usually well-liked. Eating large amounts of leafy vegetables may lead to fatigue.

* **Meat:** Meat suits this Constitution well, so regular consumption can help maintain good health. Generally, people with this Constitution do not prefer pork, but tend to eat mostly beef.

* **Wheat Flour-based Foods:** Flour-based foods are beneficial for this Constitution, making it advisable to include them regularly in the diet.

* **Dairy Products:** Milk, cheese, and yogurt are well-suited to this Constitution. However, cold milk can upset the stomach, so it is recommended to drink it warm. In fact, consuming warm foods, including dairy products, is generally more beneficial for overall health in individuals with this Constitution.

* **Fish:** Eating mackerel may cause adverse reactions such as reflux esophagitis or hives. Other fish have fewer side effects but are generally not compatible with this Constitution. Therefore, it is best to consume fish sparingly.

* **Alcohol:** Some individuals with this Constitution are strong drinkers, but they usually do not enjoy alcohol much. Others may experience severe facial redness or have a very low tolerance for alcohol, making it difficult for them to drink at all.

Diseases When the Constitutional Diet Is Violated

Digestive Diseases

Drinking beer or consuming cold foods can lead to diarrhea or stomach discomfort for this Constitution. If the lower abdomen becomes cold, it may cause diarrhea, heaviness in the legs, or back pain. Eating warm food is a strict rule for maintaining the health of this Constitution.

While milk is suitable for this body type, drinking it cold can cause stomach upset, so it's best to consume it warm. Some individuals experience stomach pain or discomfort when eating fish or seafood. People with this Constitution are often prone to irritable bowel symptoms or colon polyps. In rare cases, ulcerative colitis may occur.

Defecation

Even without major health issues, frequent bowel movements (three or four times a day) are common in this Constitution due to shorter Large intestine compared to other Constitutions. Following the Constitutional Diet can reduce bowel movements to one or two times a day, similar to the average frequency. Therefore, frequent stools in this Constitution may indicate poor physical condition, which is quite contrary to the general concept.

Lifestyle Diseases

A lack of exercise can lead to easy weight gain, increasing the risk of metabolic conditions such as high blood pressure and diabetes.

Allergies

Some individuals have sensitive skin and may develop sudden hives or itching triggered by food, drugs, dust, or pollen. After eating mackerel, some people experience reflux esophagitis or hives, while others have severe reactions where their skin turns red when exposed to cold water or air.

Dermographism, where the skin swells and turns red after being scratched, is also common. Certain individuals may exhibit atopic dermatitis-like symptoms. While the Geum-Constitution is widely associated with allergies, all Constitutions can also develop allergic reactions in the skin or respiratory system if they do not follow their Constitutional Diet and lifestyle regimen.

Lung Diseases

This Constitution, like the Mogyang Constitution, has the lowest Lung potential, making the respiratory system weaker. This can result in symptoms such as frequent phlegm production and asthma.

Others

Sweating through exercise or bathing typically improves overall health for this Constitution. Many individuals cover their lower abdomen while sleeping, even during summer, as cold abdomen can deteriorate health. Using a belly band to keep the lower abdomen warm is a crucial health tip for this Constitution.

Suyang Constitution's Characteristics

Zang-Fu Structure

(Yang Field)		|		(Yin Field)
KI·BL	LU·LI	LR·GB	HT·SI	**PA·ST**

Characteristics Related to Food

Due to the Pancreas-Stomach being at their lowest Zang-Fu potential, most individuals with this Constitution have a poor appetite and eat sparingly. However, some individuals eat well but tend to overeat, often skipping meals and then binge eating. Such eating habits frequently lead to stomach upset, nausea, or diarrhea. There are exceptions where individuals eat abnormally well and digest foods unsuitable for this Constitution without issues, and these individuals may gain significant weight or become obese.

* **Cold Foods:** Many people with this Constitution dislike or cannot tolerate cold foods. However, when young or before their stomach becomes seriously compromised, they can consume cold foods such as ice cream or cold water without issues. Younger individuals tend to handle cold foods better due to their abundant Yang Qi, regardless of their Constitution. If someone dislikes cold foods from very young age, it may indicate this Constitution (or Sueum Constitution).

In cases of fever due to illness, individuals with this Constitution often crave cold foods instead of warm foods. Even if outward symptoms suggest a need for cold foods or medications, consuming warm foods and receiving warm herbal treatments is critical for recovery. This principle is an important piece of health wisdom often overlooked in Western medicine.

* **Pork:** Pork often causes nausea, abdominal pain, or diarrhea in individuals with this Constitution, although some may—albeit temporarily—enjoy it regularly without discomfort.

* **Fish and Seafood:** People with this Constitution generally dislike fish and seafood, and consuming them often leads to stomach stasis or digestive problems. However, some individuals can eat fish or seafood without any issues. In particular, raw fish can cause sudden indigestion, severe abdominal pain, or diarrhea. Raw seafood such as sashimi, raw oysters, and live small octopus, as well as crustaceans like shrimp, crabs, and clams, are particularly harmful. They can cause severe digestive issues, including food poisoning, indigestion, and digestive discomfort.

* **Fatty Foods or Meat:** This Constitution generally dislikes fatty foods, but leaner options, such as beef or chicken with less fat, are better tolerated as long as portions are moderate. People with Su-Constitution tend to prefer and eat only lean cuts of meat. Chicken is considered the most suitable meat for this Constitution, although some individuals dislike it due to their weak Pancreas-Stomach, which are sensitive to greasy tastes and smells.

* **Vegetables:** Many individuals with this Constitution dislike vegetables, especially leafy greens, which may cause more discomfort than root vegetables.

* **Fruit:** Generally, fruit is not well-liked by this Constitution. Since fruit is often refrigerated, it aligns with this Constitution's natural aversion to cold foods. People with this Constitution tend to consume only a few types of fruits that suit them, such as apples, tangerines, oranges, and grapes. Even these should be eaten at a warm temperature to avoid digestive issues.

* **Alcohol:** Many people with this Constitution experience facial redness after just one drink and cannot tolerate alcohol well. However, some enjoy alcohol and drink it regularly without issues.

* **Advice:** To maintain good health with this Constitution, it is vital to eat a small amount of food and prioritize warm foods at all times.

Diseases When the Constitutional Diet Is Violated

Digestive Diseases

Failing to follow the Constitutional Diet often leads to digestive and absorption issues in the stomach and intestines, including symptoms such as loss of appetite, indigestion, and diarrhea. Some individuals suffer from chronic stomach problems, and prolonged poor digestion can result in severe lethargy or extreme fatigue.

Defecation

People with this Constitution typically have infrequent bowel movements, often once every few days. In a very healthy state, however, it is ideal for those with this Constitution to have daily bowel movements. Severe constipation can occur if bowel movements are delayed for too long.

Anorexia

In rare cases, individuals with a weak stomach may experience an increased appetite due to psychological factors. They may overeat but struggle with digestion or worry about gaining weight, leading them to habitually induce intentional vomiting. Repeated episodes of this behavior can result in anorexia.

Diabetes

Some individuals with Suyang Constitution have a voracious appetite and tend to overeat, which can sometimes lead to diabetes. Given that people with Suyang Constitution generally eat very small amount of food, this outcome can be surprising.

Allergy Diseases

Some individuals have highly sensitive skin, adversely reacting to most cosmetics and frequently experiencing hives, dry skin, or rashes. They are also highly sensitive to unpleasant odors and may be allergic to metals, sunlight, pollen, dust, and other irritants.

Psychiatric Illness

Headaches, tremors, obsessive-compulsive disorder, and other forms of schizophrenia may occur after severe mental shock. Excessive mental stress or prolonged deep, distressful thought can exacerbate these conditions and worsen physical health.

Hyperhidrosis

Under heavy stress, severe indigestion, or when the body's energy got all drained, individuals may experience excessive sweating. This symptom is particularly detrimental to Suyang Constitution. In some cases, sweating is localized, affecting the hands, feet, or armpits. Healthy individuals with Suyang Constitution may not sweat at all, even during intense exercise.

Premenstrual Syndrome

During menstruation, symptoms may include facial flushing and swelling, a sore and swollen throat, or heat intolerance due to fever. Appetite may increase abnormally, leading to overeating, or the body may feel sore and immobile due to extreme fatigue. These symptoms usually resolve completely once menstruation ends as if nothing happened.

Others

Ginseng, a representative herbal medicine in Korea, is especially well-suited for this Constitution. Many individuals report feeling revitalized simply by drinking ginseng tea when they are unwell.

Sueum Constitution's Characteristics

Zang-Fu Structure

(Yang Field)		|		(Yin Field)
KI·BL	LR·GB	HT·SI	LU·LI	**PA·ST**

Characteristics Related to Food

In general, individuals with this Constitution enjoy eating meat, particularly beef and chicken, which suit them well. Pork, however, is not beneficial. There is a tendency to dislike vegetables and fruits, and fish or seafood is also not particularly favored.

* **Appetite:** Some people overeat due to a strong appetite, but this often leads to sudden indigestion or stomach upset, so most individuals prefer to eat smaller portions.

* **Oily Foods:** Oily foods frequently cause indigestion or discomfort.

* **Wheat Flour-based Foods:** Flour-based foods like bread, noodles, and pizza often result in upset stomach or indigestion.

* **Milk:** Many individuals experience upset stomach or diarrhea after consuming milk, especially when it is cold.

* **Pork:** Eating pork can cause sickness for many people with this Constitution, though symptoms may not appear until the stomach is significantly upset. Once issues arise, they can escalate into severe abdominal pain and diarrhea.

* **Cold Foods:** Cold foods frequently lead to stomach discomfort. Foods that cool the Pancreas-Stomach—such as ice cream, cold water, beer, barley, melon, and watermelon—commonly cause upset stomach or diarrhea. Some individuals reportedly have disliked and avoided cold foods since childhood.

* **Spicy Foods:** Spicy foods, including peppers and garlic, generally improve digestion and physical well-being. This Constitution is particularly well-suited to spicy foods.

* **Alcohol:** While some individuals can drink alcohol well, most experience facial redness and have a low tolerance for alcohol.

Diseases When the Constitutional Diet Is Violated

Digestive Diseases

Diarrhea often occurs when eating foods unsuitable for this Constitution, consuming cold foods, or overeating beyond one's capacity. Eating excessive amounts of pork, fish, or seafood can sometimes lead to severe, prolonged diarrhea. During such episodes, energy levels significantly decrease.

Gastric Ptosis

Frequent overeating or consuming incompatible foods can cause severe gastroptosis (stomach prolapse). In such cases, the stomach may descend into the lower abdomen, and, in severe instances, it may sag as far as the bladder. Interestingly, some individuals with gastroptosis may mistakenly believe they have a fat belly coming out.

While gastric ptosis can occur in various Constitutions—including Sueum, Suyang, Geumyang, Toeum, and others—it is particularly severe in those with Sueum Constitution.

Some individuals habitually vomit; they have no issues while eating, but tend to do so after a certain amount of time has passed. Occasionally, some individuals may wake up in the morning and vomit the previous day's food.

Additionally, exposure to cold air or water can trigger diarrhea in some with the Sueum Constitution.

Some experience frequent diarrhea with little constipation, while others primarily suffer from constipation with little diarrhea.

Allergic Diseases

Allergies can manifest as hives, redness when the skin is scratched, or sensitivities to metals, dust, pollen, and similar triggers. Some individuals are allergic to crustaceans like shrimp and crab or seafood such as octopus or clams. Allergic rhinitis is also not uncommon. Although all Constitutions can develop allergies, the underlying causes differ by Constitution, emphasizing the importance of following Constitution-specific regimen.

Neuropsychiatric Diseases

Individuals sensitive to stress may experience chest tightness or palpitations, especially during prolonged stress or severe digestive issues. Those with Su-Constitution are particularly prone to psychological stressors, including worry, anxiety, and emotional shock.

Hyperhidrosis

Excessive sweating may occur in specific areas, such as the head, armpits, groin, hands, and soles of the feet. Nervousness can exacerbate sweaty palms. Conversely, some individuals may not sweat at all in certain areas of the body.

Other Symptoms

Some individuals experience significant heat in the upper body (chest or head) while their lower body (abdomen, hands, and feet) remains very cold. This imbalance is a notable characteristic of this Constitution.

Epilogue

Epilogue

Constitutional Medicine
Recognizes differences,
Yet does not permit the dominance of a certain Zang-Fu.
Constitutional Medicine dreams of harmony.

Constitutional Medicine
Affirms differences,
But does not tolerate the superiority of any Constitution.
Constitutional Medicine pursues peace.

Constitutional Medicine
Is the medicine of difference.
It is the medicine of coexistence.
It is a new humane medicine
Created to heal the world.

Born in the tears of Je-ma Lee
And in the blood and sweat of Do-won Kuon,
It is the Medicine of the earth
Developed by the people of this land

Without their sweat and tears,
Constitutional Medicine
Could not have been born at all
From the very beginning.

At this moment of reflection,
A line from Bob Dylan's song "*My Back Pages*"
Suddenly comes to my mind:

"*Ah, but I was so much older then.*
I'm younger than that now!"

Here, I have poured out the thoughts
I have accumulated over a long time
About Eight-Constitution Medicine
Since I began researching it.
And now, at this moment,
I also feel much younger.

A poem by Manhae Yong-woon Han
Gently embraces me:

"*Parting is the creation of beauty.*"

I hope this book contributes to a creation of beauty.

Body is a world of Change,
A place of eternal passing.
The journey of the Eight-Constitution Medicine
Never ends.
It's always a beginning.
Unfinished!
Yeah, it's Weiji (未濟)!

www.ingramcontent.com/pod-product-compliance
Lightning Source LLC
LaVergne TN
LVHW090257210926
848480LV00001B/50
9791199555730